DATE DUE

OCT 2 8 2011	

WHEN WINNING COSTS TOO MUCH

WHEN WINNING COSTS TOO MUCH

Steroids, Supplements, and Scandal in Today's Sports

JOHN McCLOSKEY
JULIAN BAILES, M.D.

TAYLOR TRADE PUBLISHING
Lanham • New York • Dallas • Boulder • Toronto • Oxford

Published by Taylor Trade Publishing
An imprint of The Rowman & Littlefield Publishing Group, Inc.
4501 Forbes Boulevard, Suite 200
Lanham, MD 20706

Distributed by NATIONAL BOOK NETWORK

Library of Congress Cataloging-in-Publication Data

McCloskey, John, 1973–
    When winning costs too much : steroids, supplements, and scandal in today's sports /
John McCloskey and Julian Bailes.—1st Taylor Trade Pub. ed.
        p.   cm.
    Includes bibliographical references and index.
    ISBN 1-58979-179-7 (cloth : alk. paper)
    1. Doping in sports.   2. Anabolic steroids—Health aspects.   3. Athletes—Drug use.   I. Bailes, Julian E.   II. Title.
    RC1230.M38   2005
    362.29—dc22   2004024695

Contents

Introduction   1

1 Reality Check: Kids Are Using Steroids   7
    Sidebar 1.1   Survival of the Fittest?   9

2 Follow the Leader: Kids Need Bettor Mentors,
Heroes   21
    Sidebar 2.1   Q&A with Jack Nicklaus   23
    Sidebar 2.2   A Word to Parents   26

3 Athletes to Kids: Do as We Say, Not as We Do   37
    Sidebar 3.1   Truth and Lies behind the NFL's
    "Exemplary" Drug-Testing Plan   43

4 BALCO and Beyond: The Biggest Doping Scandal in
Sports History   59
    Sidebar 4.1   What Keeps Barry Swinging   71
    Sidebar 4.2   Summary of Doping in Athens   76

5 Steroids and Designer Drugs   81

6 Supplement Boom: Big Business Spurs Big Trouble   103
    Sidebar 6.1   Fearless Youth: Why They Use
    Supplements   104

7 Solutions to the Out-of-Control Drug Problem in
Sports   111
    Sidebar 7.1   Overview of the ATLAS Program   113
    Sidebar 7.2   Q&A with Dr. Frank Uryasz   118
    Sidebar 7.3   Steroid and Supplement Legislation   126

8 Dead Serious: Catastrophic and Fatal Injuries in
Sports   137

9 The Heat Is On: Heatstroke Continues to Kill   149

10   Brain Injury: Science Waging War on Concussions   157

11   Caring for Youth Sports: Are We or Not?   177
      Sidebar 11.1   Top 10 Things Parents Don't Get About
      Kids and Sports   185
      Sidebar 11.2   Commentary: It's Inexcusable When a
      Youth Coach Breaks Rules, Our Trust   187

12   Winning at All Costs: What We're Driven to Do and
      Why   197
      Sidebar 12.1   Commentary: Winning at All Costs Is a
      Big Loss in Game of Life   202
      Sidebar 12.2   A Senior Season Lost at a Burger King   215

13   Recurrent Unexplained Deaths in Sports   221

14   Who's in Charge? Administration Is Part of the
      Problem   227

15   Struggle for Sportsmanship: Through a Ref's Eagle
      Eyes: Q&A with Barry Mano   243

16   Solutions: Winning without Losing Perspective   253
      Sidebar 16.1   Tips for Coaches, Parents, and Players   260
      Sidebar 16.2   Teaching Sportsmanship Tips   269
      Sidebar 16.3   Ethics of Competition Education
      Should Be Mandatory in All Schools   273
      Sidebar 16.4   Q&A with Terry Holland   282

17   More Solutions: Athletes Doing the Right Thing   287

      Notes   297

      Index   329

Introduction

The recent BALCO (Bay Area Laboratory Co-Operative) controversy is widely regarded as the worst doping scandal in history. We believe so because it impacts the most powerful and popular organizations in sports (the NFL, Major League Baseball, and Olympic track and field). BALCO also proved just how far science has slipped behind the cheaters in this race. This alone makes this book's critical message extremely timely and interesting to so many. But the comprehensive analysis of BALCO, as well as steroids in baseball, and the record-breaking doping violations uncovered at the Athens Summer Games are only a part of the crisis that faces modern sports.

Children in single-parent homes and those kids being raised with TV and video games as the most significant influences instead of moms and dads are reaching adolescence with far fewer role models and less respect for authority figures, rules, or the values of sportsmanship and fair competition. The problems facing sports today—trash-talking; violence toward officials; taunting celebrations; drug use to enhance performance; drugs, alcohol, and sex as status symbols for kids and recruiting tools for colleges; and cheating in every imaginable form—are getting worse, not better.

There are solutions, however. And with experience perfectly suited to identify the problems, understand their severity, and develop realistic plans to attack them, we have invested years of research and critical thinking to present what is truly a revelation of how dire the condition of competition has become.

Is it really that bad? Is it necessary to approach issues in sports so seriously? Consider the following:

- Competition for scholarships and financial rewards is causing deaths to young people at higher rates than ever. From June to September 2004, three athletes from the Houston area and one from Dallas died suddenly during or after workouts:

- ○ September 9, 2004—A Houston drill team member, Sara Krauss, age 16, dies minutes after the end of practice inside the school's gymnasium.
- ○ Aug. 30, 2004—A Houston high school football player, Ivan Okafor, age 15, collapses and later dies after practice.
- ○ Aug. 2, 2004—A Dallas high school football player, Eric Brown, age 17, dies after suffering heat-related symptoms following football practice.
- ○ June 8, 2004—A former Houston high school football player, McCollins Umeh, age 18, dies in Tucson, Arizona, after he faints 15 minutes into his first off-season workout at the University of Arizona.
- The FDA banned the weight-loss supplement ephedrine in March 2004 after 80 related deaths.
- Andro sales were also banned after sales of Mark McGwire's choice of steroid precursor sharply increased when the world learned it was the reason behind his home-run power. McGwire even stopped using it because he recognized the damage it could do to kids who could buy it over the counter.
- We know more than ever about the permanent damage caused by concussions in football, including never before understood depression, thanks to Dr. Bailes' research. We also know that NFL, college, and high school football coaches are underdiagnosing these life-threatening brain injuries.
- Despite higher levels of death and disease among Italian soccer players, American professional wrestlers, European cyclists, and bodybuilders worldwide than are normal for men in similar age groups, athletes continue to use steroids, blood-doping drugs, and supplements that are as dangerous as ephedrine. Kids know these athletes and imitate their every move. Kids are also more susceptible to the dangers of these chemicals because their bodies have not fully developed.

Doping is a deadly serious problem. And it still does not stop there. Serious social problems can also be attributed to sports:

- Rape by athletes who are conditioned to feel entitled, even untouchable.

- Violence toward girlfriends, officials, or fans at bars or in ball-parks.
- Academic fraud.
- Offering extra benefits to prize recruits.
- Authority figures abusing their positions to seek self-satisfaction instead of setting honorable examples. (See, for example, one out of every 20 college coaches, a number that could be higher or lower depending on whether you believe every basketball coach who parties with co-eds from the opposing school is caught, whether every football coach who has sex with strippers is busted, whether every player who receives cash under the table eventually has a falling out with the coach and reveals the NCAA violation, or whether every tutor hired by an athletic department to write an athlete's papers eventually comes forward with the truth. This list literally could fill its very own book.)
- Little League coaches and parents setting terrible examples—losing their tempers, lying about eligibility, overusing a 10-year-old's pitching arm, or caring more about winning games than teaching lessons and building character.
- Christian schools bending rules and boundaries to recruit the best players.
- Figure skating and boxing judges who are bought or otherwise influenced.
- Olympic committee members who take bribes to award athletes at the sacred Olympic Games.

Every parent knows it is a challenge to raise children in a world where ethics and morality are considered an option or a right rather than a vital component to a healthy and productive society. Many parents, if they were shown this ugly reality, would still think little of changing their behavior or the way they monitor their child's development. This puts the onus on coaches, other parents, older kids they look up to, league administrators, legislators, and everyone along the way to play some role in shaping kids who are being neglected. Those playing by the rules need to make sure cheaters are held accountable. Those who truly care need to aggressively pursue solutions and celebrate the successes with future leaders and role models.

With a frank discussion of the facts, this book makes its case based on a compilation of evidence and extensive primary research. The power of this book can be found in the exclusive, problem- and solution-seeking interviews with highly acclaimed sports figures and experts, including:

- Several Olympic gold medalists and other Olympians;
- The heads of the nation's most highly regarded youth sportsmanship organizations;
- The head of the National Association of Sports Officials;
- The world's most renowned experts in the fields of medicine (specifically steroids, heatstroke, and brain injury), ethics, and youth sports education;
- The head of the NCAA's drug testing and education programs;
- The creator of one of the most successful antidrug and steroid education programs in the country;
- Members of the world's antidoping agencies;
- One former NFL player;
- One former NCAA major-college basketball coach and athletic director;
- One five-time steroid-free world powerlifting champion;
- One legend of professional wrestling who now speaks out against the steroids he once abused;
- One legendary golfer who owns the record for most major victories in a sport where ethics are a way of life, not an option; and
- One legendary NBA star who challenged parents to be role models for their children and not to place such responsibility in the hands of others.

In an interview for this book in April 2004, world-renowned steroids expert Dr. Charles Yesalis said he was still informing a mostly uninformed army of journalists about steroids. He said he'd logged close to 200 interviews in less than two months with those seeking insight into baseball's "shocking" revelation during the BALCO investigation—that elite athletes were using steroids to boost their performance. This is despite the fact that athletes have been using steroids since the 1950s. And while steroids have been, since the time of their discovery, the subject of in-depth and investigative pieces by the world's news organizations, the media's watchdogs have been largely asleep in terms of alerting the public about the prevalence and dangers of steroid use and its spread to kids in high school and junior high.

Finally, Dick Pound, founding chair of the World Anti-Doping Agency, says of the struggle with performance-enhancing drugs: "The fight against doping in sport . . . is the single greatest danger that faces sport today." We agree and have compiled, in the pages that follow, an unprecedented collection of evidence behind that statement, as well as evidence of the overall erosion of ethics in sports. We also offer a comprehensive analysis of the solutions society can focus on so that one day all that is good about sports can again far outweigh that which man has meant for evil. This has not been the case these days. If this is not already clear to the reader, it should soon be.

Reality Check: Kids Are Using Steroids

Aggressive is a word sports fans love to hear. They love a baseball team that is aggressive at the plate, on the mound, and on the base paths. Fans want sports heroes to tackle aggressively, drive the lane aggressively, and attack the pin on the golf course aggressively, regardless of the hazards involved. But aggressive does not describe the way most parents and coaches of high school and college athletes educate these young stars about the dangers of steroids and so-called dietary supplements. Likewise, school leaders are not aggressive in urging parents and coaches to teach teenagers about this critical information; they do not break through the wall of perceived invincibility that young athletes build as they march toward sports fame. Most importantly, too many adults are not aggressively mentoring and monitoring today's youth. Or worse, they are taking the opposite approach—aggressively pursuing any means necessary to turn their elite athlete into the next superstar. This may involve giving up whatever it takes—time, money, or ethics—in order to obtain the best training, the latest supplements, or even the "safest" steroids, all three of which are discussed in the pages ahead.

Clear evidence of steroid use by teens has been successfully discovered and unsuccessfully disseminated for too many years. And while it may be bad for America's pastime, the recent steroid controversy in baseball has been good for America because it revealed the prevalence of the problem. Penn State professor and world-renowned steroids expert Dr. Charles Yesalis first uncovered the magnitude of this drug abuse by reporting that 300,000 people—athletes and nonathletes— used steroids per year in the late 1990s.[1] (See sidebar 1.1, "Survival of the Fittest?"). In his 2002 book, Yesalis estimated that "500,000 to 600,000" kids in the United States had used steroids in the previous year.[2] And in a December 2004 phone interview with Dr. Yesalis, he said that number has nearly doubled to 1,000,000, citing the most recent Youth Risk Behavior Surveillance System (YRBSS) study conducted by the National Institute on Drug Abuse. "And that's one million high school athletes who are cycling [steroids], because no one takes just one pill or one shot. Now if that's not enough to seriously raise our level of concern, what is?"[3]

But the abuse exceeds these statistics. A problem that is much larger and more disappointing is the number of children U.S. athletic programs fail to properly educate on this subject each year. Most experts agree, education is the key to truly reaching the greatest number of kids and to having the strongest impact on their future choices. The premise of this book goes a step further: An athlete properly educated by loving parents, caring coaches, and involved administrators—all of whom aggressively and persistently discourage the use of steroids, deplore other forms of drug abuse, supervise the sketchy world of supplement use, condone good sportsmanship, and encourage the overall pursuit of exemplary citizenship—is an athlete already on the road to success in life, not just competitive sports. Opening a newspaper or turning on *SportsCenter* these days brings the latest news about the most recent bad apple in professional or college sports. The only way to reverse this trend is to convince the next generation of stars that success does not have to be stolen. Winning does not have to come at a cost of losing our moral and ethical obligations. Aggressively pursuing sports dreams does not require the reckless endangerment of what matters so much more than sports—health, happiness, and human triumph attained without cheating.

Unfortunately, eliminating doping in sports has been a historically challenging task. Steroid use is not a new enemy. U.S. Olympic weightlifting coach Bob Hoffman accused the Soviet Union of doping at the 1952 Olympic Games in Helsinki, Finland, after the Russians won three gold medals, three silver medals, and one bronze medal. Hoffman told the Associated Press, "I know they're taking the hormone stuff to increase their strength."[4] But those claims would not be proven definitively until 2003, when former leading Soviet Union sports scientist Michael Kalinski provided evidence of a well-documented, state-supported steroid research program in his country, which recommended that its elite athletes in many sports use anabolic steroids.[5]

And long before the acronym BALCO[6] became familiar in the na-

Sidebar 1.1: Survival of the Fittest?

"'SURVIVOR' WANNABE" reads the headline over the photo on the front page of the *Houston Chronicle* on January 14, 2003. It's a shot of a smiling, good-looking young man with a tight tank top stretching to cover his fit physique. The caption beneath the photo reads: "Houstonian Daniel Lue, a tax accountant and business owner, is a member of the cast of *Survivor: Amazon*. Lue, 27, says his greatest achievement is transforming himself from a 98-pound weakling." There is nothing new about guys like Lue. He is one of countless other body-building, muscle-manufacturing stories. He's this week's episode—another illustration of a growing segment of society that is driven to look better. And in most cases, looking better means looking bigger and stronger. There is nothing wrong with that. In fact, there is everything right with lifting weights. If done naturally, it's incredibly healthy and is proven to actually make you live longer, or at least look younger.

> No form of exercise more powerfully turns back the markers of age than weight training. It increases strength, retards osteoporosis, speeds up metabolism, enhances mobility, improves posture and dramatically increases energy.[1]

It's important to note the flipside—the other growing segment of society that is not nearly as driven as Lue. These people are driving to McDonald's right now with no plans to exercise in the near future. This increasingly larger portion of the population—growing in numbers and waist size—is in far greater danger of suffering severe health problems, as are their future generations. The potential athletes among them will have a harder time getting as fit as and keeping up with guys like Lue. That competition is becoming a greater reason for young athletes to choose a shortcut to transform from a "weakling" into something much more. While Lue may not have taken performance-enhancing drugs, the evidence worldwide suggests that many in his shoes are seeking the easy way instead of the better way—a bigger, stronger or leaner, meaner body and the self-confidence that comes with it.

The sooner-the-better mentality applies to so much of what we do these days; thus it certainly seems this way of thinking would easily apply to bodybuilding and not just to professionals. Chris Redden, a medical school student who lives in Houston, Texas, and was interviewed by the *Shreveport Times* in 2002, has a lot in common with Lue, only Redden readily admitted to using steroids to gain the improved physique so many of us strive for. Not only does Redden share the same city with Lue, he no doubt shares some of his reasoning for wanting to get bigger—to be more attractive to the opposite sex. Redden began lifting weights as someone who "wasn't really serious about it."[2] Ultimately, however, he gained a purpose for pumping iron that would take him to Mexican pharmacies during two years worth of weekends in order to buy anabolic steroids legally in a foreign country and then to work on his synthetically enhanced body in a Texas gym.

Redden said that although he has since been examined by doctors, and has escaped almost all of the possible side effects of steroids, his experimentation with the drugs was abuse. "I was a healthy 18-year-old. There was really no need for me to do this. I was doing it for cosmetic uses only. I would say, yes, I probably abused them."[3] Redden was told by a casual new acquaintance which types of steroids he should take. His friend said, "'it's going to get you strong and get you big and get you abs.' It was everything I was interested in having. . . . Right off the bat, I could see that my abs were starting to come out really easily. I always had those love handles, and they just disappeared." Redden told the *Times* that he'd gained 18 to 20 pounds of muscle in the first month, while his bench press increased by 130 pounds. He was so impressed with the results and lack of immediate side effects that he told himself, "If I added on different types of steroids, I could get bigger."[4] That's how quickly these dangerous drugs can take control, especially in an increasingly harsh world that measures its men as buff or weak, and its women as fine or flabby. Redden weighed 202 pounds and couldn't bench press 225 pounds before using steroids. His weight reached 242 pounds on his 6-foot-2 frame, and his bench press ballooned to 365 at the height of his steroid use. "I was extremely amazed. I had been in the gym a year and a half previously, and I hadn't seen anything. It's just like a complete surprise, and you just want more. They hook you. You look good, and you want to look better."

But at what cost?

tion's newspapers, the letters GDR (German Democratic Republic) caused a stir in the 1970s. Dr. Steven Ungerleider, a sports psychologist, began to learn of the dangerous effects of steroids in the late 1970s when his clients told him stories of East Germany's enormous female swimmers. "They were huge," wrote Ungerleider, relaying one of the descriptions given to him. "They had shoulders like Dallas Cowboys, hair growing all over their bodies."[7] Former West German Olympic swimmer Brigitte Berendonk and her husband, Werner Franke, a molecular biologist, have been instrumental in uncovering East Germany's state-sponsored program that may have involved the doping of as many as 10,000 athletes. Their efforts helped convict the former Eastern Bloc country's top sports official and sports doctor in

1998 for causing bodily harm to its athletes. Many of the victims were minors when they were made to swallow what they believed were vitamins.[8] In 1997 Berendonk and Franke reported that Manfred Höppner, deputy director and chief physician of the East German Sports Medical Service, claimed, "many, if not all, medal-winning GDR athletes in strength- and speed-dependent events at the Olympic Games of 1972 in Munich had been treated with Oral-Turinabol."[9]

Similar large-scale drug scandals have since been confirmed in other countries, including the United States. The cheating has been persistent and continues today:

- John Ziegler, a doctor who worked with scientists at Ciba Pharmaceuticals (now Novartis) in Summit, New Jersey, created Dianabol in 1958. He later supplied the drug—the first mass-produced anabolic steroid—to the 1960 U.S. Olympic weightlifting team.[10]

- During the 1967 Tour de France, British cyclist Tom Simpson died with high levels of methamphetamine in his system, and a vial of the drug was found in his pocket. It was the first doping death to be televised.[11]

- At the 1972 Munich Games, U.S. track and field athlete Jay Sylvester unofficially polled all the track and field competitors and reported that 68 percent had used anabolic steroids to prepare for the Olympics before testing for steroids began.[12]

- Eight out of 275 athletes who were tested at the Montreal Games were disqualified after testing positive for steroids in 1976.

- Nineteen athletes were disqualified for testing positive for banned substances at the 1983 Pan American Games, the first event in which testosterone levels were tested.

- California physician Robert Kerr admitted to providing steroids for 3,000 to 4,000 patients (although other reports give a much higher number[13]), many of whom he said were celebrities and many others who were Olympic athletes. He claimed under oath to have prescribed androgenic steroids to 20 medal winners in the 1984 Olympic Games in Los Angeles.[14]

- One of the most widely publicized steroid scandals involved one man, Canadian sprinter Ben Johnson. Because American rival Carl Lewis was awarded the 1988 gold medal that was stripped from Johnson after his positive steroid test, and because of the high-profile nature of the hotly contested 100-meter dash, this doping story sparked much suspicion about these and other Olympic Games.

- In 1988 South Carolina's football program was rocked by an article in *Sports Illustrated* by former player Thomas Chaikin, who uncovered an organized steroid distribution scandal at the school. His story eventually resulted in three coaches pleading guilty to lesser charges. The case also produced multiple convictions from outside the program.

- Martti Vainio, a long-distance runner who forfeited an Olympic medal in 1984 after failing a drug test, said the use of banned substances by top Finnish athletes was common in the early 1980s.[15]

- Another doping scandal with effects reaching across the globe surfaced in 1998. A large cache of banned substances (including the endurance-boosting hormone EPO) was discovered during the 1998 Tour de France, cycling's Super Bowl. Shortly afterward, the World Anti-Doping Agency (WADA) was created. Adham Sbeih became the first U.S. athlete to test positive for EPO at the U.S. cycling championships in August 2003.

- The high likelihood that a systematic doping program is at work in China's swimming program was uncovered in 1998 by FINA (La Fédération Internationale de Natation), the sport's governing body. Six drug-related suspensions occurred at the world championships in Australia in January (four swimmers in Perth tested positive for Triamterene, a steroid-masking diuretic, and a fifth swimmer and her coach were suspended for attempting to smuggle 13 vials of the human growth hormone, Somatropin, into Australia). Most of the 28 Chinese swimmers who have been suspended for drug offenses during the 1990s train at the same regional and military training centers, implying systematic use of drugs.[16]

- The most damaging contemporary doping scandal—one that has yet to fully unravel as of the writing of this book—involves the illegal manufacturing and distributing of a "designer steroid" known as THG (tetrahydrogestrinone), which, according to a UCLA scientist who helped develop a test for the previously unknown substance, is similar in structure to the banned steroid gestrinone.[17] British sprinter Dwain Chambers, Europe's 100-meter record holder and one of his country's best hopes for a gold medal at the Athens Olympics, has been permanently barred by UK Athletics, the nation's track and field governing body, from ever competing for Britain in the Olympics. He is banned from any competition for two years, and he is the first athlete who has been punished for testing positive for THG. He leads a list of elite athletes—one that is sure to grow—who have tested positive for the drug.[18] (See chapter 4, "BALCO and Beyond: The Biggest Doping Scandal in Sports History," for more on THG).

- Six U.S. athletes tested positive in 2003 for modafinil, a stimulant related to substances banned by the IAAF (International Association of Athletics Federations): sprinter Chryste Gaines, hurdlers Sandra Glover and Eric Thomas, and hammer thrower John McEwen tested positive at the U.S. track championships in June; hurdler Chris Phillips tested positive at the World Championships in Paris in August; and sprinter Kelli White tested positive at both the U.S. and world championships. White and Gaines are coached by Remi Korchemny, one of the four men charged in the BALCO drug ring.

- U.S. sprinter Jerome Young receives a lifetime ban by the U.S. Anti-Doping Agency on November 11, 2004, following the former 400-meter world champion's second positive test for an illegal steroid. The significance of Young's second violation is that it came only five days after the International Association of Athletics Federations ruled that the 2000 U.S. men's 4x400-meter relay team, which included Young and superstar Michael Johnson, should lose all of its gold medals because Young should not have been allowed on the team after testing positive for steroids in 1999. And two other members of the same 4x400 team—twins Calvin and Alvin Harrison—were each busted for doping prior to the 2004 Athens Games (Calvin tested positive for modafinil at the 2003 U.S. Championships, and Alvin was implicated in the BALCO controversy, having been found guilty of a "non analytical positive" after the USADA found credible evidence that he used THG in June 2004). Three members of a high-profile U.S. sprint relay team brought shame to their country.

This list includes only the more memorable doping controversies in history, spanning several generations and many sports. Inevitably, similar scenarios involving athletes abusing illegal performance-enhancing drugs have spread to all levels of sports and athletes—from elite to average. But whereas the historical origins of this drug use include an East German laboratory and a California doctor's office, today's steroid use most likely begins in a simpler but more stunning place—in the impressionable mind of a child or teenager. Whether it is through their connections to the Internet, friends at school, or secondary acquaintances at local gyms and health clubs, kids are learning about steroids and leaping into the fire. The proof is everywhere, including the NCAA's 2001 drug-use habits survey, which reported that most ergogenic substance use—which includes anabolic steroids—starts in high school.[19]

Almost every modern survey conducted on steroid use arrives at the same conclusion: anywhere from 3.5 percent of teenagers (athletes and nonathletes) to 12 percent (athletes only) are using these drugs. That number drastically increases when you study only high school football players. A survey of football teams at nine schools conducted in 2000 by two University of Louisiana–Lafayette professors in 1999 and 2000 revealed that 28 percent of football players used steroids.[20] This percentage is nearly identical to that of the *Shreveport Times'* subsequent survey of 125 male athletes at seven Shreveport-area high schools in July of 2001 in which 27.2 percent admitted to taking anabolic steroids and 60.8 percent claimed to have known a local player who had tried them.[21] More evidence of the proliferation of steroids in our high schools includes the following:

- A survey of California high school students, results of which were made public on March 24, 2004, found more than 52 percent of boys and 33 percent of girls know someone who takes steroids or supplements. Five percent of girls said they had used such substances. More than 13 percent of boys and 10 percent of girls reported they used anabolic steroids or knew someone who took them.[22]
- The University of Michigan's well-regarded "Monitoring the Future" survey showed that 3.5 percent of high school seniors used anabolic steroids in 2003. The percentage had hovered between 2 and 3 percent for the first 10 years of this annual study before shooting up to 3.7 percent in 2001 and 4 percent in 2002.[23]
- The use of androstenedione (Andro), the direct precursor to testosterone, by high school seniors was reported at 4.7 percent in the

2002 "Monitoring the Future" survey. The substance has since been banned by most professional leagues and legislation is pending to make Andro and other steroid "precursors" illegal by making them subject to the Controlled Substances Act.

- According to a 2002 study led by Randall R. Wroble, teens feel pressure to take steroids and they believe the drugs are easily available. In a survey of 1,553 pre-adolescent (10- to 14-year-old) athletes from 34 states, over 2 percent felt the need to take steroids to improve performance and would consider taking them. Wroble compared his team's results to a study conducted in 1989. These athletes stated that they know where to obtain steroids (88 percent at this time versus 87 percent in 1989). These athletes also say that they are still being offered steroids (3 percent today compared to 4 percent in 1989). And those who are offered steroids often accept them (11 of 49 students, 22 percent).[24]

- A 2001 survey by the Centers for Disease Control and Prevention showed that 11.2 percent of Louisiana high school boys surveyed reported using steroids, and 5.7 percent of Tennessee high school girls acknowledged such use.[25]

- A survey of 45,000 high school students conducted by the University of Michigan Institute for Social Research in 2000 offered frightening estimates about the growing steroids problem:
  - "The rates of steroid use reported among boys in grades 8, 10 and 12 were 2.2 percent, 3.6 percent and 2.5 percent."
  - "The rate of use among 8th- and 10th-grade boys rose 50 percent between 1999 and 2000—from 1.2 percent to 1.7 percent."
  - "The rate of use among girls has remained steady since 1998."[26]

Most experts agree there is likely some level of underreporting that occurs in these surveys. Dr. Robert Voy, the chief medical officer for the U.S. Olympic Committee from 1983 to 1989, goes as far as estimating that one in six high school players use steroids to compete. What's more interesting, however, is that Dr. Voy believes that number increases to one in four in college and one in three in professional sports.[27] Though some may argue these numbers to be high, it makes sense that the prevalence of steroid use correlates with the increasing level of competition. As the stakes rise, so do the pressures of winning. The tendency to turn to steroids also rises. Perennial state championship contenders, whose top players go on to play at major Division I universities, and whose bench warmers still play on less-heralded college teams, are almost unquestionably going to have more steroid users in their locker rooms. When the rewards of a college football scholarship or a professional baseball contract begin to surface, they are very attractive, much more appealing than the risks are discouraging.

As troubling as the above research may be, the more distressing fact remains: not enough high school coaches and their principals have accepted these facts or are taking dramatic steps to effect change in young athletes. The "Monitoring the Future" survey has warned of increasingly high numbers of steroid users since 1991. That was a year after the NCAA implemented a steroid-testing plan, clearly a sign by the governing body of collegiate athletics that this was a problem in need of addressing. Consider that 14 years ago there was substantial proof that 14-year-olds were taking steroids. Yet during those years, the many improvements athletes made on the field did not coincide with the improvement coaches, parents, and others made in their obligation to prevent steroid use.

The story of three teens from Clearfield, Utah, a small city about 30 minutes north of Salt Lake City, is proof that kids are doing whatever it takes to get steroids. The three were arrested in May of 2002 after they made a run to Mexico to buy $15,000 worth of steroids. The 16- and 17-year-old boys took money from as many as 12 other students[28] and drove to Tijuana, Mexico, to purchase the drugs. Kids barely old enough to drive had the guts to drive more than 800 miles, enter a foreign country, buy drugs they knew were illegal, and transport them into the United States.[29] The incidents of kids actually getting caught are few, but only because law enforcement officials admit they cannot devote more resources to policing steroid use and trafficking, especially when they are struggling to fight the abuse of other illegal drugs that affect so many more young people. In 2003, 76.6 percent of high school seniors reported having used alcohol; 58.1 percent said they had been drunk in their lifetime; 46.1 percent had tried marijuana; 14.4 percent had used methamphetamines; and 7.7 percent had done cocaine.[30] The drug problem in the United States is obviously still rampant. These statistics give coaches responsible for the strength and conditioning of athletes even more reason to be the first to recognize when kids bulk up too quickly (see chapter 7, "Solutions to the Out-of-Control Drug Problem in Sports," for visible signs of steroid use from which parents and coaches can benefit).

Roland Eveland is the offensive coordinator for Carencro High School's football team in Lafayette, Louisiana, and he was, for years, the school's strength and conditioning coach. Bob Gobel is a high school football coaching legend in West Virginia with more than 20 years of experience, including experience as head coach for two West Virginia colleges. Charles Breithaupt is the athletic director for the University Interscholastic League, the governing body of Texas high school sports. These men, who are not unlike thousands of coaches, medical trainers, and athletic administrators across the country, are losing the war on steroids. These men, in positions of authority, are not acting on the evidence before them:

- "In 20 years" of supervising young athletes, Eveland told the *Shreveport Times* in 2001, "I've probably had 5,000 athletes that have been through the weight training program. I wouldn't think but maybe one or two of them in the whole group probably abused something else than creatine."[31]
- "The superintendents believe there's not a significant problem," said Breithaupt, who said a survey he facilitated to Texas superintendents showed no need or willingness to begin statewide steroid testing of high school athletes. "They think it can be dealt with through education."[32]
- "From what I've seen, I really don't think it's a big issue as far as abuse at the prep level," said Gobel, who told the *Charlestown* (W.Va.) *Gazette* that he has been suspicious of very few players taking steroids. "A lot of young men are aware that it's a shortcut, but it's not gonna do you any good when you go to college, because you will be tested. It seems like they're pretty much aware of that."[33]

Eveland does not think his young athletes are using steroids, but the statistics above and many more below prove that they are. Breithaupt believes the current education system is working. The coaches who were polled may be correct in thinking education is a better alternative to testing, but clearly their education programs are not effective enough. Gobel has the notion that young athletes seeking an edge in an increasingly competitive sports world have "pretty much" come to the realization that they can't use steroids, not the same steroids being used by professional, international, and collegiate athletes in every sport and at every level. The overwhelming evidence confirms that these impressionable, daring, and sometimes desperate athletes *are* "aware" of the testing, but they are even more aware of the ways to avoid being caught using them. These athletes are also aware of the artificial muscle gains that can be made and of the very high numbers of athletes across the globe who are breaking the rules and taking these steroids and other banned substances—a number they can presume is certainly much higher than the number of athletes who are caught and punished every year, which is addressed in chapter 3, "Athletes to Kids: Do as We Say, Not as We Do."

Evidence of America's steroid problem should provoke those in charge of our children to take more aggressive action in dissuading steroid use—namely through effective education. The "Monitoring The Future" study actually shows that young athletes are becoming less wary of the dangers of steroids each year. In 1998, 68.1 percent of surveyed 12th-graders saw "great risk" in using steroids, but by 2003 the rate had dropped to 55 percent. Similar findings have been reported for disapproval rates. In 1997, 90.8 percent of the respondents (identical to the figure in 1990, the first year of the survey) disapproved of steroid use. That number had steadily dropped to 86 percent by 2003.

Part of this decrease in disapproval can be attributed to the influences in the lives of the kids who responded to this survey. If their peers use steroids, and if they are not being discouraged effectively by their parents and coaches, kids won't fear the results of using steroids. Making matters worse is the fact that some parents and coaches actually encourage their young athletes to use unnatural means to become bigger and stronger, seeking athletic scholarships to make life better for the athlete or themselves. Doctors and expert researchers know how disappointing and real this situation is:

- "If you really believe in winning at all costs, and that's how you raise your kids, drug use is not illogical," Dr. Yesalis told *USA Today* in 2002. "I get about one call a year from one or two idiot parents who want my blessing to their use of growth hormone or anabolic steroids for a kid who is otherwise normal, but they want Johnny or Mary to be a superstar. The conversations are very short, and I'm not very polite. Use of these drugs by kids in sports is wrong. No discussion."[34]

- "We get calls from parents with high school athletes all the time wanting to enhance their son or daughter's performance," says Dr. Frank Uryasz, president of the National Center for Drug Free Sport and the NCAA's director of sports sciences. "Some of them are just questions about dietary supplements, but other calls are about growth hormones and other products. So we can't always rely on parents to be the voice of reason."[35]

- "I think part of it is that the coaches don't really want to know how the athletes can come back 30 pounds heavier a few months later," said Aynsley Smith, Ph.D., of Mayo Clinic's Sports Medicine Center. "Where I suspect I am seeing signs of steroid use is during screening physicals for junior college teams. Many of those players are hoping they'll still catch on at a four-year school. They look ripped, and I see lots of stretch marks, but not like they've been working hard in the gym."[36]

- "A lot of the family practice, primary care docs, are the ones getting the pressure," Dr. Edward Morgan, an orthopedic surgeon told the *Shreveport Times* in 2001. "We've really got a culture where every dad wants his son to be a professional athlete, and you've got this 'We're going to win at any cost,' and unfortunately the kids kind of get wrapped up in it."[37]

- "I see the kids in the office," said Nicholas DiNubile, orthopedic surgeon and team doctor for the NBA's Philadelphia 76ers. "The coaches look the other way; their parents want them getting that scholarship. A lot of people look away when it comes to steroids."[38]

- When 125 football players in Shreveport were asked, "Who, if anyone, has talked to you about the good and/or bad effects of supplements/steroids?" only 22 respondents said their coach. Six others cited a parent, friend, or relative, while 97 either left the question blank or answered "no one."[39]

- The 2004 California high school student steroid survey found that 18 percent of boys know coaches or other sports-related staff who promote the use of such substances.[40]

- "Who has more credibility with athletes than coaches?" asks Dr. Frank Uryasz. "When we speak on campuses, we're always telling administrators to be sure that their staff members aren't the pushers."[41]

As sad as it is that leaders of young, impressionable athletes fail to realize how much of an impact they can have on steering their kids away from steroids, it is encouraging to know there are solutions that schools can adopt that succeed despite this problem. A program called ATLAS (Athletes Training and Learning to Avoid Steroids) empowers young athletes to lead drug-prevention education. With the help of coaches and administrators, this program, highly recommended by the U.S. Department of Health and Human Services and the National Institute on Drug Abuse, is a peer- and team-based program that works. Along with ATHENA (Athletes Targeting Healthy Exercise and Nutrition Alternatives), it is thoroughly detailed in chapter 7.

Follow the Leader:
Kids Need Better Mentors, Heroes

Noted twenty-first-century philosopher Charles Barkley offers the following nugget of knowledge in his book *I May Be Wrong But I Doubt It*: "I just want guys to never ever take for granted how unbelievable our lives are, how much influence we have and how much impact we can have. I want to see guys maximize their impact after athletics, not throw it away."[1] Barkley, of course, is as wildly popular as he is abrasive and controversial, due as much to his outstanding ability as a player and his outspokenness as both a TV commentator and a leader/role model. He has seriously considered running for political office because he is genuinely concerned about social issues beyond the basketball arena. The quote from his book appears to be contradictory to his now famous proclamation in a 1993 Nike advertising campaign: "I am not a role model." But most of us know by now that Barkley's point in 1993 was an attempt to awaken a nation filled with parents who failed to be role models for their children. Of course, the commercials were also aimed at selling sneakers, deflecting criticism against professional athletes, and stirring the pot (as Sir Charles has always done in defiance of a world gone far too politically correct). Unfortunately, the public missed the intended point of the Nike ads and spent so much time "killing" Barkley because of it that they never embraced the validity of the message or the sincerity of the messenger. Without question we are in a worse situation today thanks to many parents who increasingly rely on television, video games, or someone or something else to babysit their children. The social injustice of neglectful parents ignoring the need to nurture their kids, as Barkley barked about in 1993, is a problem that continues to rage out of control and is very worthy of our time, discussion, and energy toward finding solutions. Solving the woes facing the world of sports includes identifying the larger, enveloping problems in society.

Former Oklahoma quarterback and U.S. Representative J. C. Watts connects these dots in his editorial in *The Sporting News*: "We live in a culture that has lost its way. . . . Sports at all levels, from high school to professional athletics, are being affected. . . . But no level of standards, rules, regulations or laws will prevent what we are witnessing. . . . The ultimate responsibility for instilling character in young athletes lies at the front door of their homes. Parents must take responsibility for developing the hearts and minds of their children before they send them out into the abyss of today's culture."[2] (See sidebar 2.1, "Q&A with Jack Nicklaus.")

Consider the following series of excerpts from various studies or related articles that depict the abyss Watts has accurately begun to describe, as well as a consistent, successful weapon in keeping kids from falling into the abyss—a strong, structured family:

- "In America today, [the] institutions [of marriage and family] are under attack. Social trends of the past four decades have seriously weakened marriage and family. Rampant no-fault divorce, unwed childbearing, cohabitation, single-parent families, absentee fathers, premarital and extramarital sexual relations—all have battered and weakened the American family. The crisis is real and its implications for America's future are chilling. No civilization can long endure without strong, healthy families founded on the inviolable institution of marriage as the lifelong union of one man and one woman."—Bridget Maher, policy analyst, Center for Marriage and Family Studies[3]
- "Parents in the U.S. spend less time with their children than parents do in any other developed nation in the world."—President's Council of Economic Advisors, 1999[4]
- "Families have a huge impact on the values of their children. It's not total, it's not absolute; they don't always mirror the values of their parents but it has a huge impact and parents concerned with spiritual things—and religion being the primary expression of that—generally are more concerned with ethical issues as well."—Michael Josephson, founder and president of the Joseph and Edna Institute for Ethics[5]

Sidebar 2.1: Q&A with professional golfing legend Jack Nicklaus, winner of a record 18 major PGA championships, eight Champions Tour majors, and two amateur titles.[1]

Question: What role models influenced and monitored your respect for the rules?

Answer: As I grew up, my father was my role model. My father always played by the rules, he always competed hard, he had a great work ethic and he taught me to do the same. As I grew up, playing golf at Scioto Country Club in Columbus, I was, as a youngster, thrown in with adults, so I had to learn how to behave and treat my elders with respect and deal with being a young person in an adult world. I feel as if that experience made me grow up perhaps a little quicker and it also made me understand that most of these people, who have already experienced some of the problems that youngsters face, learned to cope with them. These people became mentors to me, and from many of them, I learned how I should conduct my life. And I believe that is one of the great aspects about the game of golf: Youngsters interact regularly with adults, and things that kids are tempted by and from in today's society aren't necessarily found in that atmosphere or environment. So I was a lucky one.

And then the teacher I had, Jack Grout, taught me much of the same thing—hard work, dedication, sportsmanship, playing by the rules. All the values I consider most important I learned from my dad and Jack Grout. These were important lessons for me in my life and lessons I wish would be pushed on to all kids as they grow up. Unfortunately, it doesn't work that way. Not all sports are really involved around the adult world. And youngsters are under peer pressure. Sure, I had peer pressure and I succumbed to peer pressure in several ways. But, also because of the values I was taught from my other associations, the peer pressure wasn't a major influence on my life; the adult atmosphere was. And the sport that I was playing, by virtue of conducting yourself under the rules of the game, one learns a code of ethics that virtually no other sport has.

Q: You put a great deal of onus on your role models and the adults you surrounded yourself with.

A: I don't think a lot of kids have that. I think most of the kids today, if they had coaches and role models such as I had, those individuals would tell them what is right and what is wrong, and we wouldn't have a lot of the things that we have today. I think too much emphasis today is put on winning at all costs, and as a result, coaches compromise themselves. If they don't, they lose their jobs. The coach is put between a rock and a hard place. Frankly, there are coaches who don't allow themselves to be put in that position and they have great programs and produce good athletes and good people. Unfortunately, a lot of coaches are about what's in it for them, not the kids. The whole thing should be about the kids, not about the coaches.

Q: In your experience as a father and grandfather do you see a deterioration in the importance of sportsmanship at the sports events you watch?

A: I have 17 grandchildren—we just had our 17th—and at least 10 of them at this time are playing some sort of organized sport. I see the widest range of ethics that you could possibly see. I see some of my grandkids being taught sportsmanship; I see some of my grandkids playing a sport that is sometimes about the coach himself, which I obviously think is very disappointing. Me being a grandfather, it's not my position to get in the middle. I try to keep my mouth shut as much as possible, and, you know, that can be pretty difficult for me *(laughs)*. I do talk to their parents—my kids—and I think my five children understand the values of sportsmanship, because I think I tried to teach them the way I was taught. They are all smart and they understand when a coach is using kids. Of course, I see a coach who has given of his time to coach a little league team. But often, that coach's son or daughter is the pitcher, or catcher, and the No. 3 batter, or they are the point guard or the quarterback. Is that the right message to send the other kids?

- "From my perspective as the executive director of the Citizenship Through Sports Alliance, our organization is deeply concerned about the deterioration of values today. It seems that there is a decline in basic fundamentals. And we're concerned because sport plays such an important part in that it is such an incredible influence on young people."—John Leavens, executive director, Citizenship Through Sports Alliance[6]
- "The number one predictor of the future friends, values and morals of children is the worship life of their parents and family—worship in the home and at church."—1999 Gallup study[7]
- "Teens who do not consider religious beliefs important are almost three times likelier to drink, binge drink and smoke, almost four times likelier to use marijuana and seven times likelier to use illicit drugs than teens who strongly believe that religion is important. And teens who never attend religious services are twice as likely to drink, more than twice as likely to smoke, more than three times likelier to use marijuana and binge drink and almost four times

likelier to use illicit drugs than teens who attend religious services at least weekly."—2001 Columbia University study[8]

- "You would normally expect to see a higher percentage of religious families are going to exercise moral influence over their children. And that includes regular attendance at services, but to suggest that religion is therefore necessary in ethics is, I think, an inappropriate conclusion. . . . The children of ministers are not always good kids. The model is often as important as the preaching. So children will learn enormously from the way parents deal with situations, not just what they say. And children learn not just from how parents act when they know their kids are watching, but how they deal with temptation. A footnote to the religion issue is that kids in full-time religious schools cheat on exams at a higher rate—78 percent versus 72 percent. There are a lot of explanations for that—in private schools there's more money; they may be more highly pressured by their parents—but the fact remains that the religious affiliation itself does not produce better behavior in all areas. The Archdiocese of Los Angeles just adopted a very comprehensive plan to institute character counseling. So we've got a Catholic school system acknowledging there are challenges developing character today that may require some different strategies and approaches than the traditional ones. That's a pretty good indication that people in religious circles are in the same boat as everyone else in trying to cope with modern society."—Michael Josephson, head of the world's largest character counseling organization, the Josephson Institute of Ethics.[9]

(See sidebar 2.2, "A Word to Parents.")

And what are the problems of modern society? In her book entitled *The Family Portrait*, Bridget Maher offers an extensive list. Maher's comprehensive work describes society's moral decline, which explains the disregard of morals and ethics by athletes at all levels in modern sports. Correcting society's most serious problems obviously would have a residual effect on problems within the realm of sports, but in the absence of suddenly solving the world's evils, knowing the roots of these evils at least gives schools, youth leagues, and other pertinent organizations more knowledge of the obstacles they face. The components and requirements of success in competitive sports, such as disci-

Sidebar 2.2: A Word to Parents

One of the saddest and most tragic features of [our] "Civilization" is the awful prevalence of disobedience on the part of children to their parents during the days of childhood, and their lack of reverence and respect when they grow up. This is evidenced in many ways, and is general, alas, even in the families of professing Christians. In his extensive travels during the past thirty years the writer has sojourned in a great many homes. The piety and beauty of some of them remain as sacred and fragrant memories, but others of them have left the most painful impressions. Children who are self-willed or spoiled not only bring themselves into perpetual unhappiness but also inflict discomfort upon all who come into contact with them and augur, by their conduct, evil things for the days to come.

In the vast majority of cases the children are not nearly so much to be blamed as the parents. Failure to honor father and mother, wherever it is found, is in large measure due to parental departure from the Scriptural pattern. Nowadays the father thinks that he has fulfilled his obligations by providing food and raiment for his children, and by acting occasionally as a kind of moral policeman. Too often the mother is content to be a domestic drudge, making herself the slave of her children instead of training them to be useful. She performs many a task which her daughters should do in order to allow them freedom for the frivolities of a giddy set. The consequence has been that the home, which ought to be—for its orderliness, its sanctity, and its reign of love—a miniature heaven on earth, has degenerated into "a filling station for the day and a parking place for the night," as someone has tersely expressed it.

Before outlining the duties of parents toward their children, let it be pointed out that they cannot properly discipline their children unless they have first learned to govern themselves. How can they expect to subdue self-will in their little ones and check the rise of an angry temper if their own passions are allowed free reign? The character of parents is to a very large degree reproduced in their offspring. . . .

—Arthur W. Pink, Christian author, based on his travels in the early 1900s[1] pline, a strong work ethic, teamwork, respect for authority, respect for opponents and teammates, etc.—a lot of which we notice is disintegrating much as it is in society as a whole—can become a starting point to begin an improvement in a small but significant way. Leagues, coaches, and parents working together can take their understanding of society and its issues and target the problems with solutions that result in rewards—not just for *their* teams or *their* players but for the many other young players and fans who are involved in the same circle of influence.

No, it is not possible to decrease the teen pregnancy rate in America by teaching sportsmanship to Little League baseball players; nor will climbing divorce rates and their consequences be eliminated by coaches who successfully teach kids to respect officials. But there are small ways we *can* make a major difference. Here's one example: If we know that "family disruption and lack of parental involvement during childhood correlate with increased lying, cheating, fighting and criminal activity in children," and since we know that "children in single-parent families have a 77 percent greater risk of harm by physical abuse and an 87 percent greater risk of harm due to physical neglect," and because we know "children in single-parent families have lower grades, lower expectations about college and poorer attendance records than do children in two-parent families,"[10] we can positively influence children with divorced or disrupted families by being positive influences in fundamental areas for *all* the children on a particular team. If we know more about society's problems, we understand the importance of being role models—not only those in charge (coaches, administrators) but those who participate (parents on the sidelines, team leaders, children of coaches, high school upperclassmen, and others).

Men coach the majority of youth sports today. One third of children who live exclusively with their mothers interact with their fathers in person once a year or not at all. These children can and often do find father figures among their coaches, and there is evidence that girls need fatherly influence as much as boys do. If what ails society also ails the sports world, the problems we are dealing with may appear too daunting, but a coach who is knowledgeable about these problems is at least armed to deal with the underlying issues that can lead to breakdowns within the context of a league or team. Using

Maher's *The Family Portrait* as a source, the following list is an attempt to summarize the youth's biggest problems at present:

- Escalating drug and alcohol use and increased binge drinking.
- Increased parental adultery, a main reason for the increase in divorce and the rising cases of sexually transmitted diseases, including those that are present in nearly all cervical cancers.
- More births to unmarried women (nearly one in three), and the subsequent increase in children who will never have a father (one-fifth of white children and three-fifths of black children), and yet another high likelihood of divorce when single mothers do marry (twice as likely to divorce as were couples who did not enter marriage with children).
- Increases in cohabitation before marriage, which has a 46 percent greater risk of divorce than couples who do not live together before marriage, caused in part by increased infidelity because there is "less investment" in the sanctity of marriage.
- Increases in depression among children studied after divorces (more than one third of kids).
- An upsurge in divorce by children of divorced parents; increased suicide by these children; more abuse of children whose parents divorce; more sexual intercourse, teen pregnancies (twice as high in the United States than in any other advanced country), and STDs by these children.
- More high school dropouts who are pregnant; a higher risk of children born to teen mothers becoming juvenile delinquents and chronic criminals (males from these families are 1.7 times more likely to become chronic offenders, while the females were 2.8 times more likely).
- Increases in juvenile arrest rates for violent crimes (more than tripling from 1965 to 1992).
- Increases in teen abortions (9.5 million from 1973 to 1999 for women under age 20; one in 34 girls age 15 to 19 in 1996).
- Increases in teen suicide (between 1980 and 1998 the suicide rate among 10- to 14-year-olds doubled).[11]

Maher includes observations from a few public figures in her presentation:

- "From the wild Irish slums of the 19th century Eastern seaboard to the riot-torn suburbs of Los Angeles, there is one unmistakable lesson in American history: a community that allows a large number of young men to grow up in broken families, dominated by women, never acquiring any stable relationship to male authority, never acquiring any rational expectations about the future—that community asks for and gets chaos. Crime, violence, unrest, disorder—most particularly the furious, unrestrained lashing out at the whole structure—that is not only to be expected; it is very near to inevitable. And it is richly deserved."—Senator Daniel Patrick Moynihan[12]

- "Moral poverty is the poverty of being without loving, capable, responsible adults who teach you right from wrong; the poverty of being without parents and other authorities who habituate you to feel joy at others' joy, pain at others' pain, satisfaction when you do right, remorse when you do wrong; the poverty of growing up in the virtual absence of people who teach morality by their own everyday example and who insist that you follow suit. . . . And moral poverty, not economic poverty, is what marks some disadvantaged youngsters for a life of crime while passing over others in equal or greater material distress."—William J. Bennett, John J. DiIulio Jr., and John P. Walters[13]

Distressing. Disheartening. Discouraging. But not cause for complete despair. There is plenty of hope. Most notably there is evidence that our efforts to strengthen the family, especially the bond and communication between parents and children, can make a difference, as the following research from Maher's work suggests.

- In 2001, 79 percent of adults said parental supervision greatly affects whether or not a teenager tries illegal drugs.
- Teens' connectedness to parents, including shared activities and high parental expectations, protects against serious emotional distress and suicide, according to the 1997 Adolescent Health study of 12,000 youth.
- When compared to other strategies, Americans think that the best solution to youth violence is for married parents to stay together and to stay involved in their children's lives.

- In a 2000 poll, 78 percent supported a proposal to require married couples with children who are considering a divorce to obtain counseling before a divorce would be granted.
- Data from a 1997 longitudinal health study of 11,000 adolescents found that teens were more likely to delay sexual intercourse when they felt emotionally connected to their parents and when their parents disapproved of their being sexually active or using contraception.
- Nearly all teenagers believe that teens should be given a strong message from society to abstain from sex until at least after high school.
- In 1995, 44 percent of girls age 15-19 who said they had never had premarital sex cited religious or moral values as their main reason for abstaining.
- A 1998 poll shows that 62 percent think a divorce should be harder to obtain than it is now.
- A 1999 poll found that 64 percent of Americans think the rise of single-parent households is a serious problem.
- A 1998 poll found that 82 percent of Americans believe that teen pregnancy is a serious healthcare problem.
- In 1988, 37 percent of male teens said it was all right for a female to have an abortion for any reason, compared to 24 percent in 1995.
- In 1998, 72 percent of Americans agreed that married parents are less likely to have children who are violent and commit crimes.[14]

At the risk of grossly oversimplifying a tremendous palate of problems, Barkley was right in 1993, and he spoke the same words in 2004 in an interview for this book: "That's the solution—you gotta be better parents, plain and simple," he said. "Stop looking for cop-outs." But Barkley's message, quoted at the beginning of this chapter, is also worth an in-depth look. Professional athletes are role models who have the tremendous capability to positively affect children and teenagers. And they don't have to wait until after athletics to "maximize their efforts." They can begin to set better examples now by cleaning up their respective sports—clearly and consistently taking strong stances against drug use, working harder to seek out and discourage teammates from using performance-enhancing drugs, handling disputes with officials more professionally, and placing a priority on being a good citizen (one kids will want to look up to). Too often, kids today recognize elite athletes more because of their tattoos and temper tantrums than their character and abilities. But these star athletes have and always will enjoy "unbelievable" lives. Kids will always covet those lives. The actions of professional athletes can influence future stars as well as kids who play sports without a chance of reaching the pros. Barkley is, essentially, imploring his fellow stars to recognize God's blessings, understand how those blessings can work meaningfully in young lives, and then take action—with the same maximum effort displayed in competition—in order to help others. If it sounds as if Charles Barkley *is* a role model, it should. He still insists today: "I think all athletes are leaders and somewhat of role models, but the biggest role models are parents, not famous jocks and famous people. Most jocks and famous people are good people, but they make mistakes and the media and parents blame them [for being poor role models]."[15]

Again, Barkley is right in asking parents to do their job and for the media to minimize their influence. A majority of celebrities and sports heroes *are* good. But a majority of kids who watch celebrities and sports heroes consider them peers, and research has definitively proven the power peers have in influencing adolescent behavior. Kids want to emulate mediated peers just as they do their favorite teacher, their playground friends, or their parents. Since kids spend so much time watching television, and since TV networks strive to grab their attention, mediated peers like belly-button-baring Brittany Spears and "Be Like Mike" Jordan are as much an influence as any other peers children have. Dr. Johnette McCrery, a college professor currently studying the effects of violent video games on children, has come across this evidence in her teaching. "Many of the trends and values adopted by young people are coming from mediated figures they know only through television," McCrery says. "I remember reading in one of my textbooks that we are more likely to mourn today the death of a celebrity—for example, Princess Diana—than we are to mourn the death of a neighbor living right next door. I warn my students about replacing authentic relationships with mediated relationships because our mediated relationships can never be truly fulfilling. You must remember they are one-sided. Had I died eight years ago in a car wreck instead of Diana, she wouldn't have cried for me the way I did for her."[17] Evidence strongly linking today's teens with their television role models leaves us at the same conclusion reached during Barkley's "I'm not a role model" fallout: Athletes should not be primary role models for children, but many times they are just that. Michael Josephson, author of several books on character building, including *Parenting to Build Character in Your Teen* (2001), is qualified to offer an expert opinion on realizing how star athletes can impact young lives. The Josephson institute of Ethics makes the claim that all of its programs are "nonpartisan and nonsectarian, promoting a common language of core values called the Six Pillars of Character: trustworthiness, respect, responsibility, fairness, caring and citizenship."[17] While his organization does not seek professional athletes to be spokesmen or role models, Josephson says that athletes have an important, powerful responsibility to help lead those who follow their every move:

> I think we put too much responsibility and too much blame on the high profile people. Having said that, I don't agree with Charles Barkley's statement—and I don't know if he agrees with it anymore—that they're not role models, that they didn't sign up for it. It's not a volunteer position. . . . The problem is when we make it an either or. Wherever you are and whoever you are you have to do your share. You're either contributing to the improvement or to the dilution [of morality] by what you do. To acknowledge that is terribly important. To say they're not the primary role model is also not to say they're not a relevant or influential role model. But I am absolutely convinced that no matter how bad we might see role models from our politicians to business people to celebrities to athletes, that if [kids] have good grounding where they live, where they play, where they learn, that negative role model simply becomes an illustration of what's unacceptable rather than a temptation. . . . People become celebrities because of a talent that has nothing to do with character.[18]

Dr. Linn Goldberg, professor of medicine and the head of the Division of Health Promotion and Sports Medicine at Oregon Health and Science University, has also come to the conclusion that while kids today may emulate their sports heroes, there is no indication they will listen to warnings from superstars to steer clear of drugs of any kind. Dr. Goldberg also understands drug testing and how punishing teenagers has failed to change their behavior. He has, however, found an alternative solution that has proven to work—using peers as leaders and role models for other young athletes. Goldberg's ATLAS program is a peer-led, team-based program that has worked so well that the U.S. Department of Health and Human Services has recognized it as a "model program" in 2000, the highest award for an antidrug program. ATLAS will be discussed in detail in the drug solutions chapter of this book (chapter 7), but the premise is simple. Antidrug messages from authority figures have failed to correct the problem, but early results of the ATLAS program substantiate some often-controversial psychological research that peers can have the greatest influence in adolescents' lives. Therefore, peers can deter their peer groups from doping as well as using recreational drugs, driving while intoxicated, and stumbling into many more potential hazards of youth.

In her award-winning book, Judith Rich Harris provides perhaps the best evidence to date that peers have a bigger-than-ever impact on adolescent development.[19] And while her assertion that parents have little to no influence on certain aspects of a child's life choices is inconclusive and highly debatable, her theories are well respected by experts in the field, including those with previously opposing views. Another study shows that adolescents are most influenced by the collective desires of their peer group (more than their individual desires),[20] and yet another study reports that parents as a whole have become increasingly isolated from their children since the 1940s.[21] Psychologist Gordon Neufeld and physician Gabor Mate agree—not without resistance—with Harris's conclusions, but they urge parents to actively work to counteract the powerful peers' impact in their new book, *Hold on to Your Kids: Why Parents Matter*.[22] A review of this work in *Maclean's* summarizes the aggressive steps parents can take to do so: "The authors' tone is urgent, fuelled not just by research but also by alarming experiences with their own kids. But their advice is measured: parents must not 'abandon the field.' Maintain family outings and holidays; eat together as often as you can. Make time for activities that foster emotional intimacy."[23]

Stronger peer relationships do not justify poor parenting. To the contrary, parents should work harder to connect with and influence children despite the natural urges toward independence, which begin gaining steam during adolescence. Part of a parent's responsibility is monitoring who their children's role models are. Youth sports participants not only associate with their teammates but on a much larger scale—imagined or real—with professional athletes. Again, kids want the lives of superstars, so they imagine themselves as a part of that setting. They may attempt to model the lives of these superstars, just as they might do so for other role models they interact with daily. A parent who is involved in their child's life should not only know who their child's heroes are, but they should also be able to answer why, how much, and what are the consequences. Why are an athlete's life, abilities, and other actions "cool" or admirable? How much is the child enthralled and prone to imitate this hero? What does the child athlete gain or lose by modeling their actions after their favorite superstar? Dr. Michael Josephson says parents can capitalize by knowing more about their kids and cut out potentially poor behavior before it occurs. Spending more time with kids is the solution. "We hope part of the modeling and teaching that occurs at the level of personal interaction with a young person is to help them mediate what they see," Josephson says. "So if Brittany Spears acts in a particular way, ask questions [to children] like, 'Is that what you really want to do? Do you think that would work in your life?' "[24]

Regardless of which peers influence them, children are all prone to seek any way possible to be accepted by society. And since physical appearance is a particularly important issue to teenagers, parental interaction with their children—whether they compete in sports or not—can help parents notice the symptoms of teen steroid use (discussed in chapter 1), which is becoming an increasingly available and enticing shortcut to enhancing one's looks. A few points to consider are:

- European journalist Paul Kelso states: "There's a growing gymnasium culture of bodybuilding. And we're finding that there's more and more evidence that young people are taking drugs for no reason, really, other than vanity—to grow bigger muscles, to look better."[25]
- A 2003 Blue Cross Blue Shield Association survey found that

among the youth who knew someone using performance-enhancing supplements, 27 percent said these teens were taking the substances to "look better," an increase from 19 percent in 2001.[26]

- Because exercising is appealing to athletes and nonathletes alike, males and females are equally at risk. Dr. Charles Yesalis has said that teenage girls see the muscular appearance of today's athletes and entertainers and seek to attain similar results with steroids: "While I condemn the use of steroids to achieve that look, clearly they would affect that look in women."[27]

- And because this group of potential users—nonathletes or part-time athletes who exercise to improve their looks—are not as easy to target with educational messages from natural authority figures such as high school coaches, the importance of strong parenting is, yet again, abundantly clear.

Athletes to Kids: Do as We Say, Not as We Do

Charles Barkley may be right a lot of the time—and he may think he is right most of the time—but on the topic of steroid use in sports today, he is as wrong as he was round in Philadelphia. To his credit, he will take as much time to discuss important social matters as his schedule allows. And he has no problem stating that he is not an expert on everything: "I don't know all that much about steroids," he said in May 2004. And, once again, he is right about that. "Only five percent of athletes use steroids and 95 percent are clean, so it's not a big deal," he said.[1] But those numbers are drastically higher than most people believe, as is proven in numerous ways.

- Surveys conducted by some of the most respected sports researchers in the country indicate as many as 12 percent of athletes use steroids and at least two surveys (cited in chapter 1) show that more than twice that number of high school, college, and pro football players are doping.
- We are discovering that science continues to be at least one step behind cheaters. The designer steroid THG—the substance at the heart of the BALCO investigation that is causing an unprecedented controversy in professional baseball and in track and field—would never have been identified if not for an anonymous tip from a coach who provided the steroid to authorities who only then were able to develop the test to detect it. Because of other undetectable performance-enhancers such as Human Growth Hormone (HGH) and, perhaps eventually, gene therapy, we may never fully conquer this enemy.
- According to the U.S. Anti-Doping Agency, of the 6,890 drug tests conducted in 2003, only 22 (0.3 percent) were positive.[2] Penn State professor Dr. Charles Yesalis adds: "These results do not measure

the use of performance-enhancing strategies for which no tests are currently available. These include the use of drugs and other substances like human growth hormone, insulin, insulin-like growth factor, sodium bicarbonate and creatine, as well as techniques like blood doping."[3]

- Steroid guru Dr. Robert Kerr, a California sports physician who at one time said at least 70 physicians in the Los Angeles area alone were prescribing anabolic steroids to athletes, testified that he prescribed anabolic steroids to approximately 20 medalists at the 1984 Olympic Games. The significance here is that none of the 20 athletes tested positively for using steroids, leaving us safe to estimate that many more doping medalists were avoiding detection, totaling much higher than the oft-assumed 5 percent.[4]

- The Drug Abuse Enquiry Report concluded that there were doctors in Britain who were involved in monitoring athletes' steroid use to ensure they were within safe and undetectable ranges. And, the report added, "test centers are readily at hand at which a British athlete who has been using banned drugs in training can check in advance of competition that his urine sample will no longer disclose the presence of the banned drug."[5]

- Nine-time U.S. Olympic gold medalist Carl Lewis said in 1999: "Federations at every level are covering up drugs and covering up for people. . . . It's a joke. It's a credibility factor and it starts at the top. Sadly enough, America is right in the middle of it. . . . The commitment to find drugs is not there. There are much better ways to test than they are doing, but . . . they don't want to catch anyone in the first place."[6]

- Dr. Robert O. Voy, the former director of the U.S. Olympic committee's (USOC) drug-control program, said in a sworn affidavit that during his tenure, U.S. Olympic athletes commonly used banned drugs. And not only did the USOC fail to discourage this doping, it actually covered up positive tests. Voy submitted the affidavit in support of Dr. Wade Exum, his successor, who is awaiting a federal appeal on a lawsuit that accuses the USOC of fraud, discrimination, and routinely allowing athletes to compete after testing positive for banned substances.[7]

- In May of 2004, the accusations by Dr. Voy and Dr. Exum were affirmed when the IOC admitted the USOC failed to keep athletes out of competitions despite testing positive for banned substances. The *Orange County Register* in April of 2003 reported finding more than 100 U.S. athletes who failed drug tests and yet still competed in the Olympics and other world-class events.[8] Despite initially agreeing to explain which of these athletes claimed to have been using medication and not performance-enhancing drugs, the USOC did not do so and did not respond to several follow-up correspondences during the writing of this book.

- Dr. Elliott Pellman, the medical director for both the New York Jets and the New York Islanders, told the *New York Daily News* in 2002: "The players and the team owners have sold their souls to the devil with steroids, and I know, because I've been treating professional athletes since 1986."[9]
- The drug-testing system is flawed in many ways. Though the formation of the World Anti-Doping Agency has helped the uniformity of policies and has helped to eliminate the bureaucracy involved in previous years, significant hurdles remain. Tests consistently fail to reveal athletes who really are doping; masking agents or similar countermeasures that negate high testosterone levels and other indicators of doping remain a step ahead of the testing procedures; and it is widely known that testing is ineffective for the simple and inexcusable reason that it is often not possible to locate the athletes who are to be randomly tested when they are away from competition.

It is obvious that the small but consistent percentage of positive doping tests in sports is not indicative of the actual number of athletes who abuse these drugs (several lists of doping busts appear later in this chapter). This higher percentage of users—however small or large an increase it may be—is proof that athletes continually risk being caught because, in their minds, the potential rewards are worth the cost. "Drug testing has been a colossal flop for more than three decades," Dr. Charles Yesalis has said. "It has been the same strategy for years: We had a problem before, but now we fixed it. Well, it's not fixed."[10] Dr. Gerhard Treutlein, a professor and head of the Sports Sciences and Sports Pedagogics Department of the University of Education of Heidelberg, Germany, says the solutions have been slow to come because they are being withheld.

Condoning is much less demanding than informing people about drug abuse and rejecting drugs deliberately or passing on values effectively. Condoning and concealment seem to have been used as systematic strategies. Numerous examples illustrate this kind of behavior: the topic of drug abuse has not been dealt with in special journals; the findings of conferences on drugs have not been published; speeches have been given to manipulate the public; the reality of drug abuse has been denied and lies have been told about it; campaigns have been launched spreading false information; active commitment has been demonstrated though no positive action has been taken; athletes who were not willing to take drugs have been unsupported in their team and at nominations; and funds intended for clearing up the past and present circumstances of drug abuse have not been provided.[11]

Barkley and others are wrong if they believe that our drug-testing methods are adequate and that steroid abuse is not a big deal. Blame can be spread all around—elite athletes who dope; teammates who condone more than condemn; administrators who see dollars today instead of damages tomorrow; even fans and media who don't do enough to demand change. "The fans really don't care about doping. They want to be entertained," Dr. Yesalis says. "They view athletes as entertainers the way they view the Rolling Stones or some actor. You have a number of multibillion-dollar businesses around the world that call themselves sports. And they are very attentive to their customers. If their customers were really upset about this, things would change very quickly."[12] The lack of change means a lack of interest in finding solutions. And while these solutions are seldom sought, found, or passed on, the hope for the future of sports lies in how much improvement can be made by those willing to work at it. Teamwork, owners, commissioners, coaches, and players can make it harder to dope in professional sports. Academic and athletic leaders of colleges and the heads of other amateur sports programs can unite with their coaches, players, boosters, and sponsors to demand cleaner competition. Legislators, principals, parents, and parental figures charged with leading our adolescents can develop, fund, and implement affordable programs (e.g., ATLAS and ATHENA—see chapter 7) that exist to create better men, women, citizens, and future leaders who will continue building a stronger, straighter society as they mature.

If elite athletes do not continue to use performance-enhancing drugs—despite better testing methods and harsher penalties—kids will continue to use these drugs as well. If athletes believe "only five percent of guys are using steroids," and "it's not a big issue," as Barkley said, the problem will continue to grow.[13] It appears that not enough professional athletes, coaches, or league administrators know or care about the statistics presented in the previous chapter—12 to 16 percent of high school football players use steroids, increasing to as much as 25 percent in college and 33 percent in professional football.[14] Sports provide athletes with obvious incentives—scholarships, professional contracts, and if time and injury are not too harsh, a lengthy, lucrative career. The willingness by athletes at all levels to sacrifice health for results is a reality. As a result, performance-enhancing drugs are gnawing away at the integrity of sports today more than ever. Like the rats at Madison Square Garden, elite athletes who abuse these drugs are mostly hidden from the public, yet a small percentage of them are regularly exposed for using steroids or other banned substances. This is where the "no big deal" 5 percent comes in. Those whose job it is to root out these rodents do so on a consistent but ineffective basis. Better testing systems and stiffer penalties—though only a part of the solution—would result in fewer users and therefore fewer busts. Instead, the abuse in all sports is growing, and there is substantial evidence (cited above) that the athletes who are unlucky enough to be caught represent a fraction of those actually doping.

Even when the light is shined on these cheaters, they scurry out of sight only to return to competition after serving insignificant suspensions. The only thing worse would be no suspension at all or even no testing at all. Sadly, that is what professional baseball has sought and is still unsettled on. And as recently as 2003, the NFL's players association (NFLPA) tried to get the league to reduce penalties for using ephedra or other banned substances in dietary supplements. The NFLPA's executive director, Gene Upshaw, was trying to negotiate with the league's management council to change the policy. "(The NFL) is still at four weeks and we're at zero," Upshaw said then. "Somewhere in there is a deal."[15] An agent for one suspended player suggested that players receive a warning for a first positive test and a four-game suspension for a second positive test.[16] Fortunately, there was no deal, and the light-as-it-is penalty of four games remains in place. But the stench of dissatisfaction from the players persists as thick today as ever. In 1986, with free agency and collective bargaining agreements the hottest issues in three of professional sports' biggest leagues—the NFL, the NHL, and Major League Baseball—drug policies were difficult to agree on, with owners pushing for more and better testing and the players fighting for their privacy and right to dope. One top sports agent representing several athletes told the *Toronto Star*: "If the players try to use drug testing as a bargaining chip to gain a more liberal free-agency system, they risk disbelief, even scorn, from the public. Many people feel that something as important as (having drug-free) public figures who are major role models for millions of youngsters should be automatic and not just a commodity to be bartered at the bargaining table."[17] The penalties should be harsher at the college and professional levels, not softer. To do otherwise is to take dangerous steps in the wrong direction.

Though the NFL's policy on performance-enhancing drugs is commendable—a policy that NCAA doping czar Dr. Frank Uryasz calls the best in professional sports—the league has been playing catch-up since the start of the steroid age. In 1986 Pat Toomay, a former defensive end in the NFL for 10 years with the Cowboys, Raiders, Bills, and Bucs, said of commissioner Pete Rozelle and the NFL's lagging drug-testing program: "All of a sudden [Rozelle's] worried. Why wasn't he worried twenty years ago? Fifteen years ago? Five? It's been going on forever. What about all those guys running around on amphetamines? Painkillers? Steroids? They just didn't start hurting people last season, you know."[18] (See sidebar 3.1, "Truth and Lies behind the NFL's 'Exemplary' Drug-Testing Plan.")

Concerns about performance-enhancing drugs in the NFL were starting to surface in 1973, when George Burman, a Washington Redskins center, detailed such drug abuse, including amphetamine usage. At the time, Redskins coach George Allen said: "I know we don't have a drug problem. I'm not worried about it."[19] Almost 25 years after Allen's comments appeared in the *Washington Post*, Allen's son, Senator George Allen (R-VA), who has been an aggressive opponent to steroids in sports, wrote in April of 2004: "The growing presence of steroids in American sports is threatening the essence of the games that we so much admire. . . . We need to make sure that all young

Sidebar 3.1: Truth and Lies behind the NFL's "Exemplary" Drug-Testing Plan

The NFL's performance-enhancing drug policy is lauded as being one of the best in sports. Dr. Frank Uryasz, president of the National Center for Drug Free Sport, says, "In our industry that program is well thought of and people are confident that they take action when there are positives (in drug testing)." The league also has made an aggressive move against doping by joining the United States Anti-Doping Agency (USADA) and the University of Utah to create a new drug-testing laboratory at the school's Salt Lake City campus. According to the NFL, the laboratory will conduct state-of-the-art research into the use of and detection of prohibited steroids and other performance-enhancing substances. The NFL is certainly investing in a necessary plan to prevent further abuse, but there is much room for improvement. World Anti-Doping Agency founding chair Dick Pound says, "The NFL has made some improvements . . . [but] its program is far short of effective."[1] One reason is one most organizations face—doing nothing for so long that struggling to catch up to the cheaters is the best anyone can hope for. The NFL's leadership spent more time protecting its image than it did its players or its credibility at the outset of the fight against doping. And despite its financial commitment to the technological war against modern cheaters, it can be argued that the NFL continues to minimize the problem with its weak penalties.

When NFL commissioner Pete Rozelle said in July of 1986: "Our concern is the health and welfare of the players—those taking drugs and those injured by those taking drugs," many asked "what took so long?" Rozelle's concerns were announced at a press conference he called to announce details of the league's first performance-enhancing drug-testing program. As mentioned in chapter 3, NFL players had admitted to doping 16 years earlier. St. Louis Cardinals linebacker Dave Megyesy wrote about it in "Out of Their League" in 1970. Washington Redskins center George Burman spoke of it openly in 1973. Dallas Cowboys and New York Giants receiver Pete Gent wrote of it in his 1974 novel *North Dallas Forty*. Worse, the NFL knew doping was potentially widespread in 1974 when it issued its first penalties for violations of the league's drug policies. San Diego Chargers owner Eugene Klein, coach Harland Svare, and eight players were fined after a former player gave Rozelle multiple prescriptions for amphetamines that had been written by Dr. Arnold Mandell, a team psychiatrist. Svare later revealed that two years after he was fined, Rozelle secretly refunded his fine, another example of the league's back-room dealings kept from the public to minimize scrutiny.

Despite increasing evidence of doping, the NFL waited until 1986 to announce a drug policy. It did not begin testing until a year later in 1987, which was only for "informational purposes," and did not begin suspending players for using steroids until 1989. Effective year-round random testing was not implemented until 1990. The International Olympic Committee saw doping as an important issue and has tested medalists and other competitors chosen at random for anabolic steroids since the 1968 Games in Mexico City. Yet widespread drug use continued in the NFL for more than two decades until testing began. When a slow-moving and inadequate drug policy is actually acceptable and even praised by those in charge, who can expect the solutions to ever catch up to the problems? By not testing and suspending players immediately, the public was essentially lied to about the NFL's drug problems. It is obvious now why Major League Baseball was not embarrassed to present its joke of a drug-testing policy—one in which players were told they would be tested in several months but would not be suspended. They were warned, they had no punishment to fear, and yet at least 5 to 7 percent of them tested positively. The NFL's plan, again, praised for its effectiveness, was a preposterous precedent.

It should then come as no surprise that 18 years after the initial formation—and 14 years after its true enforcement began—the NFL today is as many steps behind as any other league. The evidence has already been presented that a vast number of athletes who are doping are not being caught, for reasons that include the controversial calculating process in which players are permitted to have up to six times the normal level of the male hormone testosterone before they are considered a "presumptively positive." Only a T/E ratio that exceeds 10-to-1 is considered "conclusively positive." The NFL (and the IOC and others that use the 6-to-1 ratio) are leaving a large enough window to cast serious doubt as to the actual number of players who are doping. In his book, *Inside the Olympics*, Pound says, ". . . there [is] no empirical evidence of such a level (6-to-1) ever being achieved naturally. Knuckles would be virtually dragging on the ground at that level."[2] (See chapter 5, "Steroids and Designer Drugs," for more detailed descriptions of the controversial T/E ratio.) As previously discussed, the integrity of the game and the health of professional football players would be better served with a lower ratio. Even when a player does test positive for absurd levels of testosterone, the minimal punishment delivered for these violations contributes to further use.

Former Pittsburgh Steelers lineman Steve Courson, who used steroids to bolster his talents and who now uses the topic of doping to boost his post-playing career, is an expert in the psychological sphere of this issue. In his written work, "Performance-Enhancing Drugs (PEDs), Image vs. Reality," Courson points to 10 "facts" athletes believe to be true that create an environment in which "non-users are the vast minority," and "the majority of world records are chemically enhanced." Courson says, "Athletes know this:"

- Their value is measured entirely by performance.
- The deception involving PEDs is more accepted than training reality.
- Drug testing has many frailties that make a level playing field impossible.
- Athletes know they have limited windows of opportunity and these drugs enhance training beyond what can be achieved without them.
- The current image of sports is unrealistic.
- Sports management and society reward performance even though it may reflect potential or even obvious drug enhancement.
- The risk factors of most of these drugs have been overstated.
- Admittance of PED use threatens job security.
- In many sports the risks of playing the sport are greater than the health risks associated with PED use.
- Many fear the inability to compete more than the risk of drug use or injury.[3]

COURSON'S CONCLUSION:

The current system tacitly encourages the use and the subsequent dishonesty of athletes in regards to PEDs. What has developed is a system where both sports federations and athletes contest the truth about the use of PEDs in an effort to further their financial and image requirements while both realize society rewards performance.[4]

The NFL may very well be the strongest warrior against doping. But it uses its status as a giant among dwarfs to hide its own loopholes and weaknesses. The NFL's tremendous financial and cultural successes make it the logical organization to serve as a leader in the next generation against doping. The commitment it is making with its laboratory at the University of Utah is among the solutions discussed in chapter 7, "Solutions to the Out-of-Control Drug Problem in Sports."

people aspiring to play football, basketball, baseball, hockey and all the other sports recognize the importance of fair play and self-discipline, and doing it without performance enhancing drugs. Strength and success, after all, do not come in a bottle."[20]

If George Allen had worried a little more about steroids in 1979, Senator George Allen would not be so worried about kids using steroids today. But he's not the only one concerned, and for good reason. Recent studies have revealed numerous mysterious deaths, leaving many unanswered questions:

- In Italy, an alarming number of soccer players have been stricken with diseases in the past 40 years, including 45 of whom (since the 1960s) have either died or are battling the rare nerve disease amyotrophic lateral sclerosis (ALS or Lou Gehrig's disease). That's 44 more than what one would normally find in a similar sample of 24,000 people. Turin-based magistrate Raffaele Guariniello, who was investigating the situation in Italy, says anabolic steroid abuse has been alleged as a factor in incidents of liver cancer among Italy's soccer players, which is also double that of statistics for the general Italian population.[21]
- In France, the country's biggest sporting event—the Tour de France—is in the center of another doping scandal, and this one is deadly. Radio Free Europe/Liberty Radio reported that from February 2003 to March 2004 eight elite cyclists in Europe died "due to heart-related reasons, some of which are known to have been caused by the use of performance-enhancing drugs."[22]
- In the United States, a *USA Today* investigation revealed that since 1997, out of the estimated 1,000 professional wrestlers age 45 or younger competing on wrestling circuits worldwide, 65 of them had died, 25 from heart attacks or other coronary problems, "an extraordinarily high rate for people that young, medical officials say. Many had enlarged hearts."[23]

How much should we be worrying? How bad is it getting? There is no color-coded system to show us (orange for high alert or red for eminent danger). But consider the following two independent research efforts that offer a glimpse of how the various types of illegal or banned performance-enhancing drugs have affected sports in the past two decades, and how there is little reason to believe the widespread abuse will stop in the next two decades.

In the spring 1987 issue of *Journal of Sport History*, current University of Texas professor and former weightlifting champion Terry Todd wrote, "If the last several years are any indication, however, [author John] Hoberman and others have good reason to be concerned about the continuing spread of drugs; the continuing technologizing of sport. Consider these recent facts:

- San Diego State University suspended its track and field program pending the investigation of steroid use among its athletes and coaching staff.
- Baylor's head basketball coach resigned after a player went public with a tape he made while discussing steroids with the coach.
- Vanderbilt University's strength coach and a local pharmacist were indicted for providing steroids to the Vandy players and for participating in a 'steroid ring' that involved numerous other East Coast colleges.
- A survey by a *Waco Times Herald* reporter revealed that steroid use existed at every school in the Southwestern conference.
- Michael David Williams, a Maryland bodybuilder, went on a crime binge while on the top end of a long cycle of steroids, robbing six homes and burning three, yet was only required to undergo outpatient counseling after his attorney successfully argued that the steroids and testosterone had altered his personality and made him unable to fully understand the consequence of his actions.
- Five Canadian weightlifters returning from the world championships in Moscow were stopped at the Montreal airport and found to be in possession of tens of thousands of doses of steroids purchased from the Soviet athletes for resale over here.
- The two top superheavyweight lifters in the world—Anatoly Pisarenko and Alexander Kurlovich—were stopped a year or so later in the same airport on their way to a Canadian competition and found to have over $10,000 worth of steroids in their luggage.
- Dr. Walter Jekot, a physician who treats athletes on the West Coast, distributed printed announcements in at least one of his three offices offering free injections of steroids in exchange for the referral of new patients.
- Brian Bosworth and 20 other collegiate football players were banned by the NCAA from participation in post-season bowls

after testing positive for anabolic steroids. The problem is clearly
not going away."[24]

- With steroid use on the rise, the NFL announced in November
1986 that it would test players for steroid use when they reported
to training camp in 1987, and it would also test college seniors at
its annual scouting combine before the draft.

- Decathlete Gary Armstrong became the seventh athlete suspended
(in 1986) for testing positive for a banned substance at a meet, joining suspended U.S. teammates Tom Jadwin (javelin), Darren Crawford and Joe Zelezniak (shot put), and Greg McSeveney, Rick
Meyer, and Art Swarts (discus).

- Two Salisbury State (Maryland) college football players were declared ineligible (December 1986) for the NCAA Division III championship game after drug tests. One tested positive for steroids and
the other for a high level of a sinus medication after the team's
quarterfinal victory. Testing at quarterfinals in Division II and
I–AA also resulted in 90-day suspensions for players from North
Dakota State (2), Concordia (1), Eastern Kentucky (2), Nevada-
Reno (2), and Georgia Southern (1).

John Maher, a reporter at the *Austin American-Statesman*, compiled the second group of facts 11 years later, spanning the year 1998.
These are the highlights and lowlights:

- *January:* World-class Chinese swimmer caught with vials containing Somatropin, a human growth hormone, and is suspended for
four years; Russian speed skater banned for life by the International Skating Union after refusing an out-of-competition test; Ro-
manian distance runner fails a drug test and is later suspended;
four Chinese swimmers test positive for Triamterene, a diuretic
used as a masking agent, and are suspended from the World Championships; U.S. bobsledder receives a three-month ban right before
the Winter Olympics, after testing positive for the stimulant ephedrine.

- *February: Sports Illustrated* article charges that as much as 20 percent of the National Hockey League's players use pseudoephedrine,
or Sudafed, for a "buzz"; New Zealand weightlifter begins serving
a two-year ban after testing positive in an out-of-competition test.

- *March:* French police find 104 syringes filled with EPO in a car owned by the Dutch TVM cycling team. Belgian judge seizes computer records of a pharmacist who sells large amounts of EPO to the Festina team doctor. Authorities later find 235 doses of EPO, 82 shots of growth hormone, numerous packets of anabolic steroids, 60 doses of testosterone, and masking agents and syringes in the vehicle of the team's trainer. A rider for Festina later admits to using EPO for two years. Another Festina rider admits he took EPO, blaming pressure from sponsors. Three cyclists are later given four-month bans.

- *April:* Two dozen Chinese athletes admit that they used performance-enhancing drugs in 1997 (competing in track and field, weightlifting, wrestling, boxing, cycling, and boating); a British shot putter becomes the first British athlete to be banned for life after testing positive for elevated levels of testosterone and failing his second drug test in three years; Sri Lankan sprinter is suspended by her country's amateur athletic association after the second of two samples test positive for the steroid nandralone; researchers in Massachusetts find that in four middle schools, 2.8 percent of the males and 2.6 percent of the females are using steroids and that children as young as 10 are taking them; a four-year suspension handed out by the Lithuanian Swimming Federation begins for a swimmer who tested positive for metandienone metabolites.

- *July:* Australian press bemoans the state of rugby as three Newcastle players test positive for banned substances; FINA doping panel hands down two-year suspensions to four Chinese swimmers for testing positive for the diuretic Triamterene; FINA suspends British swimmer for one year for testing positive for the banned stimulant Benzoylecgonine—a metabolite of cocaine; IOC president Juan Antonio Samaranch says he'd like to see the number of banned substances for the Olympics "drastically reduced"; shot putter Randy Barnes and sprinter Dennis Mitchell, president of the U.S. Track and Field Athletes Advisory Committee, are banned from competition (Mitchell for testing positive for testosterone, Barnes for androstenedione); five cyclists admit taking banned substances; Norwegian shot putter tests positive for anabolic steroids.

- *August:* Canadian sprinter Ben Johnson, stripped of a gold medal in the 1988 Seoul Olympics after testing positive for anabolic steroids, claims athletes in all sports take performance-enhancing drugs. Irish swimmer is banned for four years for manipulating her urine samples from a January test. Prosecutors alter doping products in substances seized from the TVM cycling team during the Tour de France (French newspaper later reports six TVM members used the banned substances). Prince Alexandre de Merode, chairman of the IOC's medical commission, says he is "aghast" at Samaranch's comments, stating, "People who want to reduce the list are the people who want to let doping function." He adds, "In Spain there has for a long time existed a tendency toward doping." The IOC calls for the creation of a wide-ranging Olympic antidoping agency. The *Washington Post* reports that half of all U.S. Olympic athletes picked for random drug tests aren't tested, in part because of the expense of tracking them down. The Associated Press reports that St. Louis Cardinals slugger Mark McGwire has androstenedione in his locker and that he has been using it for more than a year. A British cyclist is banned from the Commonwealth Games after failing a drug test due to high levels of testosterone; he is later banned for one year. Other athletes testing positive at the Commonwealth Games include an English weightlifter (for a too-high ratio of testosterone) and a Welsh weightlifter (for the anabolic steroid stanozolol). Offensive tackle Paul Wiggins of the Pittsburgh Steelers is suspended for four games for using androstenedione.

- *September:* The Italian Olympic Committee's laboratory comes under investigation after allegations that hundreds of urine samples of soccer players are not tested; McGwire, a user of both creatine and androstenedione, hits his record-shattering seventieth home run in a season.

- *October:* Rome newspaper reports that it is often the doctors themselves who urinate in the test tubes to protect soccer players from drug detection; the first Italian soccer player is officially named for failing a drug test; former Irish rugby player writes that the sport has been rife with steroid abuse for the last decade; German track-and-field federation suspends its top sprinter for testing positive for synthetic testosterone; Greek Basketball Federation bans former NBA player for testing positive for stanozolol; Irish rugby officials are informed that one of their players tested positive for steroids in

1997; Rome drug-testing lab run by the Italian Olympic committee flunks an IOC inspection (only 20 percent of the samples were tested for steroids and 5 percent for diuretics, and lab technicians said positive tests were ignored); Indonesian badminton player tests positive for nandrolone, and he begins serving a one-year suspension.

- *November:* Japanese snooker player, age 58, tests positive for the muscle-builder methyltestosterone and is banned for two years; South Korea withdraws its women's rhythmic gymnastics team from the Asian Games after four of six team members test positive for diuretics; a South Korean swimmer fails a drug test; New Zealand pole vaulter tests positive for stanozolol; IOC announces a drug agreement with international sporting federations (it includes a two-year minimum for first suspensions and a life penalty for repeat violators; the IOC also says it will create an independent antidoping agency for the entire Olympic movement).
- *December:* Steen Madsen's A-sample tests positive for nandrolone, and he is later given a four-year suspension by the Canadian Cycling Association. A British newspaper surveys 1,300 elite athletes and administrators in British sports, finding one quarter of all surveyed—and only 3 percent of the athletes—say their sport is clean. (Four percent of athletes believe that 60 percent or more of the athletes in their sport are using banned performance-enhancing drugs. Forty-six percent of rugby players say they've been offered drugs by teammates, other players, or dealers.) A Jordanian weightlifter is the first athlete kicked out of the Asian Games for drug use after admitting he used a banned diuretic.[25]

This massive list, though less-than-comprehensive, is disturbing because of its bulk, if nothing else. It is likely a good representation of a typical year in the world of sports. Maher's list also shows a tremendous rise in the number of doping incidents from the list Todd compiled 11 years earlier, although the consistently increasing media attention devoted to sports may be one reason for this increase. It is tough to gauge whether there still is an increase in doping today or if the same percentage of athletes are cheating, though it is quite clear that there are many more undetected incidents. While conducting the research for this book in 2003, we collected the following list—a sampling of the doping events within the previous year—which is likely well short of comprehensive:

- Former U.S. national team cyclist Kirk O'Bee was given a one-year suspension by the U.S. Anti-Doping Agency in July of 2002 for testing positive for anabolic steroids at the USPRO Championships in Philadelphia.

- English pole-vaulter Janine Whitlock and discus thrower Perriss Wilkins were suspended following positive tests for anabolic steroids in July of 2002. U.S. cyclist Tammy Thomas received a lifetime ban in August 2002 after testing positive in an out-of-competition test in March 2002 for norbolethone, an anabolic steroid. Thomas tested positive for an elevated testosterone level at the 2000 U.S. Olympic Trials and received a one-year suspension. The rules of the sport call for a lifetime ban for a second offense within a 10-year period.[26]

- Jacksonville Jaguars linebacker T. J. Slaughter was suspended for the first four games of the 2002 season for violating the NFL policy on anabolic steroids.

- Atlanta Falcons cornerback Ray Buchanan was suspended four games in September of 2002 for using anabolic steroids.

- The Nevada State Athletic Commission filed a formal complaint against Fernando Vargas for using the banned anabolic steroid stanozolol in his fight with Oscar de la Hoya in September of 2002.

- Kansas City Chiefs linebacker Lew Bush was suspended for four games in November of 2002 after testing positive for the banned stimulants ephedrine and Ma Huang.

- Carolina Panthers defensive end Julius Peppers was suspended for four games for testing positive in September of 2002 for the banned prescription diet drug phentermine.

- Baltimore Ravens wide receiver Javin Hunter was suspended for the last four 2002 regular season games due to a violation of the NFL's policy on anabolic steroids and related substances.

- Houston Texans offensive lineman DeMingo Graham was suspended at the end of the 2002 season for using ephedrine, a substance banned by the NFL.

- Denver Broncos safety Lee Flowers tested positive for the banned substance ephedra after the 2002 season.

NFL players make up a substantial chunk of this list, and not all of the players who broke the league's drug policy between June of 2002 and July of 2003 are listed. Altogether, 10 players were suspended in that period, which was immediately after the death of Minnesota Vikings tackle Korey Stringer.[27] Most of those who tested positive for ephedrine or other banned substances claimed that they did so without their knowledge. Some products containing ephedrine do not list it as an ingredient. Because of the ephedrine ban, players have avoided taking any products unless they are certain of the ingredients, so there were fewer names on the suspended list this year than last.

Anabolic steroids, on the other hand, have been banned in the NFL for decades. Players continue to use them—the reasons ranging from regaining strength lost because of injury to the blatant perception that they must seek an edge to maintain their starting job or continue playing in the league. Other professional leagues or amateur sports groups are no different. Despite the risk of huge fines and suspensions, athletes continue to believe the risk of getting caught is worth the gains earned. A penalty of missing four games at the start of an NFL season, for example, is laughable when you consider the rules were knowingly broken. There is much debate among the league's players that there are too many preseason games, and therefore too many unnecessary opportunities to be injured. No one expects to be caught for cycling steroids at the end of a season or in the summer training camp, but if the financial consequence is measured in thousands of dollars for players who make millions, and the loss of four games still leaves 12 more, not including the postseason games, the risk may very well be worth the reward. According to World Anti-Doping Agency president Dick Pound: "In the professional leagues, it almost seems as if every effort is made to get cheaters back in play as soon as possible."[28]

The number of athletes using steroids and similar drugs sends a terrible message to young athletes. An alternative viewpoint to this problem is that those who are caught doping to gain a competitive edge also appear OK with the risk of potentially influencing a kid to seek the same edge. Barkley and others are correct in assigning parents the responsibilities of primary role model and mentor in a child's life, but research has proven that as a child advances into junior high and high school, parents actually become less influential. This is not always the case, and sometimes this disconnection can be attributed to poor parenting, but it is also natural for young people to begin making their own decisions, which they will want to do independently of a parent or other authority figure. What youngsters know they can get away with and what they want to get away with are not always the same. When opportunities arise to obtain what they previously have not been able to, and if they want it badly enough, they will take a risk. And this relates to sports; if a child sees a peer or favorite athlete taking similar risks, he or she is far more likely to be influenced by what is seen as logical, justifiable, safe, or worth the risk.

The percentage of those willing to take performance-enhancing drugs *is* definitely in the minority. And some of these kids will opt for the wrong decision no matter how good a parent is; no matter how strong the antidrug education is; no matter how dangerous the risks are to one's health or future. We know this is true simply by looking at the list of names above—hundreds of elite athletes every year ignore good advice from authoritative sources. They ignore scientific evidence of the risks involved. And, sadly, they ignore the influence they may hold over a child's choice to follow a similar path of potential destruction. Some kids—and many more adults—will never listen; they'll never learn. Remaining clean isn't just the right thing to do for an elite athlete's health. Using drugs as a role model presents the possibility that young athletes will also choose the same pathway to short-term achievement.

Here are some others whose experiences and expertise offer similar findings:

- "When there is a positive drugs test for a high-profile sportsman, sales of the product that he has tested positive for go up. The best advertising that steroids manufacturers can have is to have a leading athlete test positive for their product, because it shows that the product works. So, what we are seeing is increasing evidence that—away from top-level competition of course, where cheating is the big issue—we're seeing in the UK an increasing culture of steroid use and physically enhancing drugs among young people."—Paul Kelso, reporter for the London-based *Guardian*[29]
- "It would be tremendously helpful if some sports heroes would be more visible on this issue, be willing to stand up, speak to our kids and educate them. Because kids listen to their heroes."—Nicholas

DiNubile, assistant professor of orthopedic surgery at the University of Pennsylvania Hospital in Philadelphia[30]

- "Teens are 'juicing' just like many of the sports figures they so want to emulate and coaches, parents, lawmakers and students need to wake up and start paying attention."—California State Senator Jackie Speier (D-San Francisco/San Mateo)[31]

- "Kids aren't stupid. They know what's going on. Mom and dad need to know, too. It's up to them to help their kids make safe, ethical choices."—Charles Yesalis, Penn State professor who has spent more than 20 years researching drug use in competitive sports[32]

- "I train a lot of high school athletes who are seeing LSU's (baseball) players and Mark McGwire and Albert Belle hitting the ball out of the park, and they want to do the same."—Ben Arnold, a trainer at Ron Dunigan's Professional Fitness Center[33]

- "It's not all about money, but it's a big factor. If you can sign a seven-figure contract or think you can extend your career, it would not be surprising that you get enticed by [steroids]."—New York University professor Gary Wadler, a member of the World Anti-Doping Agency committee[34]

- "Parents must be alert to the use of steroids introduced in fitness centers and occasionally by coaches. They need to look for the warning signs."—Bill Walsh, Hall of Fame NFL football coach and now a consultant with the 49ers[35]

Despite all of the evidence of their impact on young athletes, professional athletes continue to abuse performance-enhancing drugs. They are not only aware that they risk doing permanent damage to their health, reputation, and the integrity of their sport, but they are also aware of the damaging effects their use is having on children. Sadder still, some groups of athletes, such as Major League Baseball players and their union, are failing to discourage drug use by resisting steroid testing, despite pleas from Congress, the medical community, and at least one youth group. In 2000 the Boys and Girls Club of America, along with Blue Cross Blue Shield, challenged Major League Baseball players to discontinue using androstenedione. Part of the reason for concern was that Andro sales soared more than 1,000 percent to $50 million in 1998, the year McGwire hit his since-broken record of 70 home runs and admitted to using the steroid precursor. Two years later, in his letter to the players' union, Allan Korn, chief medical officer of Blue Cross Blue Shield, wrote: "Players have a responsibility to our young fans to set the right example. All the evidence indicates that these substances can be harmful to our bodies. Kids need to start hearing from their sports heroes that there is no substitute for hard work and dedication."[36] Baseball commissioner Bud Selig responded: "It remains a priority of Major League Baseball to deal effectively with the issues surrounding the use of steroids, androstenedione and similar substances."[37] Unfortunately, baseball's idea of effectively handling this performance-enhancing drug was initially to do nothing, despite conducting a study to determine its dangers. While nearly every other major professional or amateur sports organization banned Andro—the NCAA, IOC, NFL, NBA, and many more—Selig's organization chose not to. Not until Congress banned the sale of Andro for nonmedical uses in March 2004 did major-leaguers stop this form of legalized doping.

One reason the NFL banned Andro immediately was to eliminate the perception that in order to compete with those players who were using the testosterone-building substance, other players might feel forced to use a drug that has been scientifically proven to be a potential health hazard by a baseball-commissioned Harvard study. The NFL and other leagues had good reason to believe this perception was very real. Dr. Robert Kerr, "the steroid guru" who said he provided the drugs to as many as 20 medalists at the 1984 Olympics, told CBS's *60 Minutes* in 1985: "This is not cheating—not when everyone does it."[38] Australian discus thrower Werner Reiterer, winner of the 1994 gold medal at the Commonwealth Games, proved this thinking was reality and not just a theory by writing a book that revealed his steroid use. He writes: "With a heavy heart, I made a decision to . . . turn myself from a natural athlete into a normal athlete."[39]

If competitive athletes and their obsession with winning at any cost were not a severe enough of a problem, similar and respected opinions have been formed regarding doping in sports as it is linked to the greater recreational drug problems of society as a whole:

- "The conscience for the problems joined to doping is not very highly developed; too many people still think that doping concerns only the high level sport. But doping is a part of the general drug problem, of the health of the society and of the general problem if we are able to respect our limits and preserve the resources of the earth and the human body."[40]

- "The Dubin report notes the potential that performance-enhancing drugs might be 'gateway' drugs which lead athletes to more harmful abuse patterns."[41]

- "In 2000, the British Medical Association revealed that drugs such as anabolic steroids are now so common that bodybuilders have joined needle exchange schemes—originally set up for heroin users. Two years ago, Joanne Amies-Winter, Britain's strongest woman, died from a cocaine overdose. At her inquest, it was revealed that the champion bodybuilder had a cocktail of drugs in her body including Nubain (which enables bodybuilders and other weight-lifting athletes to increase their pain threshold and to get over sports injuries or allow muscles to recuperate faster after intense workouts."[42]

- A study reported in a letter to *The New England Journal of Medicine* suggests that men who abuse anabolic-androgenic steroids may begin to abuse heroin or other opioid drugs, such as prescription pain relievers, as well. Among 227 men admitted for treatment of opioid addiction in 1999, 21 (9.3 percent) reported that they had used anabolic-androgenic steroids. None of the men had used other illicit drugs prior to their steroid abuse, and most of the men said they were introduced to opioids through the dealers who supplied them with steroids and through the bodybuilding subculture.[43]

- "Five years ago when we launched the Healthy Competition program, people thought performance-enhancing drugs were only a problem for elite athletes," Allan Korn, M.D., Blue Cross Blue Shield Association's chief medical officer said in October 2003. "But today, 74 percent of the people surveyed agree that these substances pose a significant public health problem."[44]

BALCO and Beyond: The Biggest Doping Scandal in Sports History

[Barry] Bonds, the superstar leftfielder for the San Francisco Giants, the six-time most valuable player, the man who obliterated the single-season home-run record, the hitter who is in the best position to pass Hank Aaron on the all-time home-run list, is putting up numbers at an age when most major leaguers are hitting golf balls, not baseballs.

—Don Walker and Mark Maley, *Milwaukee Journal Sentinel*[1]

He's baseball's biggest star, but how he got so big is the question and the asterisk that will accompany Barry Bonds for all time. Fans in San Francisco and many more throughout the world seem to support him every step of the way, but they, too, can never erase the thoughts in the back of their minds that this superhuman hero may be a bit human after all. He may have feared that he was fading, and therefore succumbed to the pressure of seeking a boost in order to continue being the best. As of the writing of this book, Bonds has not been charged with any crime. And while he has admitted to using substances that likely were steroids, he said he did so without knowing what the substances were. After reading this book, if you still believe this to be a possibility, there is probably nothing that will change your mind short of a confession from Bonds himself. Bonds will never confess because his pride prevents such a scenario from even creeping into his mysterious mind. But the evidence will always stack up as high as his statistical accomplishments—as overwhelming as his 703 career home runs entering the 2005 season.

Unfairly or not, Bonds has become the poster player for the biggest doping scandal in sports history, one that begins with BALCO but reaches far beyond. Bonds, along with fellow major-leaguers Jason Giambi (Yankees) and Gary Sheffield (Yankees), and players Marvin

Benard (Giants), Benito Santiago (Giants), and Randy Velarde (A's), allegedly were given steroids from the Bay Area Laboratory Co-Operative by Greg Anderson, Bonds' personal trainer and friend. The original source of the allegations, according to a story broken by *The San Francisco Chronicle*, was information furnished by the U.S. government, which was investigating the nutrition supplement company on suspicion of breaking laws against steroid distribution.[2] On December 2 and 3, 2004, *The Chronicle* dropped back-to-back steroid bombs on the BALCO case—disclosing testimony by Giambi to a federal grand jury in which he admitted to using several forms of performance-enhancing drugs beginning around 2001.[3] The next day, *The Chronicle* revealed Barry Bonds' grand jury testimony in which he said he used a cream and a clear substance matching the description of two steroids known to be distributed by BALCO. Bonds, however, only admitted to having used substances he believed were safe supplements provided to him by his personal trainer.[4] There is a preponderance of circumstantial evidence to refute Bonds' claims later in this chapter.

During the summer before Bonds and Giambi's 2003 grand jury testimony was leaked, the bulk of the attention on BALCO's designer steroid, THG, shifted from baseball to some of the United States' best track-and-field stars before and during the Athens Olympics. But Bonds became the focal point of the scandal again when he hit his 700th home run on September 17, drawing closer to the only two men who have hit more home runs than he has—Babe Ruth (714) and Hank Aaron (755). Each reminder of the Giant's accomplishments invoked memories of the accusations against him. None were more believable—or more damaging—than the claims made by 100-meter world record holder Tim Montgomery, who, while testifying under oath in front of the same grand jury in December 2003, said Bonds had knowingly used the illegal THG. Montgomery, according to another *San Francisco Chronicle* report, also told the grand jury he had used THG, although he has adamantly denied doing so in every interview conducted before and after his testimony.[5]

THE BALCO TIMELINE

It has been suggested that the government's case lacks enough evidence to convict Bonds of knowingly using THG, and the reason that the federal investigation continues to move forward is that, from the outset, there has been a desire to bring down the controversial and often disliked megastar. But we believe the truth will expose Bonds, perhaps during a criminal trial against him.[6] In the court of public opinion, however, logic and skepticism are coming together and are bearing down on Bonds and the other world-class athletes in question. Using various media sources, but primarily a timeline posted on the Web site of the *San Jose Mercury News*, the following is a comprehensive look at the BALCO saga, complete with the said evidence implicating Bonds, Montgomery, Marion Jones, and others:[7]

- *June 2003:* Trevor Graham, at the time identifying himself only as a "high-profile" track coach, having previously trained Montgomery and Jones among his stable of strong runners, gives the U.S. Anti-Doping Agency a syringe with a small amount of the previously undetectable designer steroid tetrahydrogestrinone. Graham tells the USADA that several athletes are using the drug, and he names BALCO proprietor Victor Conte as the source of the organized criminal operation, in which professional athletes from several teams are being provided with the performance-enhancing substance.
- *August 2003:* Don Catlin and other scientists at the UCLA Olympic Analytical Laboratory in Los Angeles discover the makeup of the new steroid.
- *September 3, 2003:* The Internal Revenue Service, along with the Food and Drug Administration, the San Mateo County Narcotics Task Force, and a representative of USADA, raid Conte's offices in Burlingame, California, finding steroids, human growth hormone, and testosterone.
- *September 5, 2003:* The home of Bonds' personal trainer, Greg Anderson, is also raided. Steroids, $60,000 cash, and other evidence links him to the doping of several of the athletes previously mentioned in this chapter.
- *October 16, 2003:* USADA goes public with its discovery of THG. Terry Madden, USADA's chief, indicates several athletes have tested positive for the new drug.
- *October 23, 2003:* It is announced that four U.S. track-and-field athletes and British sprinter Dwain Chambers have tested positive for THG.

- *October 30, 2003:* Grand jury testimony in the case begins.
- *November 16, 2003:* Four Oakland Raiders test positive for THG.
- *December 4, 2003:* Bonds testifies before the grand jury.
- *January 20, 2004:* In his State of the Union address, President Bush calls for serious reform, saying: "The use of performance-enhancing drugs like steroids in baseball, football and other sports is dangerous, and it sends the wrong message—that there are short-cuts to accomplishment, and that performance is more important than character."[8]
- *February 12, 2004:* Conte, BALCO vice president James J. Valente, Anderson, and track coach Remi Korchemny are charged with conspiracy to distribute steroids, possession of human growth hormone, and misbranding drugs with intent to defraud and money laundering. All four plead not guilty.
- *March 1, 2004:* Multiple reports reveal that federal investigators were told that Bonds, ex-NFL player Bill Romanowski (one of four Oakland Raiders who tested positive for THG), and former A's player Jason Giambi received THG from Conte.
- *April 8, 2004:* The Senate Commerce Committee, chaired by Arizona Republican John McCain, votes to subpoena Department of Justice documents in the BALCO case. Meanwhile, federal agents seize an unidentified number of urine samples taken during the 2003 baseball steroid tests from Quest Diagnostics Inc. in Las Vegas. And, on the same day, baseball commissioner Bud Selig meets with Bonds in San Diego prior to the Giants v. Padres game. Although Selig denied it, it is reported that he was considering offering leniency to Bonds if he admitted to Selig that the slugger used steroids.
- *April 25, 2004:* The *Mercury News* reports that an IRS agent says Conte provided THG to 27 athletes (five baseball players [including Bonds], seven football players, and 15 track athletes [including Jones] are named).
- *April 29, 2004:* Hammer throwers John McEwen and Melissa Price, who tested positive for THG, receive two-year bans from competition by the U.S. Anti-Doping Agency.
- *May 1, 2004: (New York) Newsday* reports that federal investigators have the 2003 steroid-test results for all Major League Baseball players.

- *May 6, 2004:* McCain's Commerce Committee gives evidence in the BALCO investigation to the U.S. Anti-Doping Agency for use in barring athletes from competing in the Athens Olympics.
- *May 18, 2004:* The *Mercury News* reports that Kelli White, having admitted to doping, has accepted a two-year ban from USADA.
- *May 26, 2004:* The *Mercury News* reports that in 2000–2001, sprinter Tim Montgomery and four other people—Conte, body-builder Milos Sarcev, and track coaches Charlie Francis and THG whistle-blower Graham—met at BALCO to form "Project World Record," aimed at making Montgomery the world's fastest man. He would set the 100-meter world record a year later.
- *June 8, 2004:* USADA notifies Montgomery, Alvin Harrison, Chryste Gaines, and Michelle Collins of drug violations that could keep them from competing in Athens.
- *June 10, 2004:* The *Mercury News* reports that Jones' former husband, C. J. Hunter, meets with federal investigators. It is later revealed that Hunter told investigators Jones did use steroids during and after her five-medal performance at the Sydney Olympic Games in 2000, and that he helped her inject the drugs.
- *June 12, 2004:* The *New York Times* reports that Graham, Jones' former coach, has been granted limited immunity in exchange for information about the sprinter and BALCO.
- *June 16, 2004:* The *Mercury News* reports that Conte's lawyer wrote to President Bush offering to reveal what Conte knows about doping among athletes in a plea bargain of sorts. The White House later declines.
- *June 17, 2004:* Jones' lawyer says she has passed a polygraph test. The announcement comes a day after Jones calls a press conference to request a public hearing on her case, possibly before the U.S. Senate. No hearing has been held to date.
- *June 20, 2004:* The *Mercury News* reports contents of the accusations being delivered to targeted athletes by the USADA.
- *June 24, 2004:* The *San Francisco Chronicle* prints portions of Montgomery's grand-jury testimony, where he admits to taking THG and testifies that Conte told him Bonds was also given steroids.
- *July 4, 2004:* The *Mercury News* reveals Graham is the previously

unknown coach who sent the syringe filled with THG to the USADA.

- *July 8, 2004:* Hunter testifies before the federal grand jury in San Francisco.
- *August 2, 2004:* Sprinter Calvin Harrison receives a two-year sanction for his second doping offense (modafinil).
- *August 13, 2004:* The Athens Olympics open. During a six-month period leading up to the Games, more than 20 track-and-field athletes were sanctioned, implicated, or identified as the focus of an inquiry in a scandal sparked in large part by the investigation of BALCO. Twelve members of the U.S. track team were sanctioned for doping, including four for using THG.
- *August 17, 2004:* The USADA begins its drug case against Olympic runner Michelle Collins, seeking a lifetime ban against the 2000 Olympian in the 400 meters. Collins, the 2003 world indoor 200-meter champion from Raleigh, North Carolina, has never failed a drug test and refused a plea-like agreement in June. As of the writing of this book, the fate of her athletic career had not been decided.
- *August 29, 2004:* With these and many other cheaters banned from attending the Games, no Americans were sent home during the competition. Still, there were a record number of athletes—24—disqualified and/or sent home because of drug violations. Three champions were stripped of their gold medals, all from field events in track and field, and four other athletes forfeited medals.
- *November 22, 2004:* A bodybuilder with ties to BALCO (Milos Sarcev) was indicted, along with two other men, by a federal grand jury in Des Moines, Iowa, in an alleged conspiracy to import illegal steroids from Thailand. Sarcev, a former Mr. Yugoslavia, is a friend of Victor Conte.[9]
- *December 7, 2004:* The International Olympic Committee opened an investigation into Marion Jones' alleged ties to BALCO, after the company's president, Conte, stated on ABC's *20/20* that he provided Jones with banned substances and watched her inject herself with them. She continued to deny the charges, but she stands to lose her five medals from the 2000 Olympics if she is found guilty.
- *December 7, 2004:* Less than a week after the *San Francisco*

Chronicle's revelation that Jason Giambi told a federal grand jury he had used steroids provided by BALCO, and that Barry Bonds unwittingly did the same, Major League Baseball players met in Phoenix and authorized Players Union Chief Donald Fehr to make concessions in order to agree with owners on a much stronger steroid policy before spring training. As of the writing of this book, the existing MLB policy allows for five positive tests before players were susceptible to a one-year suspension or up to a $100,000 fine.[10]

For some elite U.S. track athletes who either admitted to or were suspected of doping, their noticeable decline coincided with the discovery of THG and the subsequent crackdown on doping by the USADA.

- Marion Jones won five medals in 2000 but failed to make the Olympic team in the 100, and she did not medal in Athens. She was never charged with using a banned substance.
- Tim Montgomery, the world record holder in the men's 100 (set in 2002), finished seventh in the 100-meter trials and failed to make the Olympic team. He was later charged by USADA with doping and admitted as much to a San Francisco grand jury.
- Michelle Collins, the World Indoor and U.S. Indoor 200-meter champion, dropped out of 400-meter qualifier, citing a hamstring injury. She was charged by USADA with doping.
- Chryste Gaines, sprinter and a gold-medal winner in the 4x100-meter relay in the 1996 Olympics, failed to qualify for the Olympic team in the 100-meter relay. She was charged by USADA with doping.
- Regina Jacobs, who set the indoor world record in the 1500-meter in 2003, and who broke the world indoor record in the 2-mile run in 2002, retired one month before the Olympics and three days before her scheduled hearing on doping charges.
- Calvin and Alvin Harrison (twin brothers) both won gold medals in the 4x400-meter relay at the 2000 Olympics (medals they would lose in 2004 after the Court of Arbitration for Sport determined teammate Jerome Young should have been banned from the Sydney Games after testing positive for steroids). The Harrisons both

failed to make the Olympic team in the 400-meter. Calvin was not charged with doping but Alvin was.

THE CASE AGAINST BARRY BONDS

Because the 2008 Summer Games won't take place for another three years, Marion Jones' fate is no longer among the top stories sports fans are following these days. And because Americans believe in the right of innocence until proven guilty, many baseball fans spent the latter half of the 2004 season cheering for Bonds to pass his godfather, Willie Mays, on the all-time home-run list, and then to chase down home run #700 of his career. The truth is that given the choice, about half of baseball fans would sweep the fact that Bonds used steroids under the rug rather than see one of baseball's all-time greatest players embarrassed because he might have cheated. This point was unscientifically backed up by an Internet poll on espnradio.com on September 16, 2004, where 42 percent of fans said they were rooting for Bonds to break Hank Aaron's all-time home-run record.[11] What this says about the importance society places on ethics is sad. The circumstantial evidence that Bonds might have used steroids is significant—rapid size and strength gains, swollen facial features, and statistics unprecedented in his career. The physical evidence found in the possession of Bonds' personal trainer, Anderson, adds to the case against the player:

- Federal investigators found vials containing what are believed to be human growth hormone and anabolic steroids in Anderson's apartment and sport utility vehicle.
- The government seized vials of creams, brown and white liquids, pills, and syringes.
- Containers labeled Serostim, a human growth hormone; Depotestosterone, an anabolic steroid; a bottle labeled Andriol, an anabolic steroid; zip-lock bags with pills labeled Dyazide and Aldactone, both of which are diuretics banned by many sports organizations; and more than 100 syringes, a few needles, and dozens of alcohol pads were found.
- The government also found about $60,000 in cash, much of it stuffed in envelopes with the first names of famous athletes scribbled on them, in a safe in Anderson's home. Agents also found files

with athletes' names and daily dosage schedules for steroids and human growth hormone.[12]

- In a secretly recorded conversation, Anderson admits that Bonds used an "undetectable" steroid during the 2003 season, and he was told that he would receive a warning in advance of being asked to submit a urine sample for a steroid test under the then-new Major League Baseball steroid testing policy.[13]
- In grand jury testimony leaked to the *San Francisco Chronicle* and published on December 3, 2004, Bonds admitted to paying his trainer Anderson $15,000 in cash for weightlifting services.[14]

From an article in the *Palm Beach Post*, there is clear scientific evidence that steroid-induced muscle gains can impact home-run totals:

- Men who exercised and took steroids for 10 weeks put on an average of 13 pounds of muscle and could bench press an extra 48 pounds, a 1996 study published in the *New England Journal of Medicine* found. This increase was far more than control groups who took no steroids, whether they exercised or not.
- "Bigger muscles mean the power to increase bat speed," said Jeffrey A. Potteiger, chair of the Department of Physical Education, Health and Sport Studies at Miami University of Ohio.
- Alan Rogol, professor at the University of Virginia who has studied the effects of steroids on the body, has said, "How they bulk players up is they stimulate the growth of muscle. It is probably the case that an athlete can recover more quickly for the next bout of exercise. Steroids may also give you a better attitude, or a more aggressive attitude."[15]

No evidence is greater than the numbers produced by Bonds' bat. And there is no more dubious statistic than his at-bats per home run, which jumped from 9.8 in 2000 to 6.5 in 2001. In his 10 best seasons (in terms of at-bats per home run before the 73-homer 2001 season), Bonds hit a home run every 12.8 times at bat. Even the average of his best three seasons would account for a homer in every 10.3 at-bats. Regardless of whether the number being compared is 12.8, 10.3, or 9.8, the use of performance-enhancing drugs is the only thing capable of boosting that figure to 6.5 in a single season (see list, next page). In the three years since he was accused of using steroids, his production dropped off significantly to a home run in roughly every 8.5 at-bats. And that number is only going to continue to drop along with the lasting effects of the steroids, which doctors and other steroid experts say can last years after an athlete discontinues use.

A year-by-year breakdown of the number of at-bats per home run for Barry Bonds throughout his career with the Pittsburgh Pirates (1986–1992) and San Francisco Giants (1987–2004):

Year	At-bat/HR	Year	At-bat/HR	Year	At-bat/HR
1986	25.8	1993	11.7	2000	9.8
1987	22	1994	10.6	2001	6.5
1988	22.4	1995	15.3	2002	8.8
1989	30.5	1996	12.3	2003	8.7
1990	15.7	1997	13.3	2004	8.3
1991	20.4	1998	14.9		
1992	13.9	1999	10.4		

A final, unique perspective on Bonds' case may provide some of the most convincing evidence, albeit circumstantial, that he used steroids. Interestingly, the source is the June 1, 2003, issue of *Muscle & Fitness* magazine, in an article detailing Bonds' fitness and strength. This issue was in the racks at grocery stores and pharmacies across the country when the story of BALCO first broke. In the article, Bonds describes his close relationship with Conte, noting that the BALCO president would personally call Bonds to "make sure I'm taking my supplements." And Bonds told *Muscle & Fitness* that he traveled to BALCO every three to six months from winter 2000 to summer of 2003 (between six and ten times).[16] However, Bonds has since said he met Conte "two or three times."[17] The following are some excerpts from the article:

- Bonds' imposing musculature reflects [a] new dedication to the physical arts. Working with personal trainer Greg Anderson, the superstar slugger has refined his weight training and nutrition regimens, and it shows. "Definitely, my improvements as a player are down to training and nutrition," Bonds tells *Muscle & Fitness*. "Without a doubt. It has made me a better athlete than I was before."
- But Bonds' rejuvenation owes itself to more than sets and reps.

Since winter of 2000, Bonds has worked closely with San Francisco-based nutritional consultant Victor Conte of BALCO Laboratories. Conte precisely measures the nutrient levels in the outfielder's blood, then prescribes specific supplemental regimens to correct imbalances.

- "I'm just shocked by what they've been able to do for me. . . . To have your blood drawn and analyzed can tell you what your body produces more of, what it lacks. You're able to create a program that fits for you as an individual."

- "People don't understand how important this is," he explains. "I visit BALCO every three to six months. They check my blood to make sure my levels are where they should be. Maybe I need to eat more broccoli than I normally do. Maybe my zinc and magnesium intakes need to increase, and I need more ZMA. Nobody ever showed it to me in a scientific way before, how important it is to balance your body. I have that knowledge now."

- "Victor will call me to make sure I'm taking my supplements, and my trainer Greg will sit near my locker and stare at me if I don't begin working out right away. I have these guys pushing me."[18]

Of course, Conte, Anderson, and BALCO were pushing a lot more than Bonds.

Knowing what we know now about the secret production of the designer steroid THG . . . Knowing how BALCO provided this substance to, among others, some of the world's best athletes in track and field, professional football and baseball . . .

Knowing, from Bonds' interview with *Muscle & Fitness* that Conte was as involved with Bonds' chemically enhanced training regimen as he was involved in BALCO's successful attempt to turn Tim Montgomery into the world's fastest man . . .

Knowing that Bonds' personal trainer was a steroid aficionado with access to and understanding of every possible steroid, and knowing that he had a close enough friendship with Bonds that would make it next to impossible for him not to share this expertise in an effort to maximize a player who would soon be approaching the twilight of his career . . .

Knowing what the rest of the world knows: that in 2001 a brand-new Barry, with a swollen face (one of the telltale signs of steroid use) and muscle-mass gains that one offseason of drug-free workouts could never produce, hit 73 home runs—one every 6.5 times at bat—nearly twice the offensive output of his previous season . . .

. . . it is obvious that Major League Baseball should consider stripping Barry Bonds of his home-run record. Baseball insiders who share this thinking include:

- Hall of Famer Reggie Jackson: "Somebody definitely is guilty of taking steroids. . . . Come on now. You can't be breaking records hitting 200 home runs in three or four seasons. The greatest hitters in the history of the game didn't do that. . . . Bonds hit 73 (in 2001), and he would have hit 100 if they would have pitched to him. . . . There is no way you can outperform Aaron and Ruth and Mays at that level."[19]
- Hall of Famer and home-run king Hank Aaron: "I'm sad for baseball about all of this. I played the game and we played it legitimately. Now something like this comes along and it ruins the game. All these records blown out the window. Aside from the records, though, this could be as bad as the Black Sox scandal."[20]
- Former Bonds teammate Andy Van Slyke: "Unequivocally, he's taken them. . . . I can say that with utmost certainty. Now, I never saw him put it into his body. But, look, Barry went to the bank with the robber, he drove the car, he got money in his pocket from the bag that came out of the bank. Come to your own conclusion. Did he spend the money? You decide. I think he did."[21]
- John Holway, author and baseball historian: "It's just hard for me to explain what he has done. I think there's ground for suspicion of steroids, in my opinion."[22]
- Mark Whicker, columnist at the Orange County Register, "Meanwhile, the coyotes stalk Barry Bonds, who went from 46 to 73 to 46 home runs in 2000–02 and has sparked suspicion because, frankly, he looks inflatable."[23]

BEYOND BARRY AND BALCO

Baseball's well-documented disaster of a drug policy—which has yet to suspend a player for using steroids despite the world's knowledge

Sidebar 4.1: What Keeps Barry Swinging

Barry Bonds' nutrition regimen is based on his particular needs as measured by BALCO Laboratories. BALCO president Victor Conte provided *Muscle & Fitness* magazine with the following program that he said Bonds followed during the months preceding his record season in 2001:[1]

THE NUTRITION REGIMEN:

Morning:
50 g special whey protein blend
25 g complex carbohydrates
5 g glutamine peptides
5 g New Zealand colostrum

Preworkout:
1,000 mg phenylalanine
1000 mg tyrosine
10 mg Vitamin [B.sub.6]
200 mcg chromium (as polynicotinate)
2 mg copper (as sebacate)

Post-Workout:
50 g whey protein isolates
50 g dextrose
5 g glutamine peptides
2 g arginine
200 mcg chromium (as polynicotinate)
1.5 g magnesium creatine
1.5 g creatine monohydrate
5 g New Zealand colostrum

Afternoon:
10 mg iron (as glycinate)
200 mcg selenium (as selenomethionine)
10,000 IU Vitamin A
500 mg Vitamin C
800 IU Vitamin E
400 IU Vitamin D
25 mg Vitamin [B.sub.1]
25 mg Vitamin [B.sub.2]
25 mg Vitamin [B.sub.6]
500 mcg Vitamin [B.sub.12]

400 mcg folic acid
500 mg omega-3 fatty acids
250 mg d-glucosamine sulfate
350 mg n-acetyl d-glucosamine
200 mg omega-6 fatty acids
150 mg chondroitin sulfate

Evening:
50 g special whey protein blend
25 g complex carbohydrates
5 g glutamine peptides
5 g New Zealand colostrum

Before Bedtime:
3 capsules ZMA, which contain 30 mg zinc
    (as monomethionine/aspartate)
450 mg magnesium (as aspartate)
10.5 mg of Vitamin [B.sub.6], 200mg L-theonine,
    50 mg 5-HTP

of doping for nearly four decades—is one of the biggest examples of the failure by professional leagues and elite amateur organizations to stop this abuse. The dangerous levels of acceptance of these drugs did not begin with BALCO. As a part of his Alcoholics Anonymous 12-step program, former Houston Astro and San Diego Padre Ken Caminiti admitted he used steroids when he won the National League's Most Valuable Player Award in 1996. In his revelation to *Sports Illustrated*, Caminiti said such drug use was widespread in the game, estimating as many as half the players were on steroids. Caminiti died October 10, 2004, in the Bronx, New York, of a drug overdose. Coronary artery disease and an enlarged heart (common side effects of steroid use) were listed as contributing factors in his death, which came days after admitting he had violated the terms of his probation by testing positive for cocaine.[24]

Caminiti's statistics bear obvious resemblance to Bonds' numbers. In the five years prior to 1996 (averaging 511 at-bats per year), Caminiti averaged hitting one home run per 30.8 at-bats. In 1996 he hit a home run every 13.7 at-bats. And just three years before his breakout 40-homer season, he reached 41.7 at-bats between home runs. Because it is rare for a player to admit to using steroids, his statistics are one of the few examples of the advantage extra power can provide when it comes to home runs. The statistics are even more dubious for former Baltimore Orioles outfielder Brady Anderson, suspected of taking steroids in 1996 but never admitting so. In four seasons of playing regularly (averaging 548 at-bats a year) prior to 1996, Anderson hit a home run every 35.3 at-bats, including 34.6 in 1995. The following season he blasted 50 home runs—one every 11.6 at-bats. Jose Conseco has admitted to being a steroid addict during a career in which he hit 462 homeruns. He upped the estimate of players using steroids to between 80 and 85 percent.

In addition to these player estimates, a poll of 556 big-leaguers conducted by *USA Today* in June 2002 found 89 percent believe there is some steroid use in the game, and 10 percent believe more than half of their peers are users. Many other respected players have spoken publicly about the problem, including former Cy Young award-winning pitcher Curt Schilling, who at the time played for the Arizona Diamondbacks. "Steroids are incredibly prominent in the game, I don't think there's any question about that," he said in 2002. "The fact of the matter is it has enhanced numbers (of hits, home runs, and other statistics) into the stratosphere. . . . Is it a problem? It depends on what you consider a problem. It certainly has tainted records, there's no doubt about that."[25]

Dr. Frank Uryasz says that devoting large amounts of resources to steroid education for Major League Baseball players is not going to be effective. These players know the risks of taking steroids, yet despite those risks, they fall into the categories of the athletic population who either won't take them to avoid detection or continue to take them because it's worth the risk of being caught. Because of baseball's lack of a steroid policy, there has never been a risk. And because the policies in place now are a joke, the risk is minimal. Use of the illegal drugs continued in 2003 despite a thick blanket of scrutiny covering the sport. After every player on each team's 40-man roster was tested, and after 240 more players were tested again randomly, at least 5 to 7 percent of major leaguers tested positive. The labor agreement (which runs through the end of the 2006 season) made it clear that players would be tested, yet roughly 80 professional players used steroids anyway (we don't know exact figures because MLB would not disclose the exact percentage). The punishment? Nothing, or at least nothing individually. Collectively, major league players now face slightly harsher penalties if they are caught because the minimum percentage of positive tests in 2003 triggered the league to implement its first steroid-testing policy.

The World Anti-Doping Agency founding chair, Dick Pound, shares our views and that of many others: that MLB's drug policy is a joke. Actually, Pound says in his book that it is ". . . worse than a joke. It is a travesty. It amounts to almost the complete abandonment of responsibility with respect to health of the participating athletes. Moreover, it is an insult to the intelligence of the public. . . . To make [testing] a part of the struggle between labor and management . . . is to all but guarantee that progress will be difficult."[26] Baseball's weak policy and slow progress is one reason Baltimore Orioles pitcher Steve Bechler died from supplement use containing Ephedra when he was trying to lose weight during spring training. Minnesota Vikings offensive tackle Korey Stringer and three other football players died from heatstroke in 2001. Three of the athletes—Stringer, University of Florida running back Eraste Autin, and Northwestern safety Rashidi Wheeler—had traces of Ephedra in their system when they died. A study by Dr. Julian Bailes et al., performed for the NFL Players Association and released prior to training camp in 2002, linked Ephedra to an increase in heatstroke deaths and helped lead to the NFL's ban on ephedrine. Within the following calendar year, a handful of NFL players were suspended for violating the team's banned substance policy because they used Ephedra. Bechler died during that period, yet baseball did not ban the substance. Instead, the FDA put a ban on the sale of the substance in every state, which took effect on April 12.

THE DIRTIEST AND CLEANEST GAMES EVER

Nearly 3,000 total drug tests were conducted during the 2004 Athens Games, according to the International Olympic Committee (IOC). This number is nearly a third of the 10,500 athletes who competed in these historic Summer Olympics. The final tally recorded 22 athletes who tested positive for performance-enhancing drugs at the Games, and a total of 29 athletes who were either kicked out of the Games or told in the weeks leading up to the event that they were not permitted to participate. The announcements began four days before the Games began and ended on the final day, when an athlete missed his deadline to submit another sample because of suspicion of tampering (see sidebar 4.2). Throughout these Olympics, as a number of cheaters were caught, organizers and high-ranking officials from countries, sports federations, and antidoping organizations applauded the efforts and the results.

Similar to today's professional sports leagues, the world's amateur athletics federations have stood passively for too long, watching athletes abuse performance-enhancing drugs. These organizations have done nothing to stop steroid abuse except for in-competition testing. "The undeniable message was that they did not, obviously, care about the problem," says Pound, who adds that the cavalier attitude in professional sports has carried over to the amateur level. "The owners of professional teams are in business. . . . What is important is that (their athletes) be on the field on game days. If they need drugs to do so, so be it. . . . The message is all too clear and the amateur athletes are influenced by it."[27] Pound, not unlike former USOC drug-control program chiefs Drs. Robert O. Voy and Wade Exum (see chapter 3), also has a clear message, and he is not afraid of losing friends in the Olympic hierarchy by calling on his peers to clean up their sports. Pound, who campaigned for the presidency of the International Olympic Committee, was and will continue to be outspoken and critical (sharing in our opinions) of how slow the IOC has been to react to the war on PEDs. Pound says that early Olympic drug testing "was a sincere effort, but depended solely on scientific measurement to determine whether or not there was doping. There was no consideration of the humanistic or ethical dimension. This lack of an ethical basis was responsible for [the decision-makers] . . . seem[ing] to look for every possible reason not to find that an offense had occurred . . . [and] seeming to protect the cheaters at the expense of the athletes."[28]

President Bush's decision to urge professional sports leagues to wipe out steroid use in his State of the Union speech was a motivating moment in what has been a long, frustrating battle just to be heard. All of America's professional sports organizations need to take a look at rededicating themselves to a fight that is important for many reasons, none more important than the children they try to hook every day. As Pound puts it, "This is a helpful presidential position on an issue that could have [a] profound effect on generations of Ameri-

Sidebar 4.2: Summary of Doping in Athens

Athletes who either tested positive for banned drugs during the Athens Olympics or broke antidoping regulations either immediately before or during the Games:

POSITIVE TESTS:

- *Irina Korzhanenko, shot put (Russia):* Tested positive for banned steroid stanozolol. She was stripped of her shot-put gold medal and expelled from the Games.
- *Ferenc Gyurkovics, weightlifting (Hungary):* Tested positive for steroid oxanfrolone. He must give back the silver medal he won in the 105 kg weightlifting category.
- *Leonidas Sampanis, weightlifting (Greece):* Tested positive for high testosterone levels. He was stripped of his bronze medal in the 62 kg category.
- *Olena Olefirenko, rowing (Ukraine):* Tested positive for a prohibited stimulant. Her quadruple sculls crew were disqualified and lost their bronze medal.
- *Mabel Fonseca, wrestling (Puerto Rico):* Tested positive for stanozolol and was expelled from the Games. She had finished fifth in the 55 kg freestyle class.
- *Anton Galkin, 400 meters (Russia):* Tested positive for stanozolol and was expelled from the Games. Did not make it past semifinals.
- *Aleksey Lesnichiy, high jump (Belarus):* Tested positive for anabolic agent clenbuterol and was excluded from the Games. He was last in the qualifying round.
- *Albina Khomich, weightlifting (Russia):* Tested positive for a banned steroid and pulled out of the Games.
- *Olga Shchukina, shot put (Uzbekistan):* Tested positive for anabolic agent clenbuterol. She finished last in the event.
- *Sanamacha Chanu, weightlifting (India):* Tested positive for banned diuretic furosemide. She finished fourth in the 53 kg category.

DOPING VIOLATIONS

- *Robert Fazekas, discus (Hungary):* Fazekas was caught trying to tamper with his urine sample. He had to give back his gold medal and was expelled from the Games.

- *Zoltan Kovacs, weightlifting (Hungary):* Kovacs refused to take a doping test. He was expelled from the Games where he was competing in the 105 kg category.
- *Costas Kenteris and Katerina Thanou, athletics (Greece):* Training partners who missed doping tests the night before the Athens Olympics could not take another test because they were in the hospital after a mysterious motorcycle accident. They pulled out of the Games and have since been charged with doping violations by the International Association of Athletics Federations (IAAF). Their coach, Christos Tzekos, was also charged with illegally importing and selling banned substances.

PENDING

- *Adrian Annus, hammer (Hungary):* Annus failed to give another urine sample after concerns over the legitimacy of his first sample arose. (Hungarian teammate Robert Fazekas, above, was caught tampering with his sample.) He was ordered by the IOC to return his gold medal. He has vowed to fight the International Olympic Committee in court.

OTHERS

- Slovak shot putter Milan Haborak tested positive for a banned substance and left the Olympics, according to a report from the Slovak SITA news agency on August 15, 2004.

The following weightlifters tested positive for anabolic steroids before the Athens Games began:

- Pratima Kumari (India)
- Nan Aye Knine (Myanmar)
- Wafa Ammouri (Morocco)
- Victor Chislean (Moldova)
- Zoltan Kecskes (Hungary)
- Shabaz Sule (Turkey)
- Kenyan boxer David Munyasia was barred by the IOC after testing positive for a banned stimulant in an out-of-competition test.
- Four days before the start of the Games, two Greek baseball players, a Swiss cyclist, a Spanish canoe team member, and an Irish distance runner were banned because of doping.
- American sprinter Torri Edwards had her two-year drug suspension upheld by an arbitration panel during the Games. She tested positive for a stimulant at an April meet.

- U.S. sprinter John Capel did not run on the 4x100 meters relay team because of a positive test for marijuana on August 9, 2004. Marijuana carries a public warning.[1]
- U.S. cyclist Tyler Hamilton, who won a gold medal in the time-trial event in Athens, has since tested positive for blood doping on two separate occasions. An initial doping test done after the Athens Olympics indicated Hamilton had used a blood transfusion, but because his backup specimen mistakenly was frozen, there weren't enough red blood cells to analyze and he was cleared by default. However, a second test at the Tour of Spain turned up the same suspicious results. The Russian Olympic Committee has filed an appeal with the Court of Arbitration for Sport seeking to give Hamilton's gold to Vyacheslav Ekimov, who was second in the Athens time trial event.[2]

cans."[29] With President Bush's support, the United States has been a leader in the worldwide effort to destroy doping, becoming the first of 137 original signatory states in the Copenhagen Declaration on Anti-Doping in Sport. According to the USADA, as of September 21, 2004, 153 governments have signed the declaration, which includes the understanding that the World Anti-Doping Code will be followed.[30] The code, created and administered by WADA, has a chief aim to ". . . harmonise [sic] doping controls among national and international sporting bodies."[31]

As for President Bush's stance on this issue, a White House aide involved in the drafting of the speech told *Sports Illustrated* that the topic is very near the President's heart. "We were talking about a portion of the speech—the moral integrity of social institutions," the aide recalls. "We had stuff on high school drug-testing. The President said, 'What about the moral messages sent by adults?' He brought up the issue of steroids. . . . He has a unique perspective on this. His father played baseball. He was a team owner. He doesn't like fake home-runs."[32]

Those who have fought against doping know there is nothing fake in the President's thoughts or the words in his speech. There is political motivation that is greater than the desire to restore moral integrity to the sport of baseball, to professional football, and to the greatest amateur athletic event in the world, the Olympic Games. Unfortunately, under Juan Antonio Samaranch, these great Games took several steps backward in efforts to discourage doping. In what would become one of Samaranch's very few public missteps, he once expressed to a reporter that only performance-enhancing drugs that harm athletes should be banned. Pound points out in his book that Samaranch was also unwilling to promptly announce doping violations that happened at these Games because they were damaging to his image. There is a similar hesitancy among professional sports commissioners, who throughout history have publicly denounced doping but have never backed up their talk with aggressive acts. Most notably, these commissioners have never penalized cheaters severely enough. But no matter how it is disguised, the drug problem in baseball, in the Olympics, and in many other elite sports organizations is as ugly as the truth is to Barry Bonds.

Steroids and Designer Drugs

Julian Bailes, M.D.

Aspiring and seasoned athletes have always been attracted to the allure of outside factors influencing their potential for success. In a certain way, it has been consistent with human nature to wish to accomplish set goals and to exceed one's normal capabilities. In athletic endeavors, the spirit of competition runs strong and oftentimes may predominate. Many athletes will strive for better performance and, through their training, will reach for any method which they feel may give a competitive advantage. Among the many factors which enter into the life and training of an athlete, especially one who is seeking to achieve lofty accomplishments, are the use of dietary supplements and drugs.

This is not a new trend; in fact, since ancient times there has been the recorded use of such agents to improve training, stamina, and ultimate physical performance. From the ancient Greeks who consumed hallucinogenic mushrooms and other herbs to the Roman gladiators who used stimulants such as strychnine to the Incas who enjoyed the perceived benefits of the cocoa plant to the soldiers throughout the ages who ingested high concentrations of caffeine and other substances to increase their alertness and endurance, many humans sought to gain advantage in performance through the use of exogenous substances.

By the nineteenth century, the use of foreign substances to improve athletic performance was occurring regularly. Stimulants, and especially cocaine, were often felt to give advantage to the determined athlete. In the later part of the nineteenth century, the term *doping* appeared, a derivative from the word *dop,* which was an opiate mixture given to improve the performance of racehorses. Soon the use of performance-enhancing drugs (PEDs) was common in high-level athletic training and activity, including the consumption of high levels of protein and stimulants such as cocaine, nitroglycerine, amphetamines, and other substances. Since then, doping has come to mean the utilization of foreign substances to enhance or improve training and competitive performance for athletes.

Utilizing foreign substances to improve athletes' appearance and performance has become extremely complex. There are numerous reasons for this phenomenon. While human nature continues to drive athletes toward greater performance, competition may push the elite performers, and those striving to become elite, toward new and further boundaries. Attempting to gain competitive advantage in training and contests, athletes may turn to ingestion of foreign substances or pharmacological means to achieve advantage. In addition, the allure of media coverage, publicity, and financial rewards is greater than ever. With the growth of scientific, medical, and pharmacological knowledge, there has also been an explosion of public information, especially on the Internet. This has led to extensive networking and free access to much information that was previously esoteric or not available to athletes and their advisors. Organizations representing amateur athletes, such as the International Olympic Committee (IOC) and the National Collegiate Athletic Association (NCAA), and those bodies representing professional sports have been forced to take an active role in the definition, prohibition, and testing for PEDs. However, this area has been fraught with confusion concerning what is legal versus illicit, natural versus unnatural, scientific versus random, and competitive versus unethical. At times it has been difficult for athletes, coaches, trainers, and even physicians to distinguish between doping or cheating versus legitimate, extensive preparation. It has been debated whether substances were being consumed to enable performance, to maximize genetic and training potential, or to restore worn and tired bodies. Also, there have been allowances for a single individual to have higher serum levels of the male hormone testosterone, based on a theory that they constituted the "high normal" range. There also has been uncertainty as to whether many substances are allowed and may exist in a gray area, versus those that are definitively disallowed or illegal.

HISTORY

The modern era of doping began with the recognition that anabolic steroids may provide distinct benefit in size, strength, and stamina. While testicular tissue was consumed and transplants were performed by surgeons internationally, the biochemistry of testosterone did not allow an incorporation into normal human physiology with resultant benefits until the molecule was synthesized in the laboratory. While it had been known since ancient times that castration of the male resulted not only in infertility but also in a loss of secondary male sex traits, several human physiology discoveries were necessary to develop our understanding of the function of testosterone and related molecules. In 1989 A. A. Berthold performed experiments in roosters that proved that the testes liberated a substance into the bloodstream leading to the development of roosters' sexual characteristics, including the formation of the comb and wattle.[1] This discovery led to the ultimate understanding of endocrinology, in which hormones are liberated into the bloodstream and cause their effects without nervous system intervention.

In the early part of the twentieth century, rapid development preceded our understanding of male reproductive physiology. This ultimately brought about the extraction and isolation of androsterone, which not only stimulated the capon comb but also was found in the urine of human males. Experiments across species recognized the substance isolated from the testes (testosterone) was the more active substance and was transformed in the body to several other related steroid compounds. In fact testosterone is capable of being transformed in approximately 600 related compounds, all given the classification of androgens. These are all variations in the ringed chemical structure of cholesterol. In 1935 testosterone had been chemically isolated and synthetically made in the laboratory. There is a complex biochemical capability within the human body to convert testosterone, through tissue enzymes, into hundreds of other molecules, including estrogen.

Many experiments followed, spurred by the excitement that testosterone and its related androgens have many desirable properties, including the ability to synthesize new tissue.[2] In addition to promoting the male secondary sexual characteristics, androgens were embraced because of their positive effects on anabolism (tissue growth characteristics). In addition, anabolic steroids had growth and development implications for nearly every organ in the body. As attempts were made to harness the positive or anabolic effects of testosterone, there was interest in eliminating the androgenic effects in women and children (which were undesirable because of virilization).

It soon followed that both oral and injectable forms of testosterone were utilized by the medical community, particularly in treating diseases that would benefit by a positive nitrogen balance and greater protein synthesis. It became appreciated that doping was regularly occurring and could confer a distinct advantage to the user. Dr. Otto Rieser, in his 1933 sentinel work "Doping and Doping Substances," advocated a campaign against doping or artificial means to gaining performance advantage in athletic competition.[3] The utilization of testosterone as an ergogenic benefit was first reported by German athletes in the 1936 Berlin Olympics.[4] Immediately following, it was reported that German soldiers in World War II had consumed steroids for stimulation and aggressiveness,[5] although this was never proven. The muscle-building effects of anabolic steroids were described as effective not only in those with a disease but also in healthy men and women. Before being utilized by humans, testosterone is suspected to have been first used in a racehorse to great benefit.

Although not completely documented, it was insinuated that California bodybuilders began experimenting with testosterone compounds in the early 1950s.[6] At about the same time, anabolic steroids were being used by weightlifters in the USSR. In 1958 the Ciba Pharmaceutical Company formulated and marketed methandrostenolone (Dianabol) which was utilized by weightlifters and other athletes who were in strength-dependant activities and sports, particularly football. Anabolic steroids have had an illustrative history in the treatment of patients with numerous medical conditions, including metastatic breast cancer, protein loss (catabolism) as the result of severe infections, burns, trauma, post-surgery situations, anemia, reproductive disorders, and the human immunodeficiency virus/acquired immunodeficiency syndrome (HIV/AIDS).

By the late 1960s, an emphasis upon developing greater muscular size and strength was deemed desirable in football. Greater facilities for weight training along with professional strength coaches were incorporated into college and professional football teams, and a trickle-down effect occurred at the high school level. In the 1970s, Olympic track-and-field event athletes reported up to 68 percent prior steroid use, with 61 percent within six months of the Olympic games.[7] While the NCAA disallowed the use of anabolic steroids beginning in 1973, testing was not implemented until 1986, thus allowing steroids to become firmly entrenched in the culture of American football.[8] Throughout the years numerous major college football programs began to emphasize weight training with increased strength and speed. It was well known that steroid use became prevalent in all levels of collegiate football. Subsequent studies have consistently shown that at least 10 percent of college and 6 percent of high school football players have admitted to steroid use.[9] However, the rate of steroid use has varied between studies depending, in particular, on whether the inquiries were in the form of self-report or a projection of the perceived use by competitors. In the latter, these indirect survey techniques yielded suspected use by 29 percent of college football players.[10] In 1967 the IOC adopted a drug-testing policy that outlawed the consumption of specific PEDs. In 1982 the National Football League (NFL) instituted drug testing for its players, assaying for anabolic steroids in 1987. The NCAA instituted its drug-testing program in 1986, while Major League Baseball did not begin to regularly screen for drug use until 2003.

Anabolic steroids have come to be used by three general classes of athletes. The first and most common use is by individuals who desire to be stronger with greater capacity for strength, lean body mass, and speed. When combined with weightlifting, experienced athletes can achieve strength as well as weight gain with an average 10-pound increase in body weight after approximately one month of high dose steroid consumption. This is primarily due to the greater accumulation of protein and muscle size and function.[11] Anabolic steroids appear to block the catabolic effects of glucocorticoids, which are normally released during intensive training periods, allowing these athletes to train more intensely and more often. They also are believed to increase the number of oxygen-carrying red blood cells in the body, an obvious benefit for any athlete, especially those involved with endurance activities. So not only do anabolic steroids benefit athletes who are involved in strength-related sports, but they also improve performance for athletes with high-intensity and long-duration training and competition.

In addition, there are other users who consume anabolic steroids for the perceived positive effect on their appearance.[12] The combination of steroid use and continued, simultaneous, intensive weight training, especially in experienced or pretrained individuals, results in significant increases in muscle size, strength, and body weight.[13] The long-term effects, and particularly the physiological permanent changes, the retention of prior gains, as well as the physiological effect on females and their athletic performance, have been inconclusively debated. While the number of serious adverse or fatal events with steroids has been low, the permanent or serious health effects are also uncertain. Areas of concern are the effects of the long-term steroid use upon the heart, liver, serum lipids, reproductive function, atherosclerosis, the immune system, and the psyche.[14] The systematic administration of anabolic steroids to Olympic athletes in the German Democratic Republic is the best-known example of state-sponsored pharmaceutical competition. The exposed files, containing the highly sophisticated and rampant use of testosterone and its derivatives in both males and females, led to trials and punishment for many of the principals. This sad saga, including the instances of liver and heart disease and the masculinization of many young girls, is detailed by Steven Ungerleider in his 2001 book *Faust's Gold*.[15]

The use of anabolic steroids has been practiced and to a great extent perfected over the last 40 years. In common parlance, the athlete is "juicing." Ordinarily athletes have used anabolic steroids in "cycles" lasting 6 to 12 weeks or for even longer durations of up to eight months. Often they will consume more than one steroid at a time, a practice called "stacking." In addition, they will stagger the different anabolic steroid compounds, taking them in either overlapping or stop-and-start fashion in an effort to avoid developing a tolerance, which they term "plateauing." During the period of cycling, they may also "pyramid" their dosage, moving from a low to a higher dose, often with a gradual tapering at the end of this period. A particularly dangerous trend is using steroids in combination with insulin (nicknamed "slin"). By injecting the latter, some athletes, particularly bodybuilders, feel that there is a synergistic effect with steroids resulting in enlarged muscle bulk, possibly by increasing the amount of glycogen, which is the stored form of glucose. Insulin, short acting and naturally produced by the body, is virtually undetectable by drug tests. It is extremely difficult to manage insulin as it controls the glucose level in the bloodstream on a moment-to-moment basis. Life-threatening hypoglycemia, coma, and death may result from improper use.

A sophisticated modern user can consume multiple anabolic substances. An exemplary case is that of A.L.W., a 32-year-old who focuses upon fitness and noncompetitive bodybuilding, and who has been using steroids and related compounds for four years. A.L.W. describes his growth in strength, muscle mass, and lean body weight; significant mood elevation; and increased sexual drive during his periods of PED use.

He regularly "cycles" in the following manner: His first eight week round is called a "mass" phase in which he takes 1,500 milligrams of testosterone enathate (veterinarian grade) on Monday and Thursday by intramuscular injection, 75 mg of Anadrol (oxymetholone) orally daily, and during the last two weeks 50 mg of Clomid (clomiphene) orally for its anti-estrogen effects. During this first phase, his diet will be enlarged with up to six or seven high protein meals daily. He will perform heavy weightlifting sessions five or six days a week, focusing at least one day upon maximum lifting to exhaustion for each major muscle group. The second round lasts for four weeks and is termed his "mass-cutting" phase. During this time he will inject 400 mg of Deca-durabolin (nandrolone) twice weekly to reduce fat but keep his newly gained muscle mass. His diet will reduce overall calories, continue to be high in protein, and he will increase his repetitions in weight lifting and add more aerobic workouts.

The third phase is "cutting," in which A.L.W. attempts to lose any excess water and fat attained previously. He injects 200 mg of Equipoise (boldenone undecylenate) weekly with 15 mg of Winstrol (stanozolol) daily, both of which provide relatively slow absorption, little water retention, and gained mass maintenance, giving the muscles a hard and cut appearance. Toward the end of the 16-week "cutting" phase, he will add human chorionic gonadatropin (HCG) at a dose of 2,000 I.U. injected intramuscularly or subcutaneously. This is believed to stimulate the atrophic testes to become active again, reducing their lag time, and helping to prevent muscular mass losses from occurring. The diet will consist of fewer calories, optimally none from simple carbohydrates or sugars. He will continue weightlifting training as often as he can, with slightly lower weight but increased repetitions. At the end of this seven-month cycle, he will (somewhat begrudgingly) discontinue the use of all PEDs, work on attempting to maintain his gains, perform aerobic activities, and fight off the attendant state of depression until he can resume his cycling.

The federal government and nearly all states have legislation that controls the manufacture, distribution, and possession of anabolic steroids. In addition, the prescribing of anabolic steroids is also legally controlled. The Federal Food, Drug, and Cosmetic Act (FFDCA) was amended in conjunction with the Anti-Drug Abuse Act of 1988 to stipulate that possession or distribution of anabolic steroids with the intent to distribute without a valid prescription would be classified as a felony. The Anabolic Steroids Control Act was passed in 1990, which made anabolic steroids a Schedule III drug of the Controlled Substances Act under the auspices of the Drug Enforcement Administration (DEA), which controls the manufacture, distribution, prescription dispensing, and movement of steroid medications manufactured in and exported from the United States. The majority of anabolic steroids used in the United States are illegally imported, primarily from Mexico, while other European countries, particularly in Eastern Europe, have also been found as steroid sources.[16] In addition, the potency, purity, and consistency of anabolic steroids available on the black market have been questioned.

BETA-2 AGONISTS

Another classification of drugs known as Beta-2 Adrenoceptor Agonist (beta-2 agonist) has gained increasing popularity as a PED. These compounds were previously developed for the treatment of bronchial asthma in their ability to cause dilatation of the bronchials and improved breathing patterns in asthmatics. In initial application in the cattle industry, it was felt that the desirable qualities of meat for human consumption were enhanced with these drugs. However, creative athletes came to use this class of drug to increase muscle bulk, while simultaneously decreasing body fat, without the side effects of steroids.[17] These beta-2 agonist drugs stimulate the tissues involved in growth, especially skeletal muscle. While not causing the adverse effects of stimulation of the beta-1 receptor, which involves cardiac muscle, the beta-2 stimulation was noted to result in growth in skeletal muscle mass in livestock. Several of the popular beta-2 agonists are believed to work primarily through limiting muscle protein breakdown, and these drugs became known as the so-called repartitioning agents for their ability to increase skeletal muscle mass while simultaneously diminishing body fat stores.[18] These agents are looked upon as desirable by athletes involved in strength and endurance sports, particularly in bodybuilding and weightlifting. They not only have potent muscle-building characteristics but they also appear to reduce adipose tissue, thus becoming popular with athletes in those sports that include weight restrictions when competing for specific weight classifications.

One of the most popular beta-2 agonists is clenbuterol, which has been marketed under many brand names, including Clenbumar, Cesbron, Spiropent, Clenasma, Protovent, and others. Clenbuterol achieved initial notoriety during the 1992 Summer Olympic Games in Barcelona, Spain, when two athletes were implicated as testing positive. There have not been many studies demonstrating its efficacy or safety in humans; however, it has been reported that clenbuterol, combined with diuretic use, has been responsible for the deaths of several notable professional body builders.[19] The optimal dosage that causes the desired result, likewise, is still unclear.[20] It does have, however, significant lipolytic (fat breakdown) effects and is thermogenic, meaning it produces excess body heat. Whether it has been complicit in recent, increased trends in heatstroke deaths in athletes is unknown. Chronic beta agonist use may potentially adversely affect the cardiovascular system; muscles; glucose and insulin metabolism; electrolyte levels; and the central nervous system, including causing nervousness, insomnia, headaches, and psychosis. With the exception of strictly defined medical use, primarily for asthma and related disorders, beta-2 agonists are strictly prohibited by the IOC.

GROWTH HORMONE

Human growth hormone (GH), also called somatotropin, is a polypeptide which is involved in the control of multiple metabolic and growth functions of the human body. It has significant effects on carbohydrate, protein, and fatty tissue metabolism. It is secreted from the anterior pituitary gland throughout the day; however this occurs in an irregular and pulsatile fashion with a significant rise during sleep. Although it was initially isolated from the pituitary gland of human cadavers in the 1920s, the big break came when recombinant human growth hormone was synthesized in the laboratory in 1985. The initial market was for GH-deficient children of short stature and body development; however the market and application soon expanded greatly.

The pulsatile liberation of somatotropin is controlled by two regulatory agents of the hypothalamus portion of the brain, *growth hormone releasing hormone* (GHRH), which is inhibited by *somatostatin* release. The constant balance of these two regulatory hormones determines the amount of GH secreted into the bloodstream. Multiple factors, including age, gender, fitness level, exercise level, stress, and the interaction with other hormones, influence the release of GH. The lack of sufficient GH has led to abnormally short or dwarfed individuals. The condition in which the pituitary gland produces excess GH is termed *acromegaly*. This condition is associated with increases in body electrolyte, mineral and water retention, and a multitude of facial, skeletal, and organ growth hypertrophy resulting in gigantism.

GH has numerous physiological effects upon the metabolism of glucose, the production and sensitivity of insulin, and the metabolism of fat, including its deposition, mobilization, and distribution. The most alluring action of GH, however, is its effect on muscle protein synthesis. GH causes increased deposition of amino acids into protein, which ultimately creates the building blocks of muscle growth and increased strength. Recent studies, particularly those by Yarasheski and colleagues, have shown that while there may be a decrease in fat composition of the human body, increases in muscular size or strength were not unequivocally documented.[21] There remains much to learn concerning GH and related compounds, but at the present time it appears that dosing and the effects of proper cycling are difficult and the results in ergonomic gains nebulous. In addition, it has been difficult to test for exogenous GH administration due to the normal, cyclical, and fluctuating level in humans. Two factors limiting its popularity are that GH is very expensive and is believed to be active only in injectable form.

BLOOD DOPING

Attempting to manipulate the content of human blood, particularly by increases in the concentration of hemoglobin, have been postulated for some time. Especially in endurance sports such as cycling, running, rowing, or cross-country skiing, the extended use of the large muscle groups of the arms and legs requires the delivery of high volumes of oxygen from the lungs to the peripheral musculature where it is utilized. A person's ability to deliver oxygen to the peripheral musculature is complex and dependant upon many factors, including blood volume, hemoglobin concentration, the acclimation and training of the individual, pulmonary and cardiac efficiency, and many others. Erythropoietin (EPO) is a glycoprotein produced in the kidneys and liver in response to a normal or an abnormal oxygen pressure in the body. As the availability of oxygen to the kidney, for instance, is diminished, the production of EPO is increased. Any condition that causes this perceived drop in oxygen will lead to increased production, which also varies greatly among individuals and during the course of the day. EPO has been synthesized using recombinant DNA methods and has been used to treat patients with numerous conditions in which they do not have sufficient blood oxygen carrying capacity.

Since the 1980s, EPO has been used by endurance athletes, particularly cross-country skiers and cyclists. In 1988 the French Tour de France cycling team and other athletes admitted to the use of EPO to enhance their physiological performance. In 1996 the International Ski Federal (FIS) and the International Cycling Union (ICU) began testing for hemoglobin concentrations and disallowed competition for those athletes with excessive levels. This is in great part due to the athlete's general health risk as high EPO values can cause an increased threat of clot formation within the body. In 1989 the IOC named EPO as a prohibited substance. In addition to testing with both direct and indirect methods for recombinant EPO in the athlete's system, hemoglobin values, which are ordinarily very stable and constant over time, can also be followed in athletes.

Blood doping is a technique in which blood is removed from an individual and the red blood cells (RBCs), which contain hemoglobin and carry oxygen, are separated from plasma, frozen, and stored in glycerol. Several days before competition, the RBCs are washed with saline and reinfused into the same individual. It has been found that increasing hemoglobin concentrations can positively affect oxygen delivery and consumption at the peripheral musculature, thus increasing performance, especially in endurance athletes. Increases have been documented in both maximal aerobic power and a prolongation of the time until exhaustion. Using sophisticated hematological and DNA-testing methods, evidence of blood doping can be detected, but it is not practical because of serial testing requirements. The IOC banned blood doping for performance enhancement in 1984, and several athletes have been suspected in violation or have confessed to using blood doping to improve their athletic performance. However, no practical methods are currently in place for detecting blood doping. In addition, it is likely that the development of artificial blood substitutes or plasma expanders or other oxygen-carrying molecules may be a temptation in the future.

There has been a suggestion that the body's physiological response to motherhood may confer benefits to the female athlete, a process known as pregnancy doping. Some notable accomplishments have occurred after athletes became mothers, including instances of Olympic gold medal–winning moms. Several changes occur during pregnancy, including an increase in blood volume and RBC count, enhanced heart rate and amount of blood pumped with each heartbeat (stroke volume), more efficient sweating, and an improved ability to carry additional weight. There are also many psychological factors, such as mental toughness, endurance, pain tolerance, and others. In the past, rumors circulated that some Eastern European athletes took advantage of the purported positive effects by becoming pregnant immediately prior to important contests.[22] However, there has not been any controlled study series analyzing the various factors surrounding pregnancy or whether there is a true and measurable effect on well-trained athletes.

DIURETICS

A diuretic is a pharmacological agent that works on the kidney to affect the amount of water and salt reabsorption, resulting in an ultimate increase in urinary volume. There are several types of agents that act on various parts of the kidney. Most of these are powerful substances that can cause immediate and significant changes in electrolyte and urine volume, affecting the entire fluid distribution within the body. Diuretics have become a widely abused agent by athletes. One of the most common applications is in such sports as wrestling, boxing, judo, and bodybuilding and weightlifting, which have weight limits that must be met. In addition to extreme dieting, these athletes will often attempt to reduce body weight immediately prior to weight qualification by rapidly depleting body water. In addition, diuretics have been used to attempt to dilute the urine so that PEDs or their breakdown products cannot be easily detected. Diuretics can have serious, unwanted consequences, including the reduction of performance and strength, cardiac and respiratory sufficiency, and a decrease in sweat and blood flow to the periphery, thus increasing the propensity for heat-related illness. Serious electrolyte depletion, with potential cardiac effects, is also a possibility. Other side effects include muscle cramps or soreness, fatigue, numbness, tingling, and drowsiness. Diuretics have been banned by the IOC, USOC, and NCAA and are readily detectable by urine-drug screening.

STIMULANTS

Amphetamines are biological amines that stimulate the sympathetic and central nervous systems. They cause nerve endings to release more norepinephrine, and some act directly on the same norepinephrine receptors. There are numerous amphetamines or amphetamine-like drugs, all with similar effects causing an increase in heart rate, blood pressure, respiratory rate, and metabolism. In the brain, they lead to increased amounts of liberated catacolamines and greater arousal and alertness. Numerous studies over many years have demonstrated the ability to increase heart rate and endurance with amphetamine use. There are deleterious effects upon both the central nervous system and the cardiovascular system. Amphetamine use or toxicity has been reported to cause stroke, heart attack, sudden cardiac death, psychosis, and other adverse effects. Amphetamine use has been significantly curtailed as these drugs are easily detected within urine and human hair, where their by-products exist indefinitely.

Amphetamines are nervous system or brain stimulants that were first synthesized in the 1930s. Prior to that time, soldiers, athletes, and members of the general public used cocoa leaves as a form of stimulant. While the initial use of amphetamines was as a nasal decongestant, it was soon noted that several other effects, particularly a perception of increased alertness, led to their burgeoning popularity. World War II troops were supplied with amphetamines and, following this epoch, soldiers introduced them into various athletic competitions. By the 1960s there were deaths of several prominent athletes, including the Danish cyclist Knut Jensen and the British cyclist Tommy Simpson, which were attributed to amphetamine use. The IOC went on to make stimulants including caffeine, ephedrine, and amphetamines the first class of drugs to be prohibited. Random drug testing of athletes began in the 1968 Winter Olympics in Grenoble, France. The abuse of amphetamines has declined in the ensuing years; however, much of the controversy surrounding these compounds has to do with their availability in common, over-the-counter cold remedies containing ephedrine, pseudoephedrine, or phenylpropanolomine.

Sydnocarb is a Russian drug, which, although originally used to treat psychiatric diseases, has been abused as a stimulant.[23] In the 1996 Atlanta Olympic games, several Russian athletes were discovered to be using a designer drug amphetamine (Bromantan), a derivative of amantadine, which has the same effects as phenylethylamine. Track-and-field athletes have tested positive for steroid use combined with the stimulant modafinil.[24] In addition to the "new and improved" amphetamines, such as Bromantan, the use of more traditional amphetamines, such as "Greenies," has reportedly continued at a high rate. Prior to their 2002 ban, the use of stimulants, such as ephedra compounds, was estimated in active NFL players to be 75 percent and by Major League Baseball players at 50 percent.[25] Often the athlete would feel that, while steroid use was cheating and gave an unfair advantage, the ingestion of amphetamines was acceptable and just gave them an edge.

Caffeine is a ubiquitous and accepted substance with worldwide consumption by both athletes and nonathletes alike. It is used daily by many athletes in preparing for a multitude of sports events. Caffeine has been shown to have a positive effect on metabolism, peak performance, and endurance. It is a central nervous system stimulant, causing improved wakefulness, vigilance, and activity levels. It has been shown to increase the concentration of several brain neurotransmitters such as serotonin, dopamine, norepinephrine, and glutamate. This increases activity levels and neuronal firing mechanisms. According to the IOC, caffeine is a "controlled or restricted substance." By legalizing up to 12 micrograms of caffeine per milliliter of urine, athletes who normally consume caffeine in their diet may continue such consumption prior to a contest. This allows continued use of caffeine at a normal level of consumption. Abnormal or disqualifying concentrations in the urine indicate that the athlete has taken caffeine in a tablet or capsule form in an effort to affect his performance positively.

THG

Tetrahydrogestrinone, or THG, is a newly synthesized "designer" anabolic steroid. THG is believed to have entered the market in 2003. This anabolic steroid was first suspected when a coach from the U.S. Outdoor Track and Field Championships provided a tip to the U.S. Anti-Doping Agency (USADA). This led to the design of specialized testing methods to determine the presence of the previously undetectable substance by the Olympic Analytical Laboratory at UCLA. It has been linked to the Bay Area Laboratory Co-Operative (BALCO) and to several high-profile Olympic athletes, including a British sprinter.[26] Several prominent baseball players and four members of the Oakland Raiders were reported to have tested positive for THG. They were not suspended, reportedly because THG was not a prior known banned drug. While initially unknown, once identified it was added by the Food and Drug Administration to the list of illegal substances and has been banned by the IOC, NFL, NCAA, MLB, major league soccer, and FIS.

THG is made by modifications to the chemical structure of trenbolone, a popular black market steroid, which is also used by cattle farmers to increase the bulk of their animals, and gestrinone, which has estrogenic properties and is used in the treatment of endometriosis. THG had been attractive for its undetectable state and its potency, but it is believed to have a high degree of liver toxicity. It provides us with our most recent example of so-called designer drugs in which the chemical modification of existing steroid molecules creates a substance that is not discovered during previous, routine urine testing, but yet has substantial anabolic properties. For many this alarming discovery points to the seriousness of the problem, with the creators of such a PED being conspirators in developing a potent and undetectable substance, one that gives obvious advantage over the competition. In addition, it emphasizes the magnitude of the problem facing sports and the USADA.[27]

FUTURE DESIGNER DRUGS

As modern athletes reach the limits of human physiological performance and as training methods and durations become of greater length and vigor, the tendency toward using pharmacological agents to achieve an advantage during competition will continue. However, this will always remain a form of cheating. In addition to attempting to exploit uncertain areas and newly marketed or synthesized compounds, there may always be a tendency for an abuser to stay one step ahead of regulations and current testing methods.

While some of these changes may be predictable and follow previous trends, such as the development of newly synthesized and undetectable anabolic steroid compounds, other advances may be unanticipated. For example, the concept of "gene doping" may involve exploitation of the human genome project and utilization of gene therapy to insert new genes into a cell to replace a defective or absent gene that may be causing medical problems. In addition, it may be tempting and technically possible to insert a gene that improves or enhances natural performance. Naturally occurring substances, such as testosterone or EPO, may be genetically stimulated for excessive production and may not be detected as an exogenous PED. The use of stem cells, with their great degree of plasticity, may allow them to differentiate into potent cells that provide greater advantage. Growth factors, artificial blood or blood substitutes, improved oxygen delivery systems, and older drugs whose detection is masked or prevented are all future possibilities.

DRUG TESTING

The detection of the presence of foreign substances in the human body originated with modern medicine's need to measure the type and concentrations of medications for guiding treatments and the responses of various organs to therapeutic interventions. Originally, and still today, physicians can obtain assays for the amounts of therapeutic agents such as antibiotics, anticonvulsants, cardiac drugs, and other medications to adjust dosage and to limit toxicity. In addition, the detection of unknown medications and illicit drugs is possible through a variety of toxicology screening tests using blood and urine samples, for instance when a person is brought to a hospital emergency department following an accident or a collapse without known cause. Initially, in the 1950s, a few European cyclists and track athletes were suspected of using certain drugs; however, by the mid-1960s it became possible to test for stimulants. Beginning with the 1968 Olympics, and then later at the 1972 Munich and Sapporo Olympic Games, studying the drug habits of elite athletes became possible. Steroids were first tested for at the 1976 Montreal Olympic Games, because by that time reliable measurements had been created, but they were only possible for a limited number of the competitors due to the lengthy assay procedures.[28]

During the 1980s, the identification of steroid use, especially among Olympic athletes, began to escalate, and in 1983 the testosterone to epitestosterone ratio test made its debut. American discus thrower Ben Plunknett became the first athlete to have his world record erased after being caught for steroid use. Athletes were also caught using beta-blockers, EPO, and probenecid, a medication normally used by patients with gout, but which has the ability to mask steroids by diluting their release into the system. A seminal event was the stripping of the gold medal from Canadian sprinter Ben Johnson after he was identified as having used the potent anabolic steroid stanozolol in 1988. The following year, the World Anti-Doping Agency (WADA) was established and sanctioned as an independent authority for the standards and testing of athletes. By 2003 it had grown to be accepted by 105 countries, all major sports federations, and its list of prohibited substances numbered over 200.

Through the efforts of many, and especially the International Olympic Committee (IOC) and its Medical Commission, the ability to test for illicit or prohibited drugs proceeded to more sophistication. The history of drug testing, especially at the Olympic level, has been storied and complex. There have been innumerable efforts to make the methodology more sound, scientific, and accurate, while simultaneously conspiratorial athletes have experimented and broken the rules for the use of exogenous substances. Screening procedures have involved the use of radioimmunoassay (RIA) techniques, gas and liquid chromatography, immunosorbent assays, and other methods to survey large numbers of drug samples. Once positive tests have occurred, more sophisticated but also more costly and time-consuming methods are utilized to confirm the specific compound detected. Gas and liquid chromatography and mass spectrometry are the primary measurement techniques that have been used to provide certainty about the detected substances. In brief, a solvent is employed to help separate the molecule from its presence within the athlete's urine, and once extracted it is next collided with electrons that separate the ions in a characteristic fashion that identify the particular signal intensity of a substance. This is compared to the chemical signature of a known reference sample taken from another person who has consumed the same substance as a testing control. These and other emerging high technology methods promise to help with verification of exogenous substances and to assist with the common dilemma of attempting to discern whether a normally occurring, endogenous substance, such as testosterone, growth hormone, or others, is occurring at an abnormally high concentration.

Although the blood is the usual medium tested in medical practice for both endogenous and exogenous molecules, such as hormone and medication levels respectively, drug testing in athletes has become nearly exclusively urine based. There are many reasons for this method, including that urinary sampling is not invasive; that is, a needle is not required. This prevents unnecessary trauma to the athlete and avoids any potential for transmission of needle-borne diseases, such as infectious viruses. The urine also contains breakdown products of the substances, or metabolites, which, if known, are more readily apparent than in the original compound, and in higher concentrations. However, blood testing will always be a possibility, especially when measuring certain hormones or natural substances, such as EPO. Also, blood tests may sometimes be useful when measuring pharmaceutical or synthetic portions of molecules, such as the esterfied version of testosterone.[29]

There are many issues involved with drug testing that make this effort Herculean, such as the constant specter of newly emerging unknown substances, the abuse of certain naturally occurring hormones or body chemicals, normal variability between humans and within human cyclic physiology, and the consumption of masking agents, to name a few. Many hormones, such as human GH, growth hormone releasing hormone, EPO, insulin, epitestosterone, and others, are naturally occurring but have been abused by competitive athletes. Many of these large polypeptide molecules cannot be detected with current laboratory technology, while "normal" levels have not been conclusively established for others. For instance, EPO has been abused mainly by endurance athletes who want to increase their concentration of hemoglobin, which is the blood's oxygen carrying molecule. However, it is not feasible to test for EPO directly, and therefore, its effects are assayed by measuring the blood hematocrit, which is the concentration of hemoglobin containing red blood corpuscles. A value greater than 50 percent causes a three-week suspension in most federations. The main purpose of the new or designer drugs is to create a substance with masking or obscuring molecular fragments that interfere with the standard detection methods. In other situations, the consumption of meat treated with banned drugs may cause that substance to become detected, even without the athlete's knowledge. Examples, which include clenbuterol, Zeranol, Nandrolone, Trenbolone, and others, have been discovered and only indirectly consumed through ingestion of animal meats.[30]

An area of controversy has revolved around the testing of athletes for anabolic steroid use. The IOC, NFL, and other agencies have developed a ratio of 6 to 1 (6:1) as the upper limits of allowable testosterone (T) to epitestosterone (E) levels. While the ratio in most people is normally 1:1, the governing bodies are allowing for those individuals who may naturally have a higher concentration of T.[31] In addition, there has been an occasional proven case of a ratio as high as 9:1 without exogenous steroid administration. Therefore, most organizations will not pursue an athlete unless the ratio is 10:1 or higher.[32] There has not been much documentation of using both T and E simultaneously (perhaps because it is more difficult to take both T and E, which would possibly cause levels of other tested steroids to skyrocket) because there is more legal difficulty to prove both T and E use, or possibly it has been done by expert abusers but just not discovered as the two ratios have simultaneously increased. In addition, it is emphasized that urinary testing is an analysis for normally produced endogenous substances, so there are always expected variations in a wide range of "normal" between individuals. The various agencies have been forced, perhaps because of not only physiological differences but also legal challenges, to be liberal in their allowance for variations. In addition, there are several known reasons why high T:E may occur, such as alcohol use prior to the urinary test, bacterial growth or high pH in the urine sample, naturally occurring low E levels, monthly female normal T:E fluctuations depending on menstrual cycle, oral contraceptive use, and endocrine disease, among others.[33]

There is no doubt that cycling, or other forms of cheating, occurs. One example is the application of transdermal patches to the scrotum, the skin of which has a higher concentration of the enzyme reductase, which quickly converts the T to another form, dihydrotestosterone (DHT), an andogenous molecule that is normally not tested for. Another method would be to use any form of controlled released T, perhaps in an injectable, fat-soluble form, so that the peak T levels would not occur, thus not be as likely to exceed the 6:1 ratio. However, the IOC is aware of these issues, and the NFL is just following suit. There is still room, as you can see, depending on the daring and creativity of the athlete, to potentially beat the system. Currently there is experimentation with more sensitive methods of detection, such as isotope ratio mass spectroscopy, which analyzes the type of carbon atoms within the molecules of T detected, which can distinguish natural T from animal and plant sources derived from the diet as opposed to the synthetic form of carbon from pharmaceuticals. Undoubtedly, there will continue to be further development in both the testing and circumvention areas of anabolic steroid use.

There are, however, innumerable other issues related to drug testing, which have been well detailed by Richard Pound in *Inside the Olympics: A Behind-the-Scenes Look at the Politics, the Scandals, and the Glory of the Games.* The difficulties of amateur and Olympic sports obtaining cooperation from professional sports for commitment, accuracy, timing, and reliability of testing are serious and perhaps downright obstructionist. These problems will certainly continue as the business of professional athletics dominates all discussion and negotiation for improvements in assessing sports for doping.[34]

CONCLUSION

There is a rich history of man's efforts to improve his athletic prowess and performance by utilizing exogenous substances that have come to be known as PEDs. In early years, naturally occurring substances were ingested; however, a transformation to synthetic PED has taken place, with the newly emerging designer drugs synthesized with the intent of not only illegally providing a competitive advantage but also circumventing accepted testing methods. For centuries, there has been the natural tendency by competitors to excel at any cost, and modern times have seen the continuation of that philosophy combined with more sophisticated forms of doping.

There are many issues to consider in order to better define and improve upon this age-old problem. Paramount is the question of whether society's yearn for great performances is truly a tacit approval for the use of any means, including exogenous substances, PEDs, and others, in order to achieve them. Is drug testing effective, or are there constant loopholes that allow circumvention? Is Major League Baseball serious about a crackdown on the use of PEDs and their impact upon the game? The future is uncertain; we do not know if this tendency to go to any means to gain competitive advantage will continue. In order to survive as a society that values honesty, sportsmanship, and fair competition, we must continue to search for solutions to these dilemmas that affect the youth who will become both the mundane and elite athletes in many sports.

6

Supplement Boom:
Big Business Spurs Big Trouble

"Using these supplements was like using drugs. First you start with protein, then you go to creatine and then you need both and may end up using steroids."

—Scotty Romans, 2000 Mesa Mountain View (Arizona) High School graduate[1]

"Playing baseball as a profession is a lifelong dream, and I'd do almost anything to achieve it. . . . (including Andro), the closest thing to steroids but legal."

—Harlan Malamud, 2003 Western (Florida) High School graduate[2]

"I just remember people telling me the competition we were playing . . . was doing it [creatine]. I was just trying to get bigger and stronger, and if the competition was doing it."

—L. B. Jeter, 1999 C. E. Byrd (Louisiana) High School graduate[3]

As with most of the content of this book, the comments by Romans to the *Arizona Republic*, Malamud to the Fort Lauderdale *Sun Sentinel*, and Jeter to the *Shreveport Times* are small but powerful examples of how the addiction to succeed in sports creates a "natural" pathway to potentially unethical behavior. The ultimate proof of this is found in the numerous and oft-cited surveys in which athletes have consistently said they would sacrifice five years of their life (more or less, depending on the survey) if they could be guaranteed success (winning a gold medal, receiving a pro contract, etc.). The number of "yes" responses remains disturbingly high each time the question is asked, proving the effects of steroids are not an effective deterrent. And because this thinking is so prevalent, it is safe to assume that athletes like Romans, who are dealing with increasing incentive to succeed and growing pressure to do what is necessary to stay competitive, are choosing to cheat. They see the progression from supplements to steroids as justifiable and unavoidable. Dr. Troy Potter, an internal medicine specialist at Bossier (Louisiana) Medical Center says: "These high school kids feel like they can't compete without taking it because they think that everybody else is taking it. And some kids think that if a little bit helps, then a lot will help more."[4] (See sidebar 6.1, "Fearless Youth: Why They Use Supplements.")

But even if they don't cross over from legal supplements to illegal drugs, the line they step up to by taking most supplements becomes a little more blurred every day. According to a study done by the International Olympic Committee and cited in the Anabolic Steroid Control Act of 2004, 41 percent of 624 dietary supplements studied contained either a steroid precursor or a banned substance, many of which are not disclosed on the label.[5] Consider the conclusion of the following:

- Already some health professionals believe supplements such as androstenedione are legal steroids, giving those who use them a competitive edge over those who do not.
- The *Arizona Republic* reviewed football rosters from one central

---

Sidebar 6.1: Fearless Youth: Why They Use Supplements

Rachel Olander, resource specialist at the Center for Drug Free Sport, has identified five reasons student-athletes take supplements:

- Student-athletes believe the advertisements and marketing.
- They don't believe the product is going to hurt them.
- They don't care if the product hurts them. They want to make the team, make the starting lineup, or perform at a higher level.
- They take supplements in pursuit of a better body image. They want more muscle, want to appear more "ripped" or thinner.
- They believe someone else is using them. If there's a chance it will make them half a second faster, they're going to use it.[1]

Phoenix school from 1981, 1990, and 2001 and found that the average size of a football player has increased by 26 percent.[6]

- From 1988 to 1998, the number of NFL athletes weighing more than 300 pounds increased from 27 to 235.

- As was discussed in the previous chapter, steroid precursors such as androstenedione may stunt growth as well as cause acne, breast enlargement, liver and heart problems, and personality disorders, all side effects of steroids.

If it looks like a steroid, works like a steroid (in gaining quick, substantial mass and strength), and has the side effects identical to those of steroids, then what else is it? "These are real drugs, and if you want to sell real drugs, you have to document them like real drugs," says Madelyn H. Fernstrom, a pharmacologist and director of the UPMC Weight Loss Center. "This is not like selling garlic. Not all dietary supplements are created equally."[7]

Like the steroids statistics discussed in previous chapters, the prevalence of such supplement use and the accompanying dangers should scare unsuspecting parents into learning more about them. This has not yet happened. Kids are using supplements parents do not even know exist, let alone are readily available to teens at the local mall or even through high school and college coaches. The following list includes some examples of how widespread supplement use is today:

- In a 2001 Cornell University study, 44 percent of 12th-grade male athletes in a suburb of New York reported using creatine.[8]

- A 2001 survey of seven Shreveport, Louisiana, high schools reported 49.2 percent of football players had used at least one type of sports supplement.[9]

- From 1992 to 2002, creatine sales grew by more than 900 percent.[10]

- Creatine sales soared from $30 million in 1995 to nearly a billion dollars in 2002.[11]

- Champion Nutrition reported its Andro sales jumped 1,000 percent in the four months (in 1998) following McGwire's revelation that he used the supplement. Expected sales of $30 million industry-wide surged to $40 million that year even though the McGwire story did not hit newsstands until August.[12]

- U.S. consumers shelled out some $76 million in 2002 for just three so-called dietary supplements: androstenedione, kava, and yohimbe, the only ones for which sales figures were available, according to the *Nutrition Business Journal*.[13]

- Based on projections from a nationally representative survey released by the Blue Cross Blue Shield Association, approximately 1.1 million young people between ages 12 and 17 have taken potentially dangerous performance-enhancing supplements and drugs.[14]

- Just as alarming, 76 percent of 12- to 17-year-olds could not identify any negative side effects that might result from using steroids, ephedra, and other similar substances.[15]

- "Most [creatine users] either did not know how much of the supplement they were taking or reported taking amounts that were more than the recommended doses."[16]

These facts and the research presented in chapter 7 bear out that unsupervised supplement use can be just as hazardous as taking steroids. And while there is no definitive proof that creatine is safe, helpful, harmful, or benign, the potential long-term effects are enough to warrant a more cautious approach.

A concurring source on this topic is Richard Kreider, Ph.D., a professor at Baylor University who coauthored *Creatine: The Power Supplement*. Kreider states that "All studies suggest it's safe and effective. There is no data in adolescents or children that suggests there's a problem, however there's not as much data in that population as there is in college-age kids, so some have suggested caution." He says research shows that creatine is best used by those engaged in activities requiring short bursts of energy, such as serious weight training. "Our thought is that if the person is involved in intense training, is eating a good diet and they're well-informed about the supplement and their parent or trainer or physician can supervise them or give them guidance, then—at least the high school athlete—I don't have a problem with them taking creatine."[17] Another expert who supports the responsible use of creatine is Rick Collins, a lawyer and an authority on anabolic steroids who maintains the Web site SteroidLaw.com. Collins says, "There really are no long-term studies in terms of the safety of creatine, and the short-term studies show that creatine is safe for use. Teenagers don't really think about long-term consequences."[18]

In addition to what we have learned through research for this book, we have personal knowledge of creatine's effects through our own use or experiences.[19] This experience revealed that taking recommended dosages and remaining hydrated was not only safe but also helped to increase muscle size and strength. The use of this supplement was accompanied by a healthy diet (heavy in protein) and a consistent, rigorous workout regimen. Our conclusion is that a lot of hard work can result in significant but limited gains. Young people are using creatine at such a high rate, as indicated by these and numerous other studies, which is cause for concern if these numbers come as a surprise to those monitoring the health of young athletes.

But even informed parents cannot ensure that supplements are safe. Keeping untested substances out of kids' hands can be difficult because restrictions on supplements have been slow to come by. The now-banned substance ephedra was linked to more than 80 deaths and nearly 1,500 complaints of harmful side effects before Congress finally banned its sale in 2004. Only after the deaths of NFL player Korey Stringer, Major League Baseball pitcher Steve Bechler, Northwestern's Rashidi Wheeler, Clinton Central (Indiana) High School's Travis Stowers, and the University of Florida's Eraste Autin were ephedra sales banned. Supplements similar to ephedra are not likely to be banned soon, which means more unregulated use and more expected problems. Some other reasons to be weary of the supplement industry include the following:

- *Consumer Reports* called the Food and Drug Administration's supplement division "understaffed and underfunded, with about 60 people and a budget of only $10 million to police a $19.4 billion-a-year industry. To regulate drugs, annual sales of which are 12 times the amount of supplement sales, the FDA has almost 43 times as much money and almost 48 times as many people."[20]
- Sports supplements are the fastest-growing segment of the supplement industry, thanks in part to Mark McGwire's use of Andro resulting in the subsequent explosion of its use among young athletes.
- Mike Perko, author of "Taking One For The Team: The New Thinking on Young Athletes and Dietary Supplements," says: "We live in a culture that says 'if it's legal, it must be OK for me to do.'

Since 1994, the supplement industry has been self-regulating. That means you can buy supplements anywhere—a discount store, a gas station, at the mall. To most people, that says, 'This is harmless. It's not going to hurt me.' Even in the face of facts to the contrary, many people still think that."[21]

- Ed Etzel, associate professor of sports psychology and psychologist at West Virginia University, agrees. "Supplements are now part of the entire culture of Olympic, professional and college sports. People have for years—going back to the beginning of time—looked for ways to do better, to get ahead. And supplements have become a pervasive part of that. There's really a culture of trying to perform better, and there's certainly marketing that fosters this and a culture of sport that fosters this. In my opinion, Americans are fans of a quick fix. So on some simplistic level, our supplement use makes sense."[22]

- Etzel also notes that some supplement use is due to peer pressure. "It's become the cool thing, the trendy thing to do. There's an 'extreme' theme that's very popular these days, and if you look at many supplements, their marketing somehow makes use of that word. There's certainly an adolescent population of sensation seekers who pursue that, and it also goes with the mentality of 'Well, it won't kill me.' "[23]

- Dr. Stephen Barrett, a consumer advocate and retired psychiatrist who heads Quackwatch, an organization dedicated to exposing health fraud, warns parents and others that supplements may not be what they appear. "The real problem is, we have a dishonest marketplace with a lot of low-quality products, a lot of coaches who don't understand the science, and a lot of kids who are anxious to do their best."[24]

- A study by Teenage Research Unlimited reveals that 27.6 million teenagers spent an average of $93 a month on personal items in 1989, for a total of nearly $31 billion. And teens do the shopping in 70 percent of the households with working mothers. These young shoppers often have access to their parents' credit cards and are buying more through the mail, a medium that offers a cloak of anonymity under which quacks thrive. Black-market steroids are often produced in another country or by clandestine domestic manufacturers under questionable conditions and may be contaminated.[25]

One major reason kids begin and/or continue to use potentially dangerous supplements is that parents and coaches often are endorsing these products. Coaches are frequently acting more on their urge to win than on their responsibility to mentor. "These coaches are trying to compete with other schools they know are using it, and they have to really care about the kids to tell them not to take it," says Bossier City Medical Center's Potter. "These coaches are approached all the time by people who manufacture this stuff. They want to supply the coaches with it."[26] The National Federation of State High School Association's policy statement, written in 1998, states: "In order to minimize health and safety risks, maintain ethical standards and reduce liability risks, school personnel and coaches should never supply, recommend or permit the use of any drug, medication or food supplement solely for performance-enhancing purposes."[27] And the distributing of creatine by collegiate officials has been banned by the NCAA since 2002. In fact, in some states it is illegal. In Texas, for example, it is a Class C misdemeanor for a school district employee to sell dietary supplements or other performance-enhancers to students. Many high schools and colleges have official policies banning coaches from selling or endorsing supplements, but many others have loose policies or only prevent a coach from making a profit or from selling it on campus. Because kids look up to coaches, they might hesitate to tell a coach "no" when asked to use it.

Coaches do not necessarily have to sell or even endorse supplements in order to have a negative impact on their players. Simply stressing the importance of gaining size and strength can lead kids to seek the fastest means to these goals. Barbe (Louisiana) High School baseball coach Glenn Cecchini implemented a weightlifting program during the 1997 season. Over the next four years, the Buccaneers won three of the next four Class 5A state titles, the state's highest classification. Cecchini says consistency—his team lifts three times a week during the off-season and twice a week in season—is the muscle behind the powerhouse he has built. "I think what separates us with the strength training is we do not miss. We never, ever miss. It's made a huge difference. If we didn't do what we do, I think we'd be good, but I don't think we'd be as good. Would we have won state [in 2001] or not? I don't think so."[28]

Wanting to win championships is not a bad thing. Failing to set the parameters by which those championships can be attained is an invitation for hazardous consequences. Learning which supplements are safe and knowing the limits to prevent overuse are extremely important pieces to this puzzle, and children should not be allowed to make these determinations by themselves. Our culture shows that success in sports and our body image are important to both young men and women. According to an article in the *San Francisco Chronicle*, which scrambled to increase its expertise in this area in the months following the BALCO revelations, a recent study found more than half of boys age 11 to 17 chose as their physical ideal an image so unrealistic that it could be attained only by use of steroids.[29] Coaches who push for athletic results must assume that supplements, and eventually steroids, will become a choice—an increasingly popular and accessible one—in their quest to be the best. And parents of teenagers who can't stand the way they look and can't wait for an opportunity to improve themselves must realize that children will do almost anything to fit in to a world seeking perfection at any cost. It is tough to develop a strategy that defies the seemingly sensible truth: that doping is and forever will be a part of sports. But the solution lies in a more aggressive offensive by adults in order to overcome the potentially out-of-control actions of kids.

Solutions to the Out-of-Control Drug Problem in Sports

The use of performance enhancing substances, beginning with steroids and other anabolic agents, will likely continue until real and meaningful change occurs with respect to the attitudes and expectations of athletes, coaches, and the public. Future developments using nefarious methods of producing previously undetectable or non-prohibited substances will be a temptation for the cheater and the perversely motivated athlete as well as for their families and support personnel. The potential for further pharmacological discoveries, which elude detection while providing advantages to the competitive athlete, will continue and will provide a constant challenge for all athletes, game officials, federations, and professional sports societies. The allure of "designer drugs" will be a ubiquitous specter for many years to come. More sophisticated methods of synthesis and detection avoidance, as exemplified by the recent THG scandal, may require that blood testing be performed, despite resistance in the past to such invasive monitoring methods. There is hope that new technology in measuring techniques will add precision to urinary or blood testing by increasing sensitivity and specificity for all prohibited substances. If gene doping becomes a reality, then routine sampling of bodily fluids may not detect any exogenous substance, and, instead, a tissue (such as muscle) biopsy may be necessary to ascertain if alteration of native genes has occurred.

USE PROGRAMS THAT WORK

Linn Goldberg, M.D., and Diane Elliot, M.D., at Oregon Health and Science University in Portland, developed a revolutionary program that has been implemented in nearly half of the United States. It represents the type of collaboration between science, psychology, and sports that must occur if society is to tackle the tough problem of steroids in sports effectively. Goldberg believes a lot of the thinking about this issue is outdated. It may also be unscientific and uneducated. An example is one group's recommendation that high school steroid testing is the answer, and that drug use will be discouraged by kicking players off of teams for positive tests. Not so, Dr. Goldberg says:

> No. 1, high school athletes are not college athletes—they don't have scholarships; they're very different. And there's no [scientific] proof that NCAA testing reduces use. No 2, you're going to isolate these kids further if you abandon them. They've got fragile psyches. You'll make them more depressed if you kick them off the team. . . . The last 20 years have taught us that scare tactics don't work and role models don't work [without other means of reinforcement]. If you're thinking this method works, you're really going back in time and ignoring the last 20 years of scientific evidence. Testing is not a bad idea. It may be that a combination [of testing and education] will work. I am working with the former director of NIDA [National Institute on Drug Abuse] to put ATLAS in the schools that already have drug testing to see if testing can enhance ATLAS. But testing alone won't work. What happens when these athletes graduate? What happens in the summer, when you can't test?[1]

Goldberg's program (see sidebar 7.1) is inexpensive and effective. A total of 23 states and Puerto Rico have purchased ATLAS and ATHENA. Goldberg describes his program: "It's about $4 per student. There is a coach's manual that costs $280. It has all the overheads, all the curriculum, it has the background, and it has how to train your squad leaders and the materials to do the evaluation. [Schools] can photocopy the materials as many times as they want. A coach can either hand it off to another coach or pay $15 to photocopy the entire book. Then there's a squad leader's manual and that includes the 10-session curriculum that's in the coach's manual. So one out of about six to eight students gets one of those. So for a couple of dollars they can photocopy that (it's about 70–80 pages). And then each student receives three booklets for a total of $3.95—the ATLAS Program workbook with the 10-session curriculum; the training guide for exercise training; and a sports menu, which goes through not only the drugs, but also what to eat and how to monitor their

Sidebar 7.1: Overview of the ATLAS Program

Program Features

Content	Activities (Table 4)	Frequency	Time	Setting	Time of Day	Parent involvement	Peer training
Based on athlete risk and protective factor research	Inter-active games, role-play, goal-setting	Once/week	45″ per session*	School	Flexible (usually before team practice)	Homework and parent team meeting	90-minute session with coach/instructor

ATLAS Curriculum Content

Session 1: Sport Nutrition and Exercise
Activity 1: Different styles of strength training and expected results (10″)
Activity 2: Fats, carbohydrates, and proteins (12″)
Activity 3 and 4: Effects of Natural testosterone vs. manufactured anabolic steroids (AS) (17″)
Activity 5: Instructor review (6″)

Session 2: Exercise/Anabolic Steroids Effects
Activity 1: Strength training (8″)
Activity 2: Weight room safety (6″)
Activity 3: Finding maximum strength (6″)
Activity 4: Word search re: AS effects (6″)
Activity 5: Match game re: training, AS and sports nutrition (5″)
Activity 6: Strength training and nutrition quiz (9″)
Activity 7: Instructor review (5″)

Session 3: Sports Nutrition
Activity 1: Calorie and protein requirements (8″)
Activity 2: Fluid requirements (5″)
Activity 3: High and low fat food comparisons (4″)
Activity 4: How to use the Sports Menu (10″)
Activity 5: Nutrition goal setting (15″)
Activity 6: Instructor Review (3″)

Session 4: Nutrition/Advertising/ Supplements and AS
Activity 1: Nutrition goals follow-up (9″)
Activity 2: Importance of breakfast (3″)
Activity 3: Media awareness: ads designed to treat side-effects of AS (13″)
Activity 4: Advertised supplements (12″)
Activity 5: AS side-effects (5″)
Activity 6: Instructor review (3″)

Session 5: Nutrition/Effects of Alcohol and Drugs (AOD) on Sport Performance
Activity 1: Nutrition goals follow-up (5″)

Activity 2: Pre- and post-exercise snacks (10″)
Activity 3: Effects of AOD on performance (15″)
Activity 4: Drug refusal role-play (12″)
Activity 5: Instructor review (3″)

Session 6: Drugs in Sport
Activity 1: Nutrition goals follow-up (5″)
Activity 2: Student campaign development (against drugs in sports/pro-healthy nutrition and exercise) (40″)
Activity 3: Instructor review (1″)

Session 7: Nutrition and Antidrug Campaigns
Activity 1: Nutrition goals follow-up (5″)
Activity 2: Low fat substitutions (8″)
Activity 3: Student antidrug campaign presentations (29″)
Activity 4: Instructor review (3″)

Session 8: Ethics and Drugs in Sport
Activity 1: Nutrition goals follow-up (5″)
Activity 2: Ethics and sport (15″)
Activity 3: AOD and sport crossword (10″)
Activity 4: Student antidrug campaign (12″)
Activity 5: Instructor review (3″)

Session 9: Drugs in sport/strength training
Activity 1: Nutrition goals follow-up (5″)
Activity 2: Antidrug, pro-health student newspaper article creation (25″)
Activity 3: Strength training benefits (10″)
Activity 4: Instructor review and body image homework assignment (2″)

Session 10: Review and Steroid man game
Activity 1: Nutrition goals follow-up (5″)
Activity 2: Body image homework review (5″)
Activity 3: ATLAS review game (25″)
Activity 4: Team commitment/squad leader acknowledgement (10″)
(minutes/activity = ″)

nutrition. It talks about selected supplements, vitamins, minerals, what to eat at fast food restaurants, other menu planning, etc."

He continues by saying, "In drug testing, you pay someone to come into your school and test your kids. You're not even involved. You don't teach it, you don't have to monitor it. All you do is hire Drug Testing Are Us. You set up a contract with them, they come in, they do testing, and they leave. You get the results and that's it. ATLAS and ATHENA (Athletes Targeting Healthy Exercise and Nutrition Alternatives, a program for female athletes that focuses on eating disorders and other problems) involve coaches and teammates. It involves changing social influence. Teams work together; that's what they're designed to do. Most kids are on a team of some kind. It's a pro-social atmosphere. And teams in the ATLAS program had a higher winning percentage after the program. We asked them why and they said, 'We have team leaders and better communication.' And it's not only during school time, but during the workout, training, and after-school time."[2]

ATLAS's credentials/benefits:

- Substance Abuse and Mental Health Services Administration of the U.S. Department of Health and Human Services named ATLAS an exemplary program.
- The programs can be funded by the federal Center for Substance Abuse Prevention and the National Institute on Drug Abuse, which funded the original ATLAS program.
- One of nine exemplary programs, ATLAS is recognized by the Department of Education's Safe and Drug Free Schools Program.

Tested on 15 schools in Oregon and Washington, the program claimed a 50 percent reduction rate in the use of anabolic steroids as well as reduced use of alcohol, other drugs, and sports supplements.

Some of the preliminary findings of the ATLAS program in Salt Lake City, Utah, include:

- Three-fourths of the students involved in the program are less likely to use illegal drugs than before the program began.
- More than 50 percent have a decreased desire to try anabolic steroids.
- Most student athletes reported they were better able to turn down

offers of steroids, alcohol, and drugs, and they were less likely to ride with a driver who was drinking and driving.
- Student athletes recorded improved nutrition habits and 70 percent believed the program made them a better athlete.

Timothy Condin, an associate director at NIDA, said ATLAS works because it is led by students and coaches, not guest lecturers. "It helps change the culture in the athletic departments about what is acceptable," he says. "Changing the norm in their environment is one of the hardest things to do, and you can't just depend on outside information to do it."[3]

The success of the ATLAS program is obvious but not overwhelming. Convincing the country that this type of program is a success has not been easy for Dr. Goldberg: "We're professors, not marketing experts. Does it work? Well, it's been evaluated by the Department of Health and Human Services, and they found it to be a model program in 2000. There are model programs and promising programs. Promising programs look like they're going to be effective. They may work on risk factors that may reduce substance abuse or they work for the short-term but not the long-term. Model programs are those that have shown with scientific evidence the actual reduction of substance use and abuse, and they work long-term."[4]

Education has been proven to work. Character building is proving to work. A meaningful commitment to religion in the home will work. A hundred dollars multiplied by a hundred thousand athletes for steroid testing in one state alone is not going to solve a problem that begins in the brain, not in the laboratory. Cheating is always going to be a way of life. Weakening its impact at the root—in a child's development—is far more effective that trying to catch it when an elite high school, college, or professional athlete has weighed the options and continues to choose a win-at-all-costs shortcut to the same success we all seek.

COACH KIDS TO DO RIGHT—
IT IS EVERYONE'S RESPONSIBILITY

Kevin Will is a part of the solution in the fight against steroid use. In March 2004, Kevin, who played quarterback at Sacramento's Del

Oro High School, testified at a California state senate hearing addressing steroid and supplement use at high schools. His testimony confirms what several credible studies have found: Many coaches are failing to deter young athletes from using steroids. Will said, "Coaches might say you need to get a little stronger, bulk up a bit. Kids end up taking steroids because they think they have to get bigger."[5] A survey conducted in 2002 of 1,553 athletes ages 10 to 14 found that 88 percent had heard of anabolic steroids but only 64 percent had had their side effects explained to them and only 47 percent said a parent, coach, teacher, or athletic trainer was their primary source of information. The survey's results were compared to a 1989 study before anabolic steroids became illegal. In the 1989 study, 78 percent had heard of steroids, while 50 percent had been told of the side effects.[6] The study's research suggests the need for educational programs at the junior high school level administered by qualified coaches, teachers, trainers, and parents. We could not agree more. Parents, coaches, teachers, and health-care providers need to take a more active role in educating adolescents about the effects of anabolic steroids. Too often adolescents are left to compile information on anabolic steroids from inappropriate sources and consequently do not fully understand the effects associated with steroids. Here are some of the unacceptable examples:

- The study above shows 433 of the 1,553 athletes—28 percent— used a book or magazine as their primary source of information on steroids. Parents (21 percent) were second on the list, followed by coaches (17 percent).
- The same study suggests educational programs should not be limited to the direct negative effects of anabolic steroids, but they should also "provide information about behavioral modification strategies, risk avoidance and reduction of peer pressure."[7]
- The numbers in the study above confirm what was learned in an unscientific survey conducted by the *Shreveport Times* in 2001. When asked, "Who, if anyone, has talked to you about the good and/or bad effects of supplements/steroids?" only 22 of the *Times'* 125 respondents said their coach had spoken to them, while 97 either left the question blank or answered "no one." Six others cited a parent, friend, or relative.

- A Blue Cross Blue Shield telephone survey of 1,803 people—1,000 adults and 803 youths—between April 4 and 23, 2003, showed 81 percent of young people said they had never had a conversation with their parents about performance-enhancing substances, and 69 percent said they had received no information from their sports teams.[8]
- The same survey found that 70 percent of kids and half of parents surveyed were unable to identify even one negative side effect associated with performance-enhancing drugs.[9]
- A survey of over 300 high school athletes in Minnesota found that 74 percent of those students got their information on sports supplements from friends.[10]
- Dr. Frank Uryasz, president of the National Center for Drug Free Sport, says steroid use by high school students will never be completely wiped out. This statement shows the problem's severity and the importance of improving the way we communicate and educate kids. "If it's not steroids it'll be something else that will filter on down," Uryasz says. "We really have to approach this issue on a broader scale. We need to educate kids on what's right or wrong; what kind of performance-enhancement is appropriate or inappropriate. What concerns me about the whole dietary supplement issue is that it is teaching kids that performance enhancement comes out of a cream or a bottle or a pill. Once you buy into that mindset, then dietary supplements are basically anabolic steroid training wheels. They are very motivated to look better and play better. That's a good thing. But who's sending the messages on how to do that? Is your son getting the message from *Muscle & Fitness* or *Flex Magazine*, or is he getting it from coaches or mom and dad." (For more from Dr. Uryasz, see sidebar 7.2.)

LOOK FOR SIGNS OF
PERFORMANCE-ENHANCING DRUG USE

Parents and coaches should closely monitor their child's development to recognized these signs of potential steroid use:

- Rapid gains in size (and strength if parents are monitoring this)
- Yellowish pigmentation of the skin caused by jaundice of the liver

Sidebar 7.2: Q&A with Dr. Frank Uryasz[1]

Question: Where do we need the most improvement in the global issue of drug testing?

Answer: In research that will benefit us at the highest level of sport. We need more research into the detection of substances that we can't currently detect. The granddaddy of them all would be human growth hormone. We have the use of HGH at the highest level of sport and it's going unchecked. Now we don't know to what extent it's being used at the college or high school level, but certainly it is at a much lesser degree than at the professional level. It's primarily an economic issue.

It's very difficult to detect the use of these synthetic hormones that were designed to be virtually identical to the natural hormones. . . . But because of research we were able to develop a method [of testing for testosterone] that actually found that there was a slight difference in the ratio of carbon isotopes when one compares synthetic and natural testosterone. And we now have a test to determine if an athlete is using synthetic testosterone. But we only got the test because of the research that was done.

Q: What's preventing the necessary research from being done?

A: There's not very much [funding] unfortunately. The International Olympic Committee through the World Anti-Doping Agency has made some funding available, but often times those are distributed more on politics than anything else. The U.S. Federal Government has some money and it channels it through the U.S. Anti-Doping Agency, but otherwise there really aren't any significant sources of funding [for research].

I think it's an appropriate role for the government to play. Research funding has a role to play. The professional leagues and certainly the IOC has the dollars available to put money toward research. These are organizations—like the IOC—that spend a lot of money, and the Olympics still make a lot of money. There's no question they can put some resources behind research. The human growth hormone problem is the one that's worth examining. A few months before the Olympic Games you'll see the IOC announce that they have a test for HGH. They did it in Atlanta; they did it in Sydney, and now we're hearing that they have a test that's ready to go for Athens. Well, I'm dubious. If they have a test, the research and methods haven't been published. So even if you say you can detect human growth hormone, you'd have a difficult time in a courtroom defending the test.

Q: What areas of education are in need of improvement?

A: One area that is interesting is the notion that athletes are no different than students. I hear it all the time at the college level. And I think it's hooey. Athletes are a population of risk takers, especially college football players. These are guys who are willing to take risks everyday. We have to treat them differently educationally. I always hear "Oh, we're trying to integrate the population of athletes into the student body." Well they are a different population in many ways. . . . There's a lot of things that are done in sport—from the outside looking in—that are not very healthy. So we just have to remember that the athletes for the most part—at least as a population—are not persuaded by health and safety.

Q: *What is working and how do we know it is working?*

A: I like to talk about levels of deterrence. People throw out comments like, "Testing doesn't work" and "Education doesn't work." People in this industry are quoted all the time saying these things and it's just not true. If we believe every athlete is a potential steroid user and we approach it that way, there will be a group of athletes that as a result of education will make a decision to not use anabolic steroids. Education works. We know this from the NCAA, because we ask them: "If you haven't used steroids, why haven't you?" And they say, "I'm concerned about health," or "It's against my values or my belief system." They reached those decisions by education, either by their parents, schools or however they're getting it. There's a whole other level that, despite education, they might make the decision to use. That's where the role of testing impacts on this population extensively. There are a lot of athletes who choose not to use because of fear of getting caught. The next population are those who despite testing, they use and they get caught. And they get sanctioned, and some programs have significant sanctions. In Major League Baseball it ain't so significant. And then of course there's the whole population that uses that we don't catch.

Q: *How is the problem being handled at the high school level?*

A: I think the schools are doing a better job of integrating steroid education into the drug curriculum. I think probably what we lack most of all is education and strong messages about the integrity of the sport, sportsmanship, behavior in sport. We get calls from parents with high school athletes all the time wanting to enhance their son or daughter's performance. Some of them are just questions about dietary supplements, but other calls are about growth hormones and other products. So we can't always rely on parents to be the voice of reason. . . . Those kinds of messages probably come best from the home. Establishing an ethical basis for the things that you do in your life. I don't know if any research has been done on this, but if you cheat in sports you're probably cheating in other things.

I think the schools have a role to play. I see a significant role for parents to get things in perspective about your sons and daughters' participation in sports. What happens in schools regarding education about drugs has to be supported by what's going on at home. Otherwise it's going to be undermined. We also have an obligation to put it in perspective. . . . Nearly 8 percent of high school seniors used cocaine, where only about 3.5 percent had used anabolic steroids and nearly 60 percent reported that they'd been drunk. So there are a lot of issues that we need better education on. Steroid use is important to me, but it's important to keep this in perspective. If you look at the issue of mortality, we're going to lose more of our kids through the abuse of alcohol than we are from steroids.

Q: Who needs to take on more responsibility?

A: Everyone has a level of responsibility. When I talk to coaches, I tell them that I don't know any better deterrent than strong non-use messages from coaches. Coaches will tell athletes that they need to lose weight, they need to gain weight, they need to enhance their performance in whatever way they think and they leave that open-ended. What do athletes do? The take ephedrine, they take diuretics, protein powders, anabolic steroids. So we need to be very specific in our messages from coaches. What's appropriate? What's ethical? What's safe? You just can't leave that open-ended and hope that high school athletes and college athletes know what is or isn't appropriate.

There are high schools all over the country that don't have access to athletic trainers . . . [or they are] provided on Friday nights for games. And the football coach is probably teaching the health class, too. So there's a need for greater education. It's tough for coaches because often times you typically coach like you were coached and you pass down bad information from generation to generation. When I talk to coaches and colleges I always remind them that working in institutions of higher education, their coaching methods should be research-based. But you still hear coaches telling kids things about nutrition and there is no research basis for what they're saying.

I think there has to be communication back and forth from parents to the schools. They need to reach a consensus on all the dangers surrounding their son or daughter's athletic participation. There has to be clear expectations and sanctions if the athlete fails to follow through. Parents and schools have to be on the same page and that's tough. . . . We have some parents who have unreasonable aspirations for their sons and daughters. Usually the coaches are the first ones to know their kids' limitations. And often times there's a huge disconnect.

- High blood pressure
- Increases in LDL (bad cholesterol) and decreases in HDL (good cholesterol)
- Severe acne (especially more prevalent on the chest and back since teenagers are already prone to facial acne)
- Trembling
- Mood swings and/or quicker irritability (often building into fits of what is known as 'roid rage)
- In men, baldness and development of breasts
- In women, growth of facial hair, male pattern baldness, changes in or cessation of the menstrual cycle, and deepened voice
- In adolescents, growth halted prematurely through premature skeletal maturation and accelerated puberty changes

These are not all of the signs and side effects of steroid use, but they are the most recognizable to a parent involved in a child's health and development. Coaches and parents must live up to their supervisory roles by searching for the signs of steroid use, even going out of their way to find them. This has simply not been the case, even after more than a decade of scientific evidence that kids are using steroids.

TAKE THE NECESSARY STEPS TO PREVENT/ELIMINATE DOPING

The best prevention is establishing from the very start of an athlete's career an ethics and values system that parents themselves adhere to and that their kids want to follow. There will always be kids who stray, but too often this kind of early discussion and recognition of the importance of competing cleanly and fairly never takes place. (See chapter 16, "Solutions: Winning without Losing Perspective" for more on this ethical foundation.) If there are signs of drug use, talking to a young athlete about it will be much easier if these topics have been previously discussed and if the lines of communication remain as open as possible. In any case, the conversation must take place immediately and in a serious, formal setting to communicate the importance of the subject. Simply asking a child if they're using steroids is not enough. A parent must know what they are talking about, be organized in preparing specific questions, and err on the side of being skeptical—not in an attempt to bully a child into a confession or risk breaking an existing trust, but to eliminate as much doubt as possible and to be aggressive against a serious problem. If a child is able to obtain and use illegal drugs, they also will be able to deny it and explain any side effects.

If not satisfied with the answers, next steps could include speaking to other parents within a child's peer group or speaking with coaches, gym teachers, other teachers, and the child's friends to find out if they have seen the child exhibiting questionable behavior or experiencing any other side effects. If there remains significant doubt, have the young athlete tested for steroids. It is worth the effort and a loving parent-child relationship can withstand a parent's prerogative to take every caution to protect their child's health. It is important for coaches to be just as aggressive with their athletes during this process. Finally, and if necessary, a rehabilitation process must be properly administered. Schools should have these programs in place. "You need to have a rehab program if you're going to use drug testing because you're going to catch people," Dr. Goldberg says.[11]

Jeff Scudder, a health teacher at South Broward (Florida) High School, agrees that these conversations with kids must happen. "When you know that your child is willing to take a protein shake and put in those extra hours at the gym, you need to sit down and have a talk. Ask: 'What are your goals? Is someone guiding you to make sure you do this right?' It's not a reason to panic but if they are willing to take shakes, that could blossom into something more."[12]

LEARN WHAT HAS BEEN BANNED AND WHAT'S NEXT ON THE LIST

In addition to anabolic steroids, which recently included the designer testosterone-producing drug known as THG (see chapter 4, "BALCO and Beyond: The Biggest Doping Scandal in Sports History"), the federal government prohibited the distribution of supplements that contain ephedrine alkaloids because of their health risks. That ban took effect on April 12, 2004. On March 11, the Food and Drug Administration sent letters to 23 companies that make or market Andro, warning them to stop selling the pills that are converted into steroids in the body or they would risk civil or criminal sanctions. According to published reports, there are around two dozen similar supplements that Congress and Major League Baseball are examining that could be added to the list. One substance the Consumers Union (nonprofit publisher of *Consumer Reports*) deems "definitely hazardous," which is not yet banned by the federal government, is Aristolochic acid. This "potent human carcinogen" linked to kidney failure has been the subject of FDA warnings, but the products that contain Aristolochic acid—Aristolochia, birthwort, snakeroot, snakeweed, sangree root, sangrel, serpentary, serpentaria, *Asarum canadense*, and wild ginger—are available for purchase in stores or on the Internet. In addition, *Consumer Reports*' list of supplements deemed "very likely hazardous" are:

- Comfrey (also known as *Symphytum officinale*, ass ear, black root, blackwort, bruisewort, *Consolidae radix*, consound, gum plant, healing herb, knitback, knitbone, salsify, slippery root, *Symphytum radix*, wallwort)
- Androstenedione (4-androstene-3, 17-dione, andro, androstene)
- Chaparral (*Larrea divaricata*, creosote bush, greasewood, hediondilla, jarilla, larreastat)
- Germander (*Teucrium chamaedrys*, wall germander, wild germander)
- Kava (*Piper methysticum*, ava, awa, gea, gi, intoxicating pepper, kao, kavain, kawa-pfeffer, kew, long pepper, malohu, maluk, meruk, milik, rauschpfeffer, sakau, tonga, wurzelstock, yagona, yangona)

Consumer Reports' likely hazardous list includes:

- Bitter orange (*Citrus aurantium*, green orange, kijitsu, neroli oil, Seville orange, shangzhou zhiqiao, sour orange, zhi oiao, zhi xhi)
- Organ/glandular extracts (brain/adrenal/pituitary/placenta/other gland "substance" or "concentrate")
- Lobelia (*Lobelia inflata*, asthma weed, bladderpod, emetic herb, gagroot, lobelie, indian tobacco, pukeweed, vomit wort, wild tobacco)
- Pennyroyal oil (*Hedeoma pulegioides*, lurk-in-the-ditch, mosquito plant, piliolerial, pudding grass, pulegium, run-by-the-ground, squaw balm, squawmint, stinking balm, tickweed)

- Scullcap (*Scutellaria lateriflora,* blue pimpernel, helmet flower, hoodwort, mad weed, mad-dog herb, mad-dog weed, quaker bonnet, scutelluria, skullcap)
- Yohimbe (*Pausinystalia yohimbe,* johimbi, yohimbehe, yohimbine)

The substances above have been linked to dangers ranging from cancer to kidney failure, liver damage, and heart attack.[13]

CONTINUE WORLDWIDE EFFORTS TO CONTROL THE PROBLEM

In its fight against doping in the Olympics, the IOC convened the World Conference on Doping in Sport in Lausanne, Switzerland, in February 1999. Following the proposal of the Conference, the World Anti-Doping Agency (WADA) was established on November 10, 1999. WADA, headquartered in Montreal, Quebec, is structured by equal representation of the Olympic Movement and Public Authorities. Its goal is to standardize everything from a list of banned drugs to the testing-and-appeals process. WADA's complete 10-page list of banned substances is available at www.wada-ama.org/docs/web/standards_harmonization/code/list_standard_200 4.pdf.

In addition to this antidoping code used by amateur athletes around the world, President Bush signed into law legislation aimed at controlling the ballooning problem of doping in the United States.

- The Anabolic Steroid Control Act of 2004, cosponsored by Congressmen F. James Sensenbrenner Jr. (R-Wisconsin), John Conyers Jr. (D-Michigan), John Sweeney (R-NewYork), Tom Osborne (R-Nebraska), and Howard Berman (D-California), amends the Controlled Substances Act to provide increased penalties for anabolic steroid offenses near sports facilities and for other purposes. The bill also aims to update the list of illegal dangerous substances aggressively marketed as performance-enhancing drugs and increase the penalties for those who traffic them within 1,000 feet of a sports facility.[14]
- The Senate's version of the bill was cosponsored by Senators Joseph R. Biden (D-Delaware) and Orrin Hatch (R-Utah) and applies to substances that, once ingested, metabolize in the body into ana-

bolic steroids. It amends the Controlled Substances Act to clarify the definition of anabolic steroids and to provide for research and education activities relating to steroids and steroid precursors.[15]

This legislation and more like it is necessary to bolster the efforts of sports entities and leagues in wiping out doping. Unfortunately, much of the past legislation, especially that sponsored by state lawmakers, has called for expensive drug testing, which has failed to pass. There instead should be more energy devoted toward legislation that focuses on education and building morality and character. (For a comprehensive history of steroid and supplement legislation, see sidebar 7.3).

Meanwhile, there are national organizations working independently to educate participants and initiate change. Here are the two most prominent examples:

- United States Anti-Doping Agency (USADA, www.usantidoping.org)
  - This body, formed by the United States Olympic Committee in October 1999 (roughly the same time as WADA), "is dedicated to eliminating the practice of doping in sports, including U.S. Olympic, Pan American and Paralympic athletes . . . and is responsible for the testing and adjudication process for the athletes."[16]
  - USADA is focused on education. Its efforts include collaborating with Scholastic, Inc., to pilot fifth-grade educational programs in several states in 2003, and it has plans to develop a coaching education program in 2004.
  - USADA, an independent, nongovernmental organization, is also focused on research, allocating $2 million of a nearly $13 million annual budget toward various topics and communicates with WADA's scientific committee to coordinate efforts.
  - USADA has been highly active in the performance-enhancing drug legislation process, playing a key role in the development of both the House and Senate bills of the Anabolic Steroid Control Act of 2004. USADA is a founding member of the Coalition for Anabolic Steroid Precursor and Ephedra Regulation (CASPER), which is composed of the nation's leading medical, public health, and sports organizations and is focused on supporting

Sidebar 7.3: Steroid and Supplement Legislation[1]

FAILED

- *April 29, 2004:* Florida State Rep. Marcelo Llorente (R-Miami) said he plans to continue pursuing a bill in 2005 that would make schools conduct steroid tests (requiring 5 percent of student athletes to test) as a prerequisite for membership in the Florida High School Athletic Association. This after Llorente's House Bill (HB) 861 failed to get out of committee in 2004.
- *June 14, 2002:* California State Sen. Don Perata (D-Alameda) introduced a bill to force most professional sports teams to test athletes for performance enhancing drugs if they play games in California. The state Senate's Assembly Arts, Entertainment, Sports, Tourism, and Internet Media Committee has unanimously approved the bill. There is no further record of the bill after this.
- *April 7, 1992:* A watered-down version of a 1989 bill introduced by New York State Sen. John B. Sheffer II (R-Amherst) calling for mandatory testing and educational programs for anabolic steroids for all high school athletes in the state who did not pass. He also proposed that coaches who illegally distribute the drugs be banned from amateur athletics.
- *May 19, 1989:* New York State Sen. Dean Skelos (R-Rockville Centre) proposed drug testing as part of physicals required of high school athletes and stiff penalties for offenders—possibly a year's suspension from competing for athletes. There is no record of the bill moving forward after its introduction.

PENDING/OTHER

- *August 27, 2004:* The California Senate sends Gov. Schwarzenegger a bill banning performance-enhancing supplements that are currently legal in California from high school competition starting in July 2006. Senate Bill (SB) 1630 also calls for the state to compile a list of dangerous supplements (such as those listed in chapter 6 with similarities to ephedra) and mandates related education courses for coaches. The bill was sponsored by Sen. Jackie Speier (D-Hillsborough), who initially wanted to institute steroid testing for the 2006–2007 school year "once the district has determined that there are funds to pay for the tests."[2] Critics, including the authors of this book, contend that such funds, if they are to become available, would be best served in education programs (such as ATLAS, see sidebar 7.1). The final version of the bill removed the plans to test for steroid and illegal supplement use, but it requires student-athletes to sign forms agreeing to the restrictions.[3] Indications from the outset of the bill, like previous legislation, were that the funds would not be available to conduct the necessary testing for steroids.[4] Also, California has failed in the past to properly implement an organized, mandatory steroid-training policy.[5]

- *April 22, 2004:* Sen. Speier's second bill (SB 1444) would ban the sale of steroid precursors, such as androstenedione, to minors (banning the sale of the supplement creatine to minors soon could be added).[6]

- *April 13, 2004:* California State Rep. Susan Davis (D-San Diego) introduced legislation that would force supplement companies to turn over to the FDA any consumer health complaints linked to their products. The bill also would give the FDA power to require a supplement company to submit proof of a product's safety if the FDA determines there are reasonable grounds to believe it has been adulterated.

- *April 13 2004:* Sen. Dick Durbin (D-Illinois) sponsored a bill that would require any supplement that contains ingredients that act like stimulants or steroids in the body to be tested for safety before they are sold. His bill also would require mandatory reporting of serious consumer health complaints.

- *April 12, 2004:* The Food and Drug Administration's nationwide ban on dietary supplements containing ephedra took effect after a federal judge in Newark, New Jersey, rejected a manufacturer's attempt to block it.

- *April 8, 2004:* The Senate Commerce Committee decides to (and later does) subpoena Justice Department documents on alleged use of performance-enhancing drugs by U.S. Olympic athletes. The aim is to investigate and ban athletes who are found to have used steroids before the Athens Games.

- *April 8, 2004:* Sen. John McCain (R-Arizona) sponsors a nonbinding resolution last week that urged the sport's leaders to adopt stricter testing while warning that "real" legislation will follow if the players and owners fail to act. McCain said neither he nor his colleagues want to be involved in a labor dispute.

- *April 8, 2004:* Sen. Byron Dorgan (D-North Dakota) said that "real legislation" could follow the nonbinding resolution.

- *April 1, 2004:* Legislation limiting sales of steroid precursors, such as androstenedione, a substance Mark McGwire used in his record-breaking home-run year, won approval Wednesday (March 31) by the House Judi-

ciary Committee. Rep. Jim Sensenbrenner (R-Wisconsin), Judiciary Committee chairman, sponsored the House bill.

- *March 1, 2004:* Rep. Tom Osborne (R-Nebraska) joined House Judiciary
  Chairman Sensenbrenner and Ranking Member John Conyers Jr. (D-Michigan) in introducing House Resolution (HR) 3866, the Anabolic Steroid
  Control Act of 2004, which would update the list of illegal dangerous substances aggressively marketed as performance-enhancing drugs and increase the penalties for those who traffic these substances within 1,000
  feet of a sports facility. Osborne and Rep. John E. Sweeney (R-New York)
  first introduced similar legislation in October of 2002. Sweeney said there
  is greater support for the bill in Congress than in the past two years. This
  new bill would criminalize steroid precursors, including Andro and designer drugs similar to THG.
- *March 2004:* Sen. Orrin Hatch (R-Utah)[7] sponsored a similar bill in the
  senate.[8] SB1628 is in the Judiciary committee (introduced by Sen. Joe
  Biden (D-Delaware) and Sen. Hatch). The Anabolic Steroid Control Act
  of 2003 would make tetrahydrogestrinone (THG) and other steroid precursors controlled substances, would review federal sentencing guidelines
  for steroids, and would fund steroid research and education. This bill was
  introduced on October 23, 2003, and is still alive.
- *October 10, 2003:* Rep. Osborne, the former Nebraska Cornhuskers football coach, introduced a bill that would make androstenedione and other
  steroid precursors illegal by making them subject to the Controlled Substances Act.
- *March 26, 2003:* Sen. Durbin introduces a bill that would require makers
  of dietary aids containing stimulants, such as the controversial ephedra,
  to prove their products are safe before marketing them (much softer than
  the 2004 bill).
- *1990:* Sen. Biden (D-Delaware) is the author of the law that made steroid
  trafficking unlawful.
- *October 1989:* Former California Rep. Mel Levine (D-Los Angeles) introduced a bill that would place a list of steroids on Schedule II of the Controlled Substances Act along with street drugs such as cocaine. It was
  cosponsored by California Rep. Henry A. Waxman (D-Los Angeles) and
  Rep. Benjamin A. Gilman (R-New York).
- *April 29, 1988:* Rep. Donald Ray Kennard (D-Baton Rouge [now a repub-
  lican]) wrote a bill creating stiff penalties for pushers of anabolic steroids.
  It was approved unanimously by the Louisiana House of Representatives
  but failed to pass the Senate.

efforts to regulate products containing steroid precursors and products containing ephedra.

o An athlete ambassador program exists that involves current and retired athletes who are involved with education and speak to groups. These individuals agree to be subject to additional out-of-competition testing (see chapter 17: "More Solutions: Athletes Doing the Right Thing").

o "USADA believes that deterring the use of drugs in sport is necessary to preserve the integrity of sport in the United States," said Terry Madden, USADA chief executive officer. "Athletes, including children who dream of athletic success, have a fundamental right to believe that they do not need to use drugs to compete. USADA is dedicated to protecting that right and welcomes the opportunity to work with any sport that is committed to the cause of drug-free sport."[17]

- National Center for Drug Free Sport
  o Subscribers to this organization's online Resource Exchange Center (www.drugfreesport.com) include the NFL, the NFLPA, the NCAA, and AAU Powerlifting.
  o The Center offers a full range of customized drug-prevention services aimed at eliminating red tape and streamlining program delivery.
  o President and CEO Dr. Uryasz speaks to athletes, coaches, and athletic directors across the country on doping, supplements, testing, education, and other topics involving collegiate sports in all divisions. He began traveling to educate athletes on supplements and performance-enhancing drugs in 1999, the year he founded the Center.

Dietary supplements dominate most of Dr. Uryasz's discussions. "That's been the biggest change I've seen since 1999—the proliferation of supplements," he says. "What we're trying to get them to understand is there are more factors involved in the decision to use a supplement. Most of them are relying on the supplement industry for their education. We're trying to be an alternate voice and let them know that perhaps the supplement industry has ulterior motives. I tell them that the person at the GNC is not a registered dietician. His job is to sell you dietary supplements. I'm always amazed that these kids walk into the store thinking that the guys at the counter know something about dietary supplements."

While supplement use represents the biggest change, accountability might be the biggest challenge Dr. Uryasz sees in curbing drug abuse among athletes. "It's very difficult to allow the programs to police themselves. We see this at all levels. We've even had situations in college athletic departments where coaches were responsible for applying the sanction for a positive drug test. Well, human nature being what it is and the fact that a coach's job is (almost always) on the line, some athletes are treated better than others. If you're a walk-on and it's your third marijuana offense, you're gone. If you're the starting running back, you might get another chance. You have to pull those decisions out of the hands of people who have a compelling interest. The Olympics now has taken all of that out of the (individual Olympic sports) Federation's hands and put it in the WADA system. Now USA Track and Field doesn't decide sanctions for track athletes who test positive. I think that problem has taken care of itself."[18]

Collaboration is a critical component to this fight. Dick Pound, founding chair of WADA, is attempting to get everyone fighting out of the same corner. With every organization having its own rules and penalties, this has not been easy, but Pound keeps hammering away. "We all need to continue to encourage sports bodies to adopt and, more importantly, apply the code. We need to coordinate testing activities . . . and follow up on the management of those results."[19] A positive step toward solidifying a unified system is the fact that in order for countries to compete in the Athens Games, the world governing body of each sport had to agree to the world antidoping code, a product of WADA in 2003.

LIMIT THE EASE OF OBTAINING STEROIDS

A few experts comment on availability:

- Steroids researcher William Llewellyn: "There are thousands and thousands of ways you could modify a steroid to change its structure and avoid detection. It's not tremendously difficult to create something like THG. You don't need to envision a big underground lab—someone could do it in their house. You need three chemicals and a few small pieces of equipment."[20]

- Dr. Neil Roth, orthopedic surgeon and assistant professor of surgery at Columbia Presbyterian Medical Center: "Steroid use in baseball is rampant. . . . Weightlifters, bodybuilders, college athletes, professional athletes—steroids are everywhere. The baseball players are pretty honest about it, and I ask them, because when I operate I have to know, and it's common knowledge that players are using."[21]

- William Sherman, *Daily News* staff writer: "Just how easy is it to score steroids on the street? A few phone calls, and a *News* reporter quickly made two connections for $280 worth. The first lot, two bottles of synthetic testosterone with other additives, was acquired through an intermediary who said he gets the steroids from Russian hoodlums in Brooklyn. The juice, as it's called, came from Russia, according to the intermediary, and the writing on the labels was in Russian. The second lot, also testosterone, was acquired from a user/dealer who said he has a tried and true Internet source where he maintains an active account."[22]

- Stuart Stevens, an amateur cyclist: "My quest to find (steroids) . . . started . . . at Gold's Gym (in Venice, Calif.), the place that launched Arnold Schwarzenegger and other bodybuilding greats. At Gold's you can easily meet 'gym rats' who know where to find muscle-enhancing drugs, and after a few weeks of hanging out, I found myself sitting in a beat-up sports car with one of my new lifting buddies. He handed me a bottle of pills, Stanozolol, an anabolic steroid that lifters use to add muscle mass. . . . 'Where do you get this?' I said. 'A vet I know,' he answered casually. It took me a second to realize he meant veterinarian, not military veteran. 'Vets and Mexican pharmacists, that's where you get the best stuff.' "[23]

- John P. Lopez, *Houston Chronicle* columnist: "After I typed 'buy steroids' into the search engine of my computer (March 17), just one click of the mouse returned more than 425,000 hits. One Web site boasted that buying its steroids was 'easier than ordering a pizza.' Another said: 'Consult with our online doctor, who will write a free prescription, and the steroids will be yours in 48 hours.' Yet another said its steroids were 'convenient, safe and FDA approved.' Better still, said that supplier . . . the steroids 'arrive in a discreet package.' "[24]

- Ohio drug dealer arrested by FDA officials in 1985 (who requested anonymity): "There may be as many as 10 [steroid] dealers in the U.S. who grossed at least $1,000,000 [in 1986], and they'll net at least half of that. And some do more. . . . The big dealers either get it from drug manufacturing companies, from drug wholesale houses, from pharmacists, or from other big dealers and then sell it either to users or to local distributors. Most of the main dealers have two or three hungry pharmacists in their pocket. . . . Pharmacists can make more by spending a few hours a month ordering steroids for a big dealer than they can all the rest of the month running a drug store. . . . They can get Dianabol, for instance, for around $7 a bottle, and it will sell on the street for $20 or $30 or even as much as $40 and $50 on the West Coast. I can get it for $11 a bottle. . . . There must be at least 200 pharmacists in the U.S. dealing steroids on the black market. Another way the stuff gets on the market is through Mexico. . . . At least 100 guys go down regularly to buy drugs and then smuggle them across the Texas or California border. The Mexican connection is really valuable because of the devaluation of the peso. You can buy Primabolin down there for maybe 30 to 40 cents a unit and sell it up here for four dollars. Most people don't understand how easy it is to buy steroids. All you have to do is to go into almost any gym in the U.S. and inside of a day you can score. Every gym has at least one dealer."[25]

As was mentioned earlier in this chapter, legislation is pending as of the writing of this book to increase penalties against steroid traffickers. There is a need to step up the enforcement of all steroid regulations in every area—importation from Mexico, distribution at health clubs, and sales over the Internet. Realizing the significance of the infestation is the first part of the solution. Recognizing the public need to curb this problem is the second step. Lacking law enforcement resources to address the problem may be a current reality, but an organized public outcry against steroids falling into the hands of children would add pressure to increase these enforcement measures. "I'm an optimist. I think we need more government regulation, and I think it will happen," Dr. Uryasz says. "Unfortunately, you don't get that government regulation until bad things happen to good people. You don't get that flashing yellow light in an intersection until enough people get killed that somebody decides it's too dangerous."[26]

PROFESSIONAL LEAGUES MUST HAVE STRONGER POLICIES AND PENALTIES

No organization is in a better position to take the necessary, significant steps—regardless of how potentially unpopular they might be—to create a tougher policy on performance-enhancing drugs than Major League Baseball. Yet because this league is backing down to its misguided players union, the current drug-testing plan remains more preposterous than any other in professional sports. Pound says the MLB has the power and the justification—legally and within the boundaries of the sport's labor agreement—to impose a stricter policy. "MLB is in a position to say that the sport will be governed by certain rules that are designed to enhance the sport, protect the health of players and serve as an example to all. No one is forced to play in MLB, but, if someone does, then he accepts such rules."[27] For their part, Pound says, players must also insist that their league has an effective policy, "which would include no-notice out-of-competition testing and meaningful sanctions against cheaters."[28] Other leagues must also step up their efforts. Most of all, penalties are woefully inadequate. If lifetime bans for doping have been deemed an effective deterrent, sitting out four games in the NFL for a violation almost certainly should be seen as too soft (See chapter 3, sidebar 3.1, for more on the NFL's "exemplary" drug-testing plan.) Cheaters who are caught for a second violation need to be kicked out of competition permanently. If this were the case, doping violations in the NFL, MLB, and other leagues would almost be entirely eliminated. No one would be willing to throw away millions for a minimal edge, aside perhaps from those athletes on the cusp of making a team. If leagues are concerned that drug testing might weaken their overall talent, they should consider that many cheaters currently on professional rosters don't have the talent to be there. Eliminating these borderline players would be a benefit beyond the obvious one of cleaning up tainted pro sports.

AUTHORITY FIGURES AND ROLE MODELS MUST BE LEADERS

Principals and coaches may not have the ability to stop the steroid shipments from coming to kids who want it badly enough, but they can do an enormous amount to stop the kids from wanting it that badly in the first place. Kids, especially athletes, follow their leaders. They listen to, believe, and admire their football coaches. Few people beyond mothers and fathers offer more guidance and instantly command more respect than the football coach and coaches in general. It is encouraging to know that coaches do care about their kids. For this reason, it's logical to expect that with the proper guides and responsibilities in place, coaches can make a major difference in educating and influencing young athletes not to use steroids. Some coaches already do this, but not enough of them do.

Former NFL lineman Steve Courson spreads the blame for today's drug use to many (see chapter 14, "Who's in Charge? Administration Is Part of the Problem"), but in the context of seeking solutions, those in charge of ridding doping in sports today—sports management, federations, and the athletes themselves—are the key to winning this battle. Those with the power to change things must first change themselves. Some examples of what is being done along these lines and what should be done in the future include:

- International track-and-field officials have expanded the fight against drug cheats by targeting coaches, trainers, doctors, and mangers. The International Association of Athletic Federation adopted changes that threaten support personnel with the same sanctions as those of athletes caught using drugs. The new rules take effect in March.[29]
- Madison athletic director and head football coach Ray Seals directed the NFL's High School Player Development Program camp in May 2003. A total of 303 players from Houston schools attended the camp conducted at the Houston Texans' practice facility. Seals, though, said learning wasn't restricted to the field. Camp instructors offered advice on how to prepare for the Scholastic Aptitude Test, how to earn a college scholarship, and the value of balancing academics with athletics. Other NFL high school camps have covered topics such as the dangers of ephedrine and supplements, how to be a better citizen and student, and how to stay out of trouble. "It's valuable for these kids to be well-rounded," Seals said. "I hope that was made perfectly clear. We want these kids to be more than just good football players."[30] Kids did not attend the

camp to become better citizens, nor is it likely that such a camp would be well attended if citizenship were the primary focus. But, because they respect the camp and its coaches, they might listen a little closer to these important messages.

- "The elimination of dangerous performance-enhancing substances from sports requires intensive state-of-the-art research on an ongoing basis," NFL commissioner Paul Tagliabue has said. The NFL has and must show a commitment to funding this research.[31]

- Testing on demand with high-tech methods such as gas chromatography and mass spectrometry could catch the cheaters, but it's a question of political will, according to Dr. Robert Voy, the chief medical officer for the U.S. Olympic Committee from 1983 to 1989. Other doctors with Dr. Voy's knowledge have come forward to voice complaints against organizations like the USOC that have long been hindered by a conflict of interest in pursuing a clean U.S. Olympic team.[32]

- Dr. Voy has made it a goal to seek out steroid users and help them to stop using steroids. He checks young athletes for high blood pressure, liver abnormalities, and low HDLs in those who have exceptional musculature, cystic acne, premature balding, and soft testes. He tells them, "The choice is yours. I'll monitor your lab tests and help you get off steroids, but I won't aid and abet your use of them."[33]

- Dr. Wade Exum, who succeeded Dr. Voy as director of the USOC's drug-control programs, has sued the USOC in federal court in Denver, accusing the organization of encouraging the doping of athletes. Similar actions need to be fully pursued and supported by organizations that can have an impact.

- Drug-testing methods are improving but the cheaters are still winning the race. For this reason, leagues and federations should step up the penalties for those who are caught. The risk is worth the reward for athletes because the penalties for purposefully cheating are still too small. Severe penalties (e.g., missing an entire season in the NFL for using steroids [instead of four games]) would significantly decrease doping offenses.

- Instead of joining the "norm" and doping to compete, athletes should admit their use, report others who use, and join in the battle to encourage new athletes not to use.

- Instead of punishing those who admit drug use before testing positive, teams and leagues should be prepared to laud these athletes for coming forward (or perhaps a reduced penalty would still be appropriate).
- Coaches at all levels linked in any way to athletes' doping should be punished in career-ending ways (e.g., 10-year suspensions).
- Coaches need to aggressively prevent this doping from spreading, using their authority to inform athletes about alternatives and to crack down on the drug use that is happening right under their noses.
- Parents need to take a closer look at everyone and everything involved in their child's development. Like other drug prevention campaigns, this one should stress the importance of parents asking questions. It's impossible to tell if an athlete is using steroids just by looking at him, but it is easy to see if athletes are making gains, especially large gains in a short amount of time.
- Role models should support clean competition. Mark McGwire announced his decision to stop taking Andro after realizing that "young kids take it because of me. I don't like that." Nutritionists, doctors, and medical officials praised this decision. "The message Mark McGwire sends to our young people by walking away from this substance is a powerful one," said Barry R. McCaffrey, the White House drug policy director at the time.[34]

8

Dead Serious: Catastrophic and Fatal Injuries in Sports

Julian Bailes, M.D.

Every athlete who seriously trains and competes knows that there are prices to be paid, in many respects. Not only are there the necessary time and financial commitments, each with innumerable consequences to athletes and their families, but there is the ever-present risk of injury. Many sports also inherently have a risk of serious injury or death, especially those that involve speed, contact, or collisions. In addition, many factors have led to a decreased incidence of serious injury and death in athletic events. A better understanding of the human body's pathological state as it reacts to traumatic injury has improved safety in all forms of sports, during both individual and team participation.

Another way to analyze athletic injuries is to consider them in either recreational or organized forms. In the former, there are naturally fewer methods and opportunities to influence the performance of the activity by enforcement of rules and safety changes, equipment, or through coaching techniques. In contrast, organized sports have regular and systematic conditioning, training, practices, coaching, and rules enforcement, among other advantages.

In the conditioned and healthy athlete, the study of fatalities can begin with categorizing the occurrence as traumatic, non-traumatic (spontaneous), or environmentally related. Traumatic injury, which is life threatening, usually involves a spinal cord or head (brain) injury. In the various types of sports in which there is a significant risk of catastrophic injury and death, we can analyze why they occur, and how we can influence the incidence of these serious adverse events. Some of the common injuries and their risks in athletic endeavors follow.

SUDDEN DEATH

The occurrence of an acute, unexpected death in an apparently healthy young athlete is known as sudden death. This is considered as a non-traumatic or spontaneous fatality, for it does not occur as a result of a blow, collision, or other injury. For a young, prosperous, and highly conditioned athlete to die suddenly always has a great emotional impact for not only his or her family but also the school and community. The incidence of a sudden death in high school athletes participating in organized sports has been reported to be 1 in 200,000.[1] In the United States, football and basketball are the most common sports, while in Europe, soccer players are most likely to sustain sudden death. Males outnumber females by a ratio of 9 to 1; however, this statistic may reflect much greater numbers of males participating.[2]

Studies by medical authorities have disclosed that there are predictable reasons for such events.[3] The most common is known as *hypertrophic cardiomyopathy*, which causes between 20–25 cases of sudden death annually in athletes in this country. In large autopsy studies, *hypertrophic cardiomyopathy* has consistently represented one-fourth to one-third of all cases. This is a condition in which the left ventricle of the heart, the main pumping chamber to supply blood to the body, is hypertrophied (enlarged) and susceptible to electrical instability leading to ventricular tachyarrhythmias. This condition, as well as the majority of the other cardiac causes of sudden death, is usually not responsive to cardiopulmonary resuscitation (CPR).

The next most frequent cardiovascular cause of sudden death in athletes is a congenital condition in which the coronary arteries arise in an abnormal area leading to inadequate blood flow to the myocardium, the pumping muscle of the heart. During intense exercise, compression can occur between the myocardium or great vessels of the heart and the anomalous coronary arteries. Diseases of the heart valves, myocarditis (inflammation of the heart muscle), and various other more unusual cardiac anomalies, many of them congenital but undiagnosed, are additional causes.[4]

Another common form of sudden death in athletes occurs in those who did not have preexisting heart disease but instead sustain a form of trauma. *Commotio cordis* occurs when a young athlete is struck by a blow to the chest. This is often in the form of a pitched baseball, a flying hockey puck, or even physical contact, such as a karate punch or kick. It has been documented that hockey pucks may travel up to 100 miles per hour (mph) and baseballs 50 mph, even in youth play. This phenomenon may even occur during playful activity at home, at the playground, or during organized events, and it is caused by a blow to the chest, which occurs directly over the heart during its vulnerable time of repolarization after contraction. There is an ultrabrief period (15 to 30 milliseconds) during which electrical signals are not transmitted throughout the heart's electrical conduction system. If the blow occurs exactly at the vulnerable time, cardiac arrest may result, and often the athlete is not responsive to CPR efforts.[5]

Any athlete who has a history of chest pain, fainting, palpitations (extra heartbeats), difficulty with breathing, or any other cardiac symptoms, especially occurring with exertion, should be fully evaluated prior to sports participation. Studies have shown, unfortunately, that routine preparticipation screening and physical examinations do not detect the vast majority of athletes with a potentially lethal cardiac abnormality. Even tests such as an electrocardiogram (EKG) may not disclose the abnormality or diagnose an unknown cardiac condition, and more sophisticated examinations are often necessary for definitive diagnosis. Consultation with a primary care physician may lead to the involvement of cardiology specialists in order to confirm or exclude any serious risk to an athlete, and these consultations should be performed if a question arises concerning cardiac status.[6]

MECHANISMS AND INCIDENCE OF INJURY

Although almost every kind of recreational sporting activity can be associated with some type of injury to the head, eyes, or face, the most serious injury primarily involves the potential for brain injury. The most frequently reported injury, excluding facial, ocular, and scalp injuries, is mild traumatic brain injury (MTBI), also known as concussion. The frequency of all sports-related MTBI has been estimated to be up to 300,000 occurrences annually in the United States.[7] This common injury will be covered thoroughly in chapter 10. Equestrian sports account for approximately 46,000 hospital emergency department visits annually, with nearly 20 percent of equestrians experiencing injuries to the head or neck, and 70 percent of deaths related to head injuries resulting from falls.[8] About twenty deaths from horseback-riding-related accidents are reported each year in the United States, with alcohol involved in about one-third.[9] There has been an annual rate of approximately seven fatalities from skateboard activities, with 90 percent experiencing severe head injury.[10] Roller skating and in-line skating together account for about 100,000 injuries yearly, with few reported deaths and a 5 percent incidence of head injury.[11]

Bicycling is one of our most popular and ubiquitous forms of recreation, and it is enjoyed by nearly 30 million children, with the vast majority of youngsters participating. Although most injuries seen in males are to the soft tissue and extremities and are associated with traveling at high speeds, head injuries account for the most serious consequences of such activity. Recreational and commuter bicyclists sustain approximately 900 fatalities each year, approximately one-half being children and adolescents, with most dying from cerebral injuries.[12] These accidents lead to 580,000 emergency department visits and 23,000 hospital admissions, and have been estimated to cost more than $8 billion annually. There are many common characteristics of bicycle injuries, including riding in the later part of the day or evening, being in an unsafe riding environment, and not wearing a helmet. A crash with a motor vehicle is a common occurrence and relates to increased severity of the injury. As always, alcohol or substance abuse may be a factor.

Head injuries occur at a significant rate in downhill skiing as well. Many of these are serious injuries, occurring as a result of collision, often at high speed, with trees and boulders as well as other skiers. Head injury is the leading cause of fatality at most large alpine skiing resorts, causing approximately 32 deaths annually in the United States.[13] Most of these traumatic lesions are intracranial hematomas, often with associated brain tissue damage, cerebral edema, cranial fractures, and resultant brain herniation syndromes. Snowboarding participants are as prone to serious and fatal brain injury or spinal injury as skiers. The sport of snowmobiling has been associated with approximately 30 fatalities annually in the United States. Most other sports involve sporadic head injuries, with hang gliding, skydiving, mountaineering, and racecar driving being among the most dangerous. Although diving mishaps are the leading cause of spinal cord injury in sporting activities, intracranial injury is unusual. The true incidence of diving injuries may be underestimated, as many victims drown.[14]

The use of All-Terrain Vehicles (ATVs) is another popular form of motorized recreation that has become one of the most dangerous in terms of serious injuries and fatalities. The U.S. Consumer Product Safety Commission has determined that there have been an average of 357 deaths annually in the United States from ATV use. More than one-third occur in children less than 16 years old. Brain and spinal injuries account for 80 percent of the fatalities, and many are in underage children without helmets. Our study in West Virginia, a state that, until recently, had no legislation to prevent injuries, to limit road use, to require helmets, nor other safety regulations, demonstrated the highest fatality rate in the country (eight times the national average).[15] These vehicles are constructed with oversized and low-pressure tires, made for off-road riding. They require an "active rider," meaning that there must be constant shifts of weight and leaning in the direction opposite of the turn, which is counterintuitive but necessary to maintain the ATV upright. Rollover, flipping, or ejection of the rider are real possibilities and account for the majority of the injuries sustained. Lack of head protection, insufficient training or operating skill, juvenile or elderly drivers, the presence of passengers, and the use of alcohol are leading factors involved with the serious injuries and fatalities seen with ATVs. As with any motorized vehicle, there are innumerable issues that must be correctly addressed in order for safe and enjoyable operation to ensue.

In the United States, football ranks at the top in both the number of participants and the incidence of head injuries in organized sports. There are approximately 1.5 million annual participants in contact football in the United States, and it has been estimated that 4 to 20 percent sustain an MTBI each season.[16] In addition, a small number experience either cumulative effects or major head injuries annually. There are approximately five deaths (in a range of zero to seven deaths) annually in the United States attributable to head injuries in organized football from traumatic mechanisms, whereas another seven or so die without trauma as a cause (e.g. cardiac arrest, heat-stroke, or other means). Head injuries occur while playing football because of the nature of the game—headfirst collisions with opponents occur intentionally and with every play, usually during blocking or tackling.

Soccer is also a sport associated with MTBI.[17] Ice hockey experienced a significant decrease in serious head injuries and MTBI after the sport implemented the use of effective helmets.[18] Concussion has been reported to occur in as many as 7 percent of ice hockey players during a single season. Major brain injuries are rare in rugby, basketball, and baseball, and seasonal concussion rates are reported as 6, 2, and 1 percent, respectively.[19] Periodically, another sport, such as pole vaulting, may become the source of increased fatalities, as occurred in 2002, when three track-and-field athletes died from falls sustained during pole vaulting.[20] Studies of these deaths, which have averaged about one annually for the last two decades, indicate that based on only approximately 35,000 athletes competing, pole vaulting is one of our most dangerous sports. These studies have also shown consistent causes, principally that the vaulters either landed beyond the end of the intended landing cushion or mat, or fell off to one side.

Boxing has been documented to have had approximately 1,300 deaths since records were first kept. These are usually due to the boxer sustaining multiple blows to the head during a long fight, with these blows leading to brain swelling and sometimes to intracranial hemorrhage. Surprisingly, it is not usually the impressive, devastating, knockout punch that leads to death in the ring, but rather it is the accumulation of multiple, subconcussive blows, which result in the irreversible brain edema and cascade of events leading to loss of consciousness and lapse into fatal coma.

BRAIN INJURY

Our understanding of brain injury has been assisted by considering it as either focal or generalized trauma. This classification also helps our understanding of athletic head injuries. Focal brain injury usually results from a direct impact causing penetration and tearing of cerebral substance and vessels or other types of localized injury. Hemorrhages, hematomas (clots), or contusions (bruising of the brain) may also be seen. Diffuse brain injury varies from mild to more severe forms of concussion, with alteration of consciousness. Diffuse brain injury also occurs along a continuum of diffuse injury to axons (fibers) within the brain, a clinical entity characterized by shearing of white matter fiber tracts as they course from the cortex to the midbrain and brainstem. This is thought to occur especially with rotational energy forces, leading to the disruption of axons at these levels, sometimes marked by small areas of hemorrhage visualized on neuroimaging studies such as computerized tomography (CT) or magnetic resonance imaging (MRI) scans. In its most severe form, the patient who has experienced diffuse brain injury is rendered deeply and often permanently comatose, termed "a vegetative state." There are associated severe cognitive, memory, and motor deficits and a mortality rate of more than 50 percent.

BIOMECHANICS

Collisions, either with another player or with an object, are the cause of sports-related head injuries. Boxing differs from all other sports in that repetitive blows to the head, made in an attempt to disable the opponent's central nervous system, are the usual contest strategy. In football, tackling maneuvers have been implicated as the primary cause of head injury, including concussions. Soccer players sustain head impacts through collisions with other players, equipment (such as goalposts), or by grounding and striking the ball with the head during play (known as "heading"). However, this latter mechanism of injury has been considered controversial. Head injuries in hockey occur either because the player was struck on the head with a stick or puck propelled at a high speed (low-mass/high-velocity impact) or because the player struck the goalpost, sideboards, another player, or the surface of the ice (high-mass/low-velocity impact). In wrestling, the takedown, or activities associated with this maneuver, where the head is driven into the mat, is usually the cause of head or spinal injury.

Acceleration-deceleration injury, which is a linear impact, usually occurs when the person is traveling at a particular speed and strikes a solid or immovable object. On the contrary, a stationary cranium may be struck by a moving object. These two mechanisms constitute the methods of imparting injurious forces to the head of an opponent during sports participation. The resulting injury causes linear, tensile, and compressive strains that disrupt the brain tissue. Rotational (angular) movements also occur because of the brain's fixation at various points or because of the direction of force vectors. Though different forces or mechanisms may coexist in a single patient's injury, research has shown that one biomechanical feature is usually predominant. Contact sports, especially football, ice hockey, and boxing, have a high degree of acceleration-deceleration energy. When the forces are sufficient, the cerebral cortex and the reticular activating formation (the major brain nuclei that are responsible for the wakeful state) are shut down, leading to a loss of consciousness (LOC).

Blocking and tackling, checking, jabs, cross-punches, and many other techniques predominantly deliver acceleration-deceleration or linear energy to the contestant. On the other hand, mechanisms exemplified by the boxing hook punch impart rotatory forces to the mandible and head. It is thought that the rotatory component of the cranial or mandibular impacts contributes most directly to the injuries that include LOC, explaining the cause of many football cerebral concussions. In addition to the biomechanics of such injuries, recent research has elucidated the biochemical abnormalities that occur during concussion. The primary mechanism seems to be a disturbance in glucose utilization by the brain. The rise in glycolytic energy requirements has been shown, both experimentally and clinically, to be present within the first several days (usually five days) after concussive brain injury.

There is a constant risk of severe head injury in every sport, but contact sports maintain the highest exposure to significant kinetic energy and potential for central nervous system damage. The participation in contact sports provides high-speed encounters with other objects, and studies demonstrate that collisions of various types translate into sufficient exposure to potentially injurious circumstances. Noteworthy is the association of this lesion with the phenomenon of the *lucid interval* and the well-known potential for subsequent neurological deterioration that may occur.

The lucid interval happens when there has been a blow to the head, sometimes with LOC, followed by a period of wakefulness. Later a slow deterioration in brain function takes place, as bleeding and swelling occurs and progresses intracranially, possibly leading to coma or death. This has been described in baseball players and golfers struck on the head by a high-velocity ball. The classic situation is the development of an epidural hematoma that forms between the skull and brain. Although the brain itself is not initially damaged, bleeding or oozing results in a clot formation that later compresses the brain. An understanding of this clinical picture is crucial for all caregivers who work with athletes, especially athletic trainers, coaches, and team physicians. It requires an adequate observation period for delayed hematoma formation and neurological deterioration for those athletes who have been potentially injured. Many of these victims need life-saving emergency craniotomy for clot evacuation.

Traumatic subdural hematomas and brain hemorrhages account for the majority of lethal brain injuries seen in both organized and recreational athletic activities. As stated previously, we have estimated that there have been approximately 1,300 boxing deaths recorded since 1880. Serious head injury remains a risk in athletes who play football, with 132 football players possessing documented intracranial hemorrhages in the 10-year reporting period of 1975–1984. The apparent increase is also related to improved detection of clots with the advent and widespread use of advanced imaging such as CT scanning. During this period, the fatality rate from intracranial injuries in football averaged eight per year, which, on an exposure basis, is a small but nonetheless significant number of fatalities. Due to improvements in helmet design—especially better helmet materials and construction, with, for example, absorption materials placed in the inner lining, a suspension configuration, a four-way chin strap for better stability, and more secure fittings—the incidence of serious head injuries and fatalities in football has substantially decreased. As stated above, football witnessed a decline in fatalities of approximately 30 annually in 1950 to an average level of five currently. Despite various attempts at further reduction, this number has held constant for the last two decades.

SPINAL INJURY

Injuries to the spinal cord represent arguably the most dramatic and devastating events in all of sports. The public nature of the accident, taking the most vital bodily functions from an athlete in the prime of his or her life, heightens the magnitude of the catastrophe. While spinal injuries are rare in sporting events, the constant potential for their occurrence, especially in contact sports, mandates that high vigilance be maintained for such a possibility. Many injuries to the cervical spine, especially if higher up in the neck (above the third vertebral level), will result in cardiopulmonary arrest and rapid death if CPR is not instituted. This is primarily due to the fact that the nerves to the diaphragm become paralyzed and the victim will stop breathing, thus converting what was initially only a spinal injury into a fatality.

Approximately 10,000 cases of spinal cord injury occur annually in the United States, and about 12 percent of these take place during sporting activities. The majority of spinal injuries happen during unsupervised, sports-related activities such as diving, surfing, skiing, and "sandlot" games. Much more visible, however, are those injuries occurring during football, ice hockey, wrestling, soccer, rugby, and gymnastics, which constitute 2 to 3 percent of all spinal injuries. Such injuries sustained by professional athletes are of the highest profile.

For the past 20 years, there has been an estimated annual average of 40 cervical spine fractures in football players, with approximately 10 being rendered quadriplegic. However, the ongoing risk is demonstrated by four high school football players in Louisiana who sustained cervical spinal cord injuries during the 1989 football season alone. These accidents occurred in a state where, based on the national average, only one such injury would be expected during a 14-year period. A recent dramatic increase in the incidence of cervical fractures has also been reported for ice hockey players, with seven occurring in a two-year period.[21]

Diving injuries to the neck are prevalent and devastating injuries that are readily preventable. Diving injuries tend to occur in teenage males who are involved in recreational unsupervised activities in the summer months. The incidence of diving accidents has been reported to comprise between 2 and 22 percent of all spinal injuries, with the incidence increasing when the reporting center lies in close proximity to an area of high water-sport activity (frequented by younger age groups) or in times of seasonal droughts. The true incidence of diving-related spinal injuries is thought to be even higher because many are likely to have occurred in drowning victims. Many of the diving injury patients have alcohol consumption as a modifying factor in their injury and presentation. The most common mechanism of diving injuries is for the diver to strike his head on the bottom of a pool, lake, or ocean after miscalculating the water's depth or by striking another swimmer or a submerged object.[22]

TYPES OF SPINAL INJURY

Trauma to the spine in sporting events may occur via damage to the bony vertebral column, its supporting ligamentous and muscular structures, and/or the intervertebral discs. Injury to the underlying spinal cord is always possible and is seen in roughly one third of athletes with vertebral column fractures. Traumatic disruption or wall injury to the major arteries, carotid or vertebral arteries, may also occur, resulting in interruption of the brain's blood supply and stroke.

Depending upon the amount of bony injury and displacement, instability, and degree of impact, a variety of clinical appearances (syndromes) are seen. The initial insult is rapidly followed by secondary pathological phenomena, such as ischemia (lack of blood supply), hemorrhage, free-radical and other toxin release, and edema (swelling) within the spinal cord. *Complete spinal cord injury* results in a total loss of spinal cord function below the level of the lesion. The injury may lead to actual anatomical disruption of the spinal cord, which occurs in a minority of cases. More often, there is a physiological block to transmission of spinal cord impulses due to hemorrhagic or ischemic injury within the spinal cord. Improvement in patients with complete injury patterns is rarely seen, except for one spinal level of function as a result of resolution of initial segmental traumatic spinal cord swelling.

Incomplete spinal cord injury is usually expressed in one of several patterns. Various combinations of loss of either motor (movement) or sensory functions in either the arms or legs, along with bowel, bladder, and sexual control are seen. These incomplete syndromes are determined by the area of the spinal cord or its blood supply that are involved in the injury and have various manifestations.

CONCLUSION

Due to the enormous popularity of sports throughout the world, both organized and recreational athletes are subject to a variety of mechanisms that may result in serious injuries or death. As discussed, bicycling and motorized sports provide the greatest potential for such events, in large part due to the high numbers of participants. There are inherent dangers, which may not be possible to eliminate, while other factors may be modifiable, including such commonsense methods as proper protective equipment, alcohol avoidance, adherence to proper safety protocols, and others. In organized sports, rules, training, equipment, coaching, and other factors are paramount to minimize catastrophic injury or death. Additional discussion and particular recommendations to help reduce the incidence of catastrophic or fatal sports injuries are contained in chapter 16, "Solutions: Winning without Losing Perspective."

The Heat Is On:
Heatstroke Continues to Kill

Julian Bailes, M.D.

Depending upon the sport and its training requirements, environmental factors are a constant potential for adverse consequences or events. Through the years, we have found that fatalities in organized sports have followed numerous trends. Several recent, highly publicized fatalities in organized sports have prompted great concern regarding a perceived increased incidence of death due to heatstroke, and this has led us to review and analyze the available data concerning this phenomenon.

Data obtained from the National Center for Catastrophic Sports Injury Research indicates that three distinct periods of heatstroke fatality trends in American football have been evident during the past three decades. The initial period (1965–1974), which occurred prior to our adequate understanding of the risks of dehydration in sports, had 44 deaths, or 4.4 per year. With emerging scientific evidence and reports of the advantages of proper hydration before and during practices and games, the next 10-year period (1975–1984) included a total of 17 fatalities, or 1.7 per year.[1] From 1985 to 1994, a greater understanding occurred of the importance of freely available water for hydration and rehydration as well as the promotion of policies and publicity that advocated active fluid replacement, on a regular basis, with both free water and electrolytes. During this period, only six deaths were recorded from dehydration and heatstroke, for a rate of only 0.6 per year. The recent period (1995–2001), however, indicates a reversal of this downward trend, despite the widespread teaching of athletic trainers, coaches, and players. The years 1995, 1998, and 2000 witnessed four deaths each, and three fatalities were reported in 2001; all of these deaths occurred during the summer preseason American football conditioning and practice sessions. This recent increased incidence has led us to investigate whether athletes' current behavior and training regimens pose new and dangerous risks for heatstroke.[2]

This small but important increase, a result of heat-related illness in the years after the deregulation of dietary supplements, has occurred despite what we think is adequate and effective knowledge of the clinical science of dehydration and its treatment by physicians, athletic trainers, coaches, and players, and it has occurred while the number of direct injury-related football deaths generally remains constant.

HEATSTROKE: HOW IT OCCURS

The control of the body's internal thermostat is a constant and sophisticated feature of several organs, originating with the brain's hypothalamus and coordinating throughout the body. Heatstroke has a spectrum of clinical manifestations dependent on many factors, including the temperature and especially the extent of heat exposure, the humidity level, the athlete's level of conditioning and underlying health status, caloric expenditure, and volume of total-body water loss. Heatstroke results from an increase in cellular metabolism that exceeds the cardiovascular system's ability to provide adequate circulation to the major organs. This results in the internal body temperature rapidly surpassing a normal level. Dependent upon several deleterious steps leading to environmental heat gain and endogenous heat production, there is a progressive rise in body temperature, with an estimated 13 percent increase in cellular metabolism for every 1°C increase in body temperature.

Several minor heat-related states may occur, which progress to heat syncope and heat edema based on the body's ability to manage temperature rise.[3] *Heat cramps*, which are thought to occur when water and sodium depletion cause the body's pH level to rise (alkalosis) along with increased osmolality and lactate levels, result in involuntary spasms of the major muscle groups. When treated with either oral or intravenous fluid replacement and rest, heat cramps can usually be controlled and are not serious.[4]

Heat exhaustion is the intermediate step in which heat excess produces symptoms such as nausea, vomiting, intense fatigue, and hyperventilation, among others. During a rise in body temperature, signs of dehydration may not become noticeable, and brain function remains normal. Heat exhaustion is a reversible condition that is treated by the administration of fluids, removal of the person from the hot environment, and observation by qualified personnel.

Heatstroke is a critical and often irreversible state with elevated temperature, alteration of consciousness, and hot, dry skin. These victims have headache, confusion, disorientation, incoherent speech, seizure, and delirium. Progression to a comatose state may occur. Although body temperature is increased to greater than 40°C (104°F), heatstroke is not necessarily related to the degree of temperature elevation. There is ordinarily increased heart rate (tachycardia, 120–160 bpm) and hyperventilation. In some cases, heatstroke has developed without any definite warning signs. An acute phase response occurs with cells liberating heat-shock proteins and other inflammatory mediators, many effects originating at the intestinal level. As heatstroke proceeds unchecked, there is usually a rapid failure in the function of numerous organs, including the liver, kidneys, coagulation system, and final cardiovascular collapse. The initial treatment for this condition is removal of the person from the hot environmental conditions, rehydration, rapid cooling, and immediate presentation to proper medical personnel.[5]

CAUSES OF RECENT DEATHS

How do we explain these recent fatality trends in athletes? In American football players today, many have an unprecedented large body mass, often with large amounts of adipose tissue. While some recent heatstroke deaths have been in very large athletes who were starting their conditioning in extremely hot, humid conditions, not all had these characteristics. The prevalent use of certain dietary or nutritional supplements has prompted us to caution against their use, especially in heat-stressed environments. Claims of their properties are made based on the manufacturer's interpretation of the scientific literature and these supplements' purported activity on the consumer's body structure, function, and general health or well-being.[6] Since 1994, under a law known as the Dietary Supplements Health and Education Act, the U.S. Food and Drug Administration does not have strict authority to regulate the manufacture or sale of these products. Deregulation saw a marked increase in the marketing of such products and their purchase by enthusiastic consumers, which resulted in the growth of a multibillion-dollar industry. This industry has been subject to little or no governmental control or oversight with regard to the purity, consistency, potency, drug interaction, and potential side effects of these products.[7]

The consumption of numerous substances, including anabolic steroids, stimulants, and performance-enhancing agents, has become a behavior of many amateur and professional athletes.[8] Notwithstanding attempts to discourage or prohibit the use of these substances by athletes in organized sports, a certain number of athletes persist in seeking a perceived competitive advantage by the use of these substances. Dinitrophenol (aka Solfo Black, Nitrophen, Chemox) has been used as a metabolic stimulant or fat burner for some athletes who are in training and are attempting to lose weight. It has been reported to cause significant increases in body metabolism and temperature. Football, ice hockey, wrestling, and many Olympic and endurance sports are the events most often associated with the use of dietary supplements. Among football players, up to 30 percent of high school athletes and as many as 71 percent of Division I players have used creatine supplements.[9] The consumption of ephedrine alkaloids, which are derived from various species of herbs of the genus ephedra, also referred to as Ma Huang *(Ephedra equisetina)*, has increased. These substances were often manufactured in numerous products advertised to promote weight loss and increased energy with preservation of muscle mass, and they were universally available as over-the-counter preparations under brand names such as Muscle Milk (made by CytoSport in Concord, California), Ephedra Super-Caps (manufactured by D&E Pharmaceuticals Inc. in Bloomingdale, New Jersey), and Ripped Fuel (produced by Twinlab Corp. in Hauppauge, New York), and slang or "street" names, such as *bishop's tea* and *Chi powder* (or *Tien Chi ginseng* or just *Tien Chi*).[10] These preparations would also contain other amphetamine compounds, such as phenylpropanolamine, pseudoephedrine, and phentermine.

Ephedrine alkaloids are amphetamine-like compounds that have potentially significant stimulatory properties that act on the heart and brain. The serious side effects associated with amphetamines and amphetamine-like compounds, including cocaine, are centered primarily on adverse cardiovascular events, including heart attack (myocardial infarction), lethal heart rhythm disturbance, myocarditis, and severe hypertension.[11] The ingestion of ephedrine and related compounds is conducive not only to cardiac abnormalities but also to seizures and both hemorrhagic and ischemic strokes.[12] The side effects of amphetamines are aggravated by caffeine, of which the simultaneous consumption of large quantities is common in athletes.[13]

Ephedrine and related alkaloids also have been linked to an inability for the body to control temperature (thermoregulatory dysfunction), including increased metabolism, heat production, and core body temperature elevation.[14] One physiological action of these substances is the narrowing of the blood vessels of the skin (cutaneous vasoconstriction), which can diminish an athlete's ability to conduct internal heat outside by not perfusing the skin's sweat glands. The use of these substances has commonly been associated with heat cramps.[15] Amphetamines, in addition to increasing the outright risk of heatstroke, also may be detrimental in certain stressful or hot conditions because of their ability to mask fatigue, thus allowing an athlete to push him- or herself beyond a recognizable danger point.[16] For the 2002 season, the National Football League added ephedrine to the list of drugs that mandated a four-game suspension for athletes who tested positive, including pseudoephedrine (a common over-the-counter cold remedy) if it is present in large amounts. Both the National Collegiate Athletic Association[17] and the National Football League have adopted policies and educational programs to prohibit the use of ephedrine and related compounds in their athletes. Because of the numerous reports and perceived dangers, in 2003 the Food and Drug Administration moved to ban the sale or inclusion of ephedrine in dietary supplements.

Another popular performance-enhancing substance is creatine monohydrate. Creatine is marketed as an ergonomic aid and is used to enhance energy by increasing energy production, control, and efficiency. Creatine has been purported to increase skeletal muscle creatine concentration by up to 20 percent, thereby increasing the resynthesis of adenosine triphosphate during periods of peak muscular contraction.[18] The literature on creatine is somewhat controversial. There is some evidence that creatine usage causes shifts of body water into skeletal muscle cells, which, especially early in the usage of this substance, may result in a relative and unsuspected depletion in intravascular volume.[19] Reports of athletes experiencing diarrhea, muscular cramps, and heat intolerance during or after the consumption of creatine are numerous.[20] It has been reported that creatine may cause dehydration, reduced circulating blood volume, electrolyte abnormality, and heat-related illness. Two cases of renal damage that purportedly occurred secondary to creatine use have been reported.[21] McGuine and coworkers recently reported that 17 percent of high school football players who used creatine supplementation experienced undesired side effects, including gastrointestinal upset, diarrhea, muscle cramping, and dehydration.[22] Wrestlers attempting to "make weight" by pre-event fasting and dehydration also seem to be at risk. The potential for side effects due to the long-term use and/or the excessive consumption of creatine has not been investigated.[23]

Creatine has been in widespread use for over a decade and is generally a safe and efficacious dietary supplement. While numerous studies have demonstrated its positive effects as an ergonomic aid, the question remains as to whether any athlete who is about to exercise in an extremely hot or humid environment should continue to use exogenous substances. Studies have indicated that during football, soccer, baseball, and cycling trials with creatine, there were no observed trends toward abnormalities in kidney, metabolic, muscular, or fluid maintenance function. However, it is questionable if an experimental study could reproduce the multiple factors that must be in place for circulatory insufficiency to progress to multiple organ failure and thermoregulatory death. In addition, there are additional variables that must be considered, including the relative dehydration of the athlete before participation, heat acclimatization, fluid replacement, the amount of heat and humidity exposure, the intensity of exercise, the design of the athlete's clothing and/or uniform, the athlete's underlying medical or cardiac status, the simultaneous ingestion of substances or medications that may interact, excessive dosage and purity, genetic predisposition, medical care administered, and other potential factors.

Creatine's actions increase the total body water volume by enlarging the water content of muscle cells. It is unknown if this increased intracellular water content can be mobilized adequately or in a timely manner in select individuals to be available for intravascular volume support during acute heat illness.[24] This is especially true for the small number of athletes who may have simultaneously ingested other medications or herbal or dietary supplements, as well as those with recent dehydration, or those athletes who are not heat-acclimated. Athletes also may experience individual variability or have unrecognized medical illnesses or conditions. In addition, the body's attempts to compensate for heatstroke-induced impending circulatory failure have never been studied with regard to the role and interaction of exogenous substances.[25]

The exact science and body mechanisms of dehydration and heatstroke in athletes are incompletely understood. Great advances in the management of hydration, electrolytes, and the conduct of practice sessions have occurred in sports such as football during the past three decades. Progressively diminishing fatality rates due to heatstroke in athletes were seen prior to the mid-1990s. The recent and dangerous upward trend, reflected in the National Center for Catastrophic Sports Injury Research statistics for heatstroke-related deaths in American football players who engaged in summer training activities, is disturbing. These data suggest that another mechanism besides heatstroke may be involved.

All team personnel and athletes must be aware of the signs of heat-related illness, particularly during summer and preseason football practice sessions. Protocols should be implemented that limit strenuous exercise during hot weather. The early recognition of warning signs may prevent the serious consequences of heat-related illness from occurring. It has been estimated that athletes require one to two weeks to become acclimated to exercising in hot conditions, and fluid delivery remains the top priority for athletes while exercising in these environments.[26] Programmed drinking with cold liquid (especially water) seems to increase the rate of body-core cooling and gastric emptying.[27] Amateur and professional athletes alike are under pressure for peak performance, and the use of nutritional supplements is rampant. The use of these unregulated dietary and nutritional supplements may be a significant risk factor for intravascular volume depletion, and it has the potential to cause central nervous system side effects in selected or vulnerable athletes. Educating athletes about the dangers of over-the-counter supplements and their misuse and potential side effects should continue, because the use of these substances may predispose certain individuals to experience life-threatening dehydration and heatstroke.[28]

Modern athletes sustain tremendous pressures to compete and win.[29] It is known that current athletes often not only consume numerous substances but also do so in greater-than-recommended amounts. Studies have not been performed, however, to measure the effects of larger or combination doses, particularly in a heat-stressed environment. In addition, athletes often consume a cornucopia of exogenous substances, including not only anabolic steroids but also caffeine, human growth hormone, erythropoietin, clenbuterol, salbutamol, and others.[30]

While the number of non-traumatic or heat-related fatalities in U.S. football is small, these deaths are significant. While not incriminating all dietary supplements and realizing that the numbers are small, there is a constant risk of heatstroke in athletes who train and compete in heat-stressed conditions. The symptoms or signs of heatstroke may begin in a subtle way, but they have rapid onset and progression, and they constitute a medical emergency with death as a constant possibility. Discussions with many current athletic trainers will disclose that one of their greatest concerns today is the uncertainty surrounding athletes' rising use of exogenous substances. We recommend the cessation of all such substance use before engaging in training sessions during hot conditions, especially by individuals who are not heat acclimated.[31]

Brain Injury:
Science Waging War on Concussions

Julian Bailes, M.D.

The occurrence of head injuries in those involved in athletic endeavors has become increasingly recognized to affect a large number of participants and to have the potential for later deleterious effects. This is true of professional or scholar athletes participating in organized contact sports as well as for recreational athletes involved in the numerous activities that have head injury as a risk. Historical attitudes concerning the inconsequential nature of minor head injuries, such as the so-called "dinged" state in football, have been challenged, and the potential effects of these injuries are now better appreciated. There has been much publicity and media attention paid to the professional athlete who may have a career-threatening injury, but, more importantly, there are thousands of people who are at risk daily of head injury either during organized or recreational sporting activities. To put those exposed in perspective, it has been estimated that 30 million people participate in organized sports.

A characteristic aspect of contact sport athletes is that they are the only groups of patients who, by the very nature of their activities, request to be allowed to return to play and thereby to sustain other head impacts and, often, concussions. Although the incidence of serious or life-threatening brain injury has decreased in most sports, there is emerging scientific evidence that suggests that concussion, also known as mild traumatic brain injury (MTBI), may be more common and more serious than previously appreciated. The future consequences of repetitive blows to the head are now considered detrimental to many who have participated in contact sports. This is in addition to the possibility of a major injury or of death in many sports.

The incidence and severity of head injury and its impact upon the player's role in the contest vary greatly with the sport involved. Athletic endeavors are considered in categories that allow the nature of the play and the participants to be defined in terms of types of sporting events and characteristics of the players. As discussed in chapter 8, the most useful classification is that of recreational, nonorganized sports versus organized, sanctioned sports. The former can have little formal structure, fewer rules, no refereed officials, less use of protective equipment, and participation by a mixture of people under a variety of conditions, backgrounds, and training. In contrast, organized sporting events have specific requirements and regulations concerning training, rules and their enforcement, protective equipment, and physicians and athletic trainers dedicated to the prevention and care of those who are injured. Classification of sports also defines the *contact sports* as football, ice hockey, boxing, and wrestling while basketball, soccer, baseball, skiing, gymnastics, lacrosse, and others are traditionally considered *collision sports*. The former contain rules in which head and bodily impacts are expected and occur routinely on nearly every play, while the latter sports have the ever-present risk of colliding with opponents, the ground, or equipment.

EVOLUTION IN KNOWLEDGE ABOUT ATHLETIC CONCUSSIONS

By the early 1970s, it was recognized that short-term memory impairment in college football players who had not had apparent alteration of consciousness could be an expression of a MTBI.[1] These players all shared similar characteristics, such as a sense of bewilderment without marked cognitive difficulty, an inability to recall immediate events, and other signs. Sometimes they were initially able to recall an event immediately afterward, but these memories would rapidly fail, indicating that the ongoing, dynamic process of memory encoding was disrupted. The term "ding," which had previously been an aphorism for a benign brain insult, was thus first equated to being mildly concussed. Prior to this milestone, previous eras had considered concussion as an incident when a person was either unconscious, or "knocked out," or awake but in obvious disorientation and bewilderment. In other words, a concussion came to be appreciated as an injury that may occur with only subtle changes. In addition, we know that two types of football players commonly sustain MTBI: players involved in high-velocity impacts (tackling or being tackled) and those who do not see the impact coming. Examples of the latter would be the blindsided quarterback or the running back struck from the side by a tackler approaching from outside his visual field.

The recognition in the early 1980s that MTBI exists as an important clinical entity began to pave the way for an increased appreciation of concussion in sports. The heterogeneity of patient populations with MTBI and the wide spectrum of injury, especially implicating those with cerebral contusions or other structural brain lesions, led to a greater understanding of the wide clinical expression of injury in these patients. In contrast to the attitudes in earlier times, when being concussed was considered an acceptable occurrence for a contact athlete, new evidence provided proof that ongoing cerebral dysfunction could exist.[2]

The concept of MTBI or sports concussion has also evolved in recent years aided in great part by the application of formal neuropsychological and cognitive studies and by studies of patients involved in vehicular and other significant trauma.[3] Rutherford and his coworkers, in a study of 145 patients with MTBI, reported that 51 percent had persistent posttraumatic symptoms up to six weeks after their injury, while other researchers showed that a wide range (20 to 40 percent) of patients have persistent posttraumatic symptoms at three months after injury.[4] Specialized testing, focusing on attention and information processing functions, is often required for documenting ongoing deficits and has been shown to be more sensitive than other generalized testing of reaction time and intellectual function, which will often fail to adequately disclose subtle cognitive dysfunction. A routine medical history and physical examination may not show an obvious abnormality.

As stated previously, head-injured athletes comprise the only patient population who request permission to return to competition in contact sports, thus invariably subjecting themselves to multiple future instances of head impact. Many of these impacts will result in at least subclinical (not obvious) head injury. Although a single episode of MTBI seems to be well tolerated overall in the majority of athletes, long-term effects on a player's cognitive function have been thought to occur with as few as two episodes of concussion.[5] Despite aggressive use of concussion classification guidelines, good medical care, and implementing accepted return-to-play criteria, the likelihood exists that future head impacts will occur, along with the potential for additive brain injury, whether or not this injury is recognized. It has been estimated that a sports-related cerebral concussion increases the chance of a subsequent MTBI three- or fourfold.[6]

The effects of subsequent subclinical head injuries may also be more difficult to detect and may also be underreported by the athlete. Researchers have described the phenomenon of athletes who are hesitant to describe their concussion symptoms, and these researchers emphasize that, initially and later, postconcussion symptoms must be actively sought.[7] An athlete with MTBI may manifest difficulty remembering his or her assignment during a contest and thus often does a disservice to the team by attempting to participate. There is inherent difficulty in dealing with individuals who have experienced a concussion because usually the symptoms must be self-reported by the athlete. A third factor pertinent in athletes is that the presence of learning disabilities, which tend to manifest especially when a higher level of play is required, may complicate the diagnosis of MTBI, leading to a risk for more severe injury or aftereffects.[8] As athletes participate at more advanced levels in scholar or professional leagues, they represent a more heterogeneous population that arises from differing social and educational backgrounds. It is harder to diagnose concussion accurately in athletes with learning disabilities, and these athletes are more susceptible to having diminished cognitive reserve. Finally, athletes at all levels of play may incur significant stress, such as financial or other incentives and peer pressure, to return to contact sport participation. Thus, the athlete may minimize or not accurately report neurological or cognitive symptoms, even if characteristic symptoms occur and are recognized by the athlete. Former NFL star Merril Hoge has described the common scenario: "[A]n ankle or knee injury comes with certain symptoms. If my ankle or knee is bad, it is tough for me to perform my duties as a running back. The injury shows up the next day in practice. The brain, on the other hand, is very tricky. Right after a hit, the signs can be pretty obvious. You can see the glare in my eyes and you see that I'm sick to my stomach. A week later, I don't ask what happened any more. I obviously understand what happened. I'm not sick to my stomach anymore. I seem to have my orientation back but I still suffer. If you ask me to add two plus two, I don't automatically say four. I have to stop and count; one, two, three, four. I can still function. I feel better. Physically, I can play the game, but mentally I'm still not completely recovered."[9]

The incidence of MTBI in organized sports has been most reliably studied in football. Gerberich and coworkers reported a 19 percent incidence of concussion in high school football players in the late 1970s.[10] It was initially thought that the incidence of MTBI diminished after implementation in 1980 of NOCSAE helmet protection standards; however, more recent research shows that the measurement of concussion is difficult for several reasons. There are several reasons why incidence rates may vary between studies. There is variability in the way people present with concussive injury and how they are classified, making the use of different classifications of concussion confusing at times. Second, many players do not recognize the symptoms of concussion and thus do not report them to their coaches, athletic trainers, or team physicians. Also, there are numerous reasons that cause a player to want not to be identified as having sustained a concussion, such as the stigma of injury, being removed from the contest, and missing playing time. Former NFL New York Giants star Harry Carson has stated, "[P]layers look at concussions, or 'getting your bell rung,' as part of the game. Players are more concerned about the other physical injuries—the knee, the ankle, the back, or the elbow injuries. Going into the game, players know they might get injured, but they worry about body injuries rather than brain injuries. As a defensive player, I had the mentality that I was the one who was going to do the punishing; I was the one who was going to do the hitting. In my mind, I was not supposed to get hit back. One of the reasons I retired is because they started hitting me back. In football, everyone gets hit. The expression that 'football is a contact sport' is wrong. Football is a collision sport, and there are certain things that happen on a football field that players cannot control. They can try to protect themselves, but getting hit is just the nature of the game. Taking a hit that causes a concussion is not always obvious. It can be something very subtle."[11]

Barth found a 7.7 percent incidence of MTBI in college football players, whereas McCrea reported a 5.8 percent incidence in high school and college football players.[12] An extensive study by Powell and Barber-Foss of 23,566 injuries in 10 high school sports found a 3.9 percent incidence of MTBI in high school football, with wrestling, girls' soccer, boys' soccer, and girls' basketball representing a decreasing order of concussion incidence.[13] Based on their data, Powell and Barber-Foss project an estimated annual incidence of 62,816 cases of MTBI nationally in high school varsity athletics. Football accounted for 63 percent of these injuries. The incidence in ice hockey has been reported at 9 percent annually.[14] Up to 22 percent of elite European ice hockey players have sustained at least one concussion during their careers.[15] It has been reported that 27 percent of amateur soccer players had incurred one soccer-related concussion, whereas 23 percent had multiple (up to five) concussions throughout their amateur career. With 200 million Federal International Football Association–registered soccer players worldwide, this represents a major medical and public health concern.[16] It has been estimated that within a 10-year soccer-playing career, the odds are 50 percent for a man and 22 percent for a woman that a concussion will be sustained.[17] Surprisingly, there is a high incidence of concussion in horse racing jockeys.

Recent medical literature has suggested that the incidence of concussion in contact sports may be higher than previously thought. Chris Nowinski has researched the topic from the player's perspective. His work has documented that contact sports contain a higher-than-suspected rate of MTBI and that there are several understandable causes for this phenomenon. Many facets will be detailed in his upcoming book. Especially noted in football players, there are numerous reasons for underreporting symptoms, including the "mind-set" of football players and their coaches to minimize an injury or "play through" an injury. And unfortunately, this includes head injury in the form of concussion. In many instances, players believe that they will compromise their ability to remain a starter or active player on their team if they are removed because of an injury that is not obvious or seen by others, as opposed to a sprained ankle, knee, or other visible injury. Helmeted football players are not readily noticed in many cases to have had an MTBI, and everyone in attendance is accustomed to witnessing violent collisions on every play. As former NFL star Mark Kelso has stated, "concussions are serious, but they happen to everyone and they happen frequently, so players don't always treat them seriously."[18]

A recent study of Canadian professional football players showed an alarmingly high incidence of concussion, with 47 percent sustaining concussion during a single season. In addition, even at their relatively advanced age, experience, and maturity, often the players do not recognize the sometimes-subtle signs of MTBI.[19] Current studies at both the high school and collegiate levels have concurred with these reports, showing higher than previously thought incidences of concussion. Langburt's 2002 study of high school players found that 47 percent sustained a concussion annually, while Delaney and coworkers detected 60 percent of college players with concussion.[20] These concussion frequencies in high ranges attest to more sensitive detection and reporting of some very mild injuries, many of the type that the athlete will often play through. The question arises, however, as to the long-term impact of such repetitive "minor" concussions.

In summary, depending upon the method of detection, the definition of concussion used, the degree of scrutiny of the athletes, their level of play, the extent that those players recognize and can be educated concerning the symptoms of concussion, and their motivation to either report or to mask symptoms, there has been a wide range in the reported incidence of concussion in contact sports. Suffice to say, however, there is a growing awareness that this is not a benign problem and that there are innumerable factors that come into play. In fact, the Centers for Disease Control recently announced that concussions in athletic activities have now reached epidemic proportions, with over 300,000 occurring annually in the United States alone.[21] One of our greatest hopes is that continued work in this area will better define our ability to detect and manage these players in order to do two things: first, to optimize their playing time and positive experience, and, secondly, to minimize any potential for long-term deleterious effects upon their cerebral or motor function.

POSTCONCUSSION SYNDROME

The vast majority of concussions, whether they occur in the general population, for instance resultant from an automobile crash, fall, or other trauma, or in an athlete, will resolve without consequence. As stated above, however, the athletic population has nuances in that they are the only patients who ordinarily go on to sustain other head impacts. Most symptoms of concussion are self-limited and relatively minor. However, the post-concussion syndrome is not an unusual occurrence after a head injury. It is usually seen in patients who have been involved in motor vehicle accidents simply because they represent greater numbers. But it is also seen in athletes, especially those with repeated or successive concussions during the course of one season.[22]

Numerous complaints occur with post-concussion syndrome and typically include persistent headache, irritability, poor concentration, vertigo, dizziness, memory impairment, and generalized fatigue. Many factors, including motivation, psychological factors, pending litigation, educational level, and degree of injury may influence the duration, extent, and number of post-concussion syndrome complaints. Post-concussion syndrome also may present in a different fashion, including deficits in thinking and mental processing, diminishment of the sense of physical well-being, and mood disturbance. This causes diminished memory and concentration, fatigue, dizziness, depression, anxiety, and irritability. Most of these symptoms seem to run a self-limited and benign course, usually resolving by six to eight weeks after the accident.[23] The person may look, talk, and appear to act normally, and a routine physical examination by a physician may fail to disclose anything as wrong. Brain CT or MRI scans may also be interpreted as normal. Neuropsychological testing documents recovery in varying time intervals. Formal neuropsychological evaluation with a formal testing battery may be the best, and it may provide the only objective measure for documentation and serial follow-up in these patients. It can be invaluable for athletes who must perform at maximal physical levels and for the medical team attempting to decide who may safely return to play. Typically, neuropsychological tests show a reversion to normal within five to seven days following an uncomplicated sports-related concussion.

CUMULATIVE INJURY

Several high-profile professional athletes have had their careers ended by repetitive head injury, including Troy Aikman, Merril Hoge, Al

Toon, Harry Carson, Stan Humphries, Pat LaFontaine, and others. Some have stated that they have gone on to experience chronic symptoms, which they have attributed to multiple concussions sustained in their sport.[24] Their experience and that of others, many documented in the medical literature, press the question of the potential role of multiple MTBI in leading to lingering aftereffects of the game. Former NFL player Harry Carson remarked: "I didn't realize until 2 years after I had left the league that I needed help. I knew I was having problems, but I thought the problems would go away. I went to my personal physician after I retired and told him I was having trouble with my vision, my memory, and even my speech. I had the words in my mind and I couldn't translate them from my brain to my mouth. He sent me to a neuropsychologist. I went through 2 days of testing and he diagnosed postconcussion syndrome."[25]

Our work at the Center for Study of Retired Athletes has focused, among other issues, upon the potential for cumulative effects of such injuries. We have studied 2,600 retired NFL players, in conjunction with the NFL Players' Association, initially using a detailed questionnaire concerning the presence of symptoms such as memory loss, headaches, and personality changes. Our findings disclosed that there appeared to be an increased incidence, compared to age-matched controls, of not only cognitive difficulties but also depression in retired NFL players. In addition, there was a correlation between the head injury exposure, i.e. the number of concussions sustained during playing years, with the incidence of ongoing cognitive or memory symptoms.[26]

The concept of cumulative brain injury is important in the study of athletic head injury. There are two aspects to this phenomenon. First, as has been discussed above, the effects of concussion seem to be most pronounced after the athlete sustains a second concussion.[27] Second, although exact data do not exist, it seems that the temporal proximity of sustaining multiple episodes of MTBI determines the likelihood of long-lasting effects and may lead to a greater chance of having a prolonged period of post-concussion symptoms. In the immediate period, this affects the athlete's return to competition and may affect his or her personality and academic performance.

Chronic traumatic brain injury represents the additive effect of multiple subconcussive and concussive head impacts and is expressed as the long-term neurological functioning of the athlete.[28] Chronic injury in the brains of boxers was first described in 1928, in a 38-year-old retired boxer with advanced Parkinson's disease, pyramidal imbalance, and behavioral abnormalities. Mendez categorized the clinical manifestations of such boxers into cognitive, motor, and psychiatric symptoms.[29] A spectrum of clinical symptoms may exist, including early difficulty with speech and coordination, the onset of tremor and attention deficits, and psychiatric symptoms. The last, or severe, stage of chronic brain injury in boxers has been termed *dementia pugilistica*. Roberts used random sampling to study 250 retired professional British boxers, finding that 37 (17 percent) had clinical evidence of brain dysfunction likely caused by boxing.[30] Risk factors that have been purported to increase a boxer's risk of injury include being a professional rather than an amateur boxer, absorbing more punches rather than skillfully avoiding blows, greater sparring exposure, history of technical knockout or knockout, and overall poor boxing performance.[31] Using other testing modalities, the EKG of boxers may contain focal slowing localized to the frontal or temporal lobes of the brain, findings that are correlated with increased boxing exposure.[32]

Autopsy findings in the brains of men who had been boxers have shown characteristic patterns of cerebral change that seemed not only to be the result of boxing but also to underlie many features of the punch-drunk syndrome. Pathological examination has disclosed several characteristic abnormalities in the brains of boxers, including areas of cavitation (*cavum septum pellucidum*), scarring of the cerebellum, degeneration of the deep nuclei (*substantia nigra*), and regional deposition of Alzheimer's neurofibrillary tangles.[33] Extensive L3-protein immunoreactive deposits or plaques have been found in the brains of retired boxers with dementia pugilistica.

Considering genetic predisposition to injury in sports with repetitive head impacts, there is also evidence to suggest that the presence of the gene apolipoprotein E e4 allele is involved with an increased risk in people who experience traumatic brain injury.[34] Jordan and his colleagues reported a study of 30 active and retired boxers in which they found that apolipoprotein E e4 was associated with a greater severity of chronic traumatic brain injury. This study suggested that there may be a predisposition to deleterious brain damage in those boxers who had a prolonged boxing career (more than 12 professional bouts). Similar findings of a genetic predisposition were also reported for active professional football players, in which the presence of the same genetic marker indicated a higher incidence of MTBI per exposure.[35]

Chronic or cumulative traumatic brain injury may also occur in professional soccer players. Matser and his research team studied 53 active professional European soccer players using in-depth neuropsychological testing. They found evidence of chronic cognitive impairment involving planning ability, memory, and visual-perceptual processing. Forward and defensive players, those who are more likely to use their heads to strike the soccer ball, had the highest incidence of impairment.[36] Preliminary evidence also suggests that retired professional football players may have a higher incidence of ongoing post-concussive symptoms (including depression), which correlate with the incidence of MTBI during their playing years. Neuropsychological impairment, CT scan abnormalities, and EKG wave slowing have all been reported in retired Norwegian soccer players.[37]

Although the hallmarks of cerebral concussion are confusion and amnesia, the athlete with persistent effects of MTBI may demonstrate only an easy distractibility and poor vigilance. He or she may be unable to maintain a coherent stream of thought or carry out a sequence of goal-directed actions, may be emotionally labile, or may have short-term memory deficits. It is likely that significant and ongoing chronic effects exist in a portion of those athletes who have sustained multiple previous episodes of MTBI. Further research is necessary to elucidate the true occurrence and meaning of many of these findings.

CONCUSSION CLASSIFICATION

Concussion has been categorized into three types or grades for clinical purposes. One of the biggest advances in the understanding of MTBI has come through our ability to define and categorize concussions into levels of severity or grades. This has assisted us in numerous ways in understanding both the brain's reaction to such trauma and how to best manage these players medically and in respect to allowing them to return to play. Previously held beliefs concerning the identification and severity of athletic MTBI have now been replaced with more current thought based on research and experience with large groups of injured athletes; this was never available before. Several classification schemes have been proposed, with three currently in widespread use: the Colorado scale, the Cantu classification, and the Colorado guidelines.[38]

The least severe MTBI in sports is termed a mild concussion (Grade I). It is most common and involves no LOC, with confusion only being the hallmark. Cantu's classification of a mild concussion includes no LOC with confusion alone or with a brief (less than 30 minutes) period of amnesia.[39] The American Academy of Neurology (AAN) practice parameters define a Grade I concussion as having no LOC and mental status abnormalities that resolve in less than 15 minutes.[40] This type of concussion occurs to at least one or more football players in every game, if the players are thoroughly scrutinized. The athlete, who is awake and alert, surprisingly may be able to function during the course of the athletic contest. If significant disorientation, confusion, memory disturbance, dizziness, headache, or any neurological abnormality persists after the 15-minute observation period, the athlete has more than a mild concussion. One should keep in mind that concussion might be present and significant without the athlete having sustained LOC.

With the Colorado guidelines, a moderate or Grade II concussion is associated with the development of amnesia either initially or during the period of observation. There is no LOC. The athlete is usually removed from competition and not allowed to return. Cantu defined the moderate concussion as less than 5 minutes of unconsciousness or posttraumatic amnesia for longer than 30 minutes but less than 24 hours duration, whereas the AAN system indicates a person with a Grade II concussion has no LOC but only mental status changes lasting longer than 15 minutes.[41]

A severe or Grade III concussion is associated with LOC, according to the Colorado and AAN guidelines. Cantu defines a severe or Grade III concussion as one having a more than 5-minute period of unconsciousness or 24 hours or more of posttraumatic amnesia. The finding of an LOC implies the severest form of concussion for the Colorado and AAN guidelines and includes a wide spectrum of injury ranging from a brief period (a few seconds) to a prolonged time of unconsciousness. In general, a period of LOC has been considered a marker for the degree of impact (and injury) which the brain has sustained, and it gives the neurosurgeon an indication of the potential for intracranial damage. In many instances of athletic MTBI, there is what has been referred to as the "briefest LOC," which may be akin to just being stunned and nonresponsive for a few seconds. This obviously does not imply the likelihood for major brain injury as much as someone who sustains a more prolonged LOC, which can last for several minutes or hours, or even prolonged amnesia, which indicates ongoing brain disturbance.

Concussion exists on the spectrum of what is known as *diffuse brain injury*. This means that instead of a focal or small and defined area of brain damage, there is an insult to the entire brain, and it manifests usually with an alteration of the level of consciousness, the severest form being a comatose state. Therefore, someone who sustains an LOC may have a diffuse, widespread brain injury and subsequent dysfunction, or they may also have a localized injury including areas of intracranial bleeding or blood clots (hematomas). Regardless, for the personnel performing the on-field assessment, the identification of a Grade III concussion instantly elevates the concern for the possibility of major or even life-threatening brain injury and the player must be handled with suspicion and caution until this potential is ruled out. Therefore, any athlete with an LOC following head injury should be carefully scrutinized and, if not rapidly awake and proceeding toward a normal neurological assessment, may require transport to the nearest physician or hospital for further evaluation.

There has been no universal agreement on the definition and grading of concussion, and attempts at classification have tended to focus on the presence or absence of a period of LOC and amnesia as hallmarks in the grading schemes. However, concussion may present with any combination of the following signs and symptoms: a feeling of being stunned or seeing bright lights, a brief LOC, lightheadedness, vertigo, loss of balance, headaches, cognitive and memory dysfunction, tinnitus, blurred vision, difficulty concentrating, lethargy, fatigue, personality changes, inability to perform daily activities, sleep disturbance, and motor or sensory symptoms. The lack of a universal definition or grading scheme for concussion has made it difficult to evaluate epidemiological data.

THE SECOND IMPACT SYNDROME

One of the most feared complications of athletic head injury is the Second Impact Syndrome (SIS). Although this condition is rare, it may be associated with a sudden deterioration to a comatose condition in an athlete who has a repetitive head impact. Any athlete still symptomatic from a previous head injury should not be allowed to return to full practice or participation in a contact or collision sport because the brain is vulnerable. This vulnerability is not only to cumulative injury but also to the uncommon, yet potentially lethal, SIS. SIS occurs when an athlete who sustains a head injury—often a concussion or greater injury, such as a cerebral contusion—sustains a second head injury before symptoms associated with the first have cleared.

Typically, the athlete experiences some degree of post-concussion symptoms after the first head injury. These may include visual, motor, or sensory changes and difficulty with cognitive and memory processes. Before these symptoms resolve, which may take days or weeks, the athlete returns to competition and receives a second blow to the head. The second blow may be minor, perhaps only involving a blow to the chest that jerks the athlete's head back and indirectly imparts accelerative forces to the brain. Affected athletes may seem stunned but usually do not lose consciousness and often complete the play. They usually remain on their feet for 15 seconds to a minute or so but seem dazed, similar to a Grade I concussion without LOC. Often, affected athletes remain on the playing field or walk off under their own power.[42] What happens in the next few moments to several minutes sets this syndrome apart from a concussion or even a subdural hematoma or other form of brain hemorrhage. Usually, within seconds to minutes of the second impact, the athlete who is conscious yet stunned precipitously collapses to the ground and becomes comatose, with rapidly dilating pupils, loss of eye movement, and evidence of respiratory failure.

Between 1980 and 1993, 35 probable cases among American football players alone have been identified; however, the condition remains controversial, with some question as to whether it has occurred this often. It is believed to be caused by a loss of regulation in the amount of blood (blood volume) in the brain, in which the second injury causes a marked second rise leading to severe and irreversible engorgement and brain swelling. SIS is not confined to American football players as it has also been reported in ice hockey, boxing, and even downhill skiing. This can become a catastrophic condition with a mortality rate approaching 50 percent and nearly a universal persistence of neurological problems in the survivors. Therefore, prevention becomes crucially important. An athlete who is identified to be still symptomatic from a prior head injury must not participate in contact or collision sports until all cerebral symptoms have subsided, and preferably not for at least one week afterward. Regardless of the length required to reach the asymptomatic state, athletes should not be allowed to compete while they display any significant post-concussion symptoms. Despite uncertainty regarding the pathophysiological events, which lead to death and the true incidence, SIS is still occurring in the U.S.

TESTS FOR CONCUSSION

Ancillary tests have shown significant value in assisting the documentation of ongoing brain involvement after a concussion. Neuropsychological testing has come to the forefront of supplementary methods of objectifying the cognitive deficits in athletes, when the other aforementioned tests are not able to document an abnormality, providing the ability to measure, quantify, and follow persistent and evolving cognitive and higher cortical function modalities in these patients.

To be effective, neuropsychological testing must be quick to administer, reproducible, and structured for the athlete. A baseline examination performed in the preseason period and specific for the athlete is preferred, administered by a qualified neuropsychologist. Several researchers led the way in identifying the prominent role of neuropsychological testing in sports medicine. In 1989 Barth and his coworkers published their experience with using these testing methods to measure deficits in mental processing that were not obvious by either routine verbal questioning or a physical examination by a physician.[43] Maroon, Lovell, and Bailes pushed for the application of this emerging science at the NFL level, which was implemented by the Pittsburgh Steelers in the early 1990s and determined to be very effective for assessment of the degree of MTBI and monitoring the athlete's recovery and ability to return safely to play. Other researchers followed suit and now neuropsychological testing has been proven both practical and accurate for athletes of all ages and at all levels of play. Currently, neuropsychological testing is used throughout the NFL, NHL, and by many collegiate and secondary schools.

Orientation, attention, information processing, memory, and other functions are the basis for neuropsychological testing of the athlete. Neuropsychological examination provides an objective measure for documentation of brain disturbance often when all other tests, including physical and neurological examination, are normal. As a concussion resolves, improvement in the neuropsychological testing mirrors the brain's recovery. This objective measure of cognitive and mental status function is most helpful for athletes, team physicians, trainers, coaches, officials, parents, and family in understanding and following the extent of the injury. Usually, an uncomplicated concussion will revert to normal in five to seven days. Other forms of ancillary testing for athletic MTBI have been shown to be beneficial, including balance testing and sophisticated brain imaging studies, such as CT, MRI, "functional" MRI, PET scans, and other tests of ongoing metabolic function.[44] There will likely be continued evolution in our ability to image the brain as it works, and thus to be able to more precisely identify the degree of injury and the rate of recovery. This measure is critical to discern the presence of MTBI and to provide the player, parents, coach, and athletic trainer with an objective determination of the injury that all can see, especially when athletes with concussions many times outwardly appear "normal."

When an athlete has been withheld from play because of persistent effects from a mild concussion, he or she should be examined by the team physician or other appropriate medical personnel, although exact management will vary dependent upon several factors (for example, with a single mild concussion, the athlete ordinarily may return to competition after one week of being asymptomatic at rest and exertion). If symptoms persist, the athlete should not be allowed to play until they abate, and a head CT scan may be helpful in excluding any structural abnormality. With a second mild concussion in the same season, the athlete should be withheld from contact sports for two weeks, and a CT scan should be considered, especially if the concussions came in short succession. The athlete should be asymptomatic at rest and exertion, with a normal neurological examination and CT scan, before he or she is allowed to return to play. Of benefit may be the performance of a "provocative exertional" practice session, in which the athlete participates fully in his sport, including aerobic activity, with the exception of avoiding head impacts. This maneuver is often helpful in deciding whether the athlete is asymptomatic and ready for competition. Many experts recommend that the athlete be pulled from play for the rest of the season if a third concussion of any category occurs in a single season.

In the case of a Grade II concussion, generally the management consists of the athlete being removed from competition and not allowed to return. If indicated, he or she should be examined by the team physician and consideration should be given for consultation with a neurological specialist, especially if disturbances in the level of consciousness or other neurological signs develop. An athlete with a second moderate concussion in one season may be withheld for one month after being asymptomatic, and he or she should preferably have a CT scan within normal limits before returning to play. A third moderate concussion would be grounds for pulling the athlete from play for the rest of the season. Some experts suggest that at this point, consideration should be given to disallow the athlete's return to contact sports permanently. However, such athletes may often safely return to contact sports the next season.

An athlete with a Grade III concussion often requires emergent transport to the nearest facility with CT scanning capabilities, and consideration should be given for neurosurgical consultation, especially with any prolonged LOC or neurological deficit. The possibility of concomitant cervical spine injury must always be considered in an unconscious patient, and transport should be performed with cervical immobilization and maintenance of an adequate airway. Most often, unless the LOC has been very brief, for instance, less than 30 seconds, the athlete may be admitted to the hospital overnight for observation. He or she is treated according to the standard accepted procedure for closed-head injury and observed for signs of development of an expanding intracranial hematoma, brain swelling, or other abnormalities.

Any significant LOC may require neurological and CT scan examinations. If both are normal and the athlete is asymptomatic, he or she may return to competition within two weeks of being without symptoms, if the length of unconsciousness was less than one minute. With an LOC greater than one minute, which implies significant interruption of cerebral function, it is often recommended that competition be avoided for one month. A second severe concussion will usually terminate the athlete's season, and consideration should be given to ending the patient's participation in any contact sport. These recommendations are based on personal experience and that of others and are reinforced by studies that use neuropsychological and other forms of ancillary testing. These are also merely recommendations and examples of management schemes; their application may vary and all neurological sports medicine decisions must be individualized to the particular situation.

We do not have a complete understanding of the concepts, classification, and metabolic effects of MTBI. This is especially true in contact sport athletes, who, as stated previously, are exposed inherently to multiple head impacts and, at least, subclinical, or not obvious, concussions. Reports from the NFL Committee on Head Injury have suggested that their players are not at the same risk and should follow different classification and management schemes compared to other levels of play.[45] Amateur or scholar athletes may be at a different risk than professional athletes who perhaps, for such various reasons as ability level and preselection for ability to sustain head impacts without suffering from significant brain injury, are less susceptible to concussive head injury. Researchers and sports medicine specialists are still understanding more about the metabolic changes that occur in MTBI, such as glucose metabolism, which is ordinarily reversibly perturbed for about five days following a "routine" concussion. Better ways of identifying and measuring the effects of concussion are being researched but are not so helpful if players are not being identified, as some have found. This is still an ongoing, evolving area of sports medicine, with large implications for the future of numerous sports and athletes.

CONCLUSION

There have been many dedicated researchers who have devoted their careers to analysis of the numerous factors concerning MTBI in the athletic setting. As previously stated, for the person involved in a contact or collision sport in which they are liable to sustain repetitive head impacts, this poses unique challenges for not only athletes but also the medical and athletic training personnel who are attempting to advise them concerning the safety of returning to play. Medical experts have gained an increased understanding of the mechanisms of MTBI, not only how frequently it occurs, but also the biochemical reaction within the brain with a disturbance of glucose metabolism for several days in most significant concussions. Better efforts at identifying concussions when they occur, beginning with sideline evaluation, and their classification have improved our ability to manage these athletes during the vulnerable period and to predict when a return to contact or collision sports is safe. We still have much to learn concerning the nuances of each particular sport. If properly managed, such athletes usually can continue their playing careers with a minimal risk of incurring permanent brain injuries that could have long-term consequences. There is still much left to understand, however, as we anticipate future research that will improve our knowledge and appreciation of the potential for injury to the brain. In dangerous sports that entail the constant specter of repetitive head impacts, such as boxing and football, research may help reduce the potential for long-term consequences.

Caring for Youth Sports: Are We or Not?

Because time has the power to heal, youth sports in this country continue to be beaten and bruised by violence, poor sportsmanship, and the same win-at-all-cost mentality that hurts all levels of sport. The sting caused by so many wounds is only felt for a short time before the minds of the American people turn to other matters. The latest unbelievable tale is soon replaced by another in a different state and a different sport. The story of a father who tells his son to stop crying and keep pitching because baseball is a man's sport only makes the front page of the local newspaper. The horrific news of a hockey coach attacked and killed in front of kids by a father complaining that practice was getting too rough fades away by the time the sports headlines are done rolling at the end of the newscast. And every year hundreds of youth league and high school referees and umpires become the victims of assault by enraged parents, coaches, and athletes. Most of these outrageous acts are fast and furious—both in their origin and in how soon we forget about them. Even the events that become network television movies of the week—for example, a cheerleader's mom who tried to have the mother of her daughter's rival murdered in Texas—soon drift into a collection of clouded sports memories. Some memories are based on real events; others are based on complete fiction. Often it is difficult to distinguish between the two. For the past 20 years the topic of youth sports problems has spawned numerous research studies, articles by experts in scientific journals, books by sports psychologists, and investigative reports by newspapers, magazines, and every cable and network television station in the country. What do we have to show for all this concern and compassion for kids and the sports they play for fun?

- *March 2004:* Two college professors conclude from their study that incidents of "Little League Parent Syndrome" or "sport rage" are on the rise.[1]

- *August 2003:* A majority of parents (56 percent) believe their kids' sports programs focus too much on winning, with nearly half of those responding to a new national NFL/PTA survey saying that organized youth sports need to be completely revamped. And almost half of parents (44 percent) said their child had dropped out of a sport because it made him or her unhappy.[4]
- *March 2003:* "The truth . . . is there are more incidents now than two years ago," said Rick Wolff, chairman of the Center for Sports Parenting at the University of Rhode Island, in 2003.[2]
- *February/January 2003: SportingKid* magazine surveyed 3,300 parents and found 80 percent who claimed to be victims of "violent parental behavior" at kids' sports events; 84 percent said they witnessed this behavior toward children, coaches, or officials.[3]
- *November 2002:* The National Alliance for Youth Sports, a nonprofit organization based in West Palm Beach, Florida, estimated that the number of confrontations and violent acts involving parents and coaches had tripled over the previous five years.[5]
- *November 2002:* "There is a 20 percent chance that violence will break out at any youth game, and it's getting worse," said Scott Lancaster, senior director of NFL Youth Football Development and author of "Fair Play: Making Organized Sports a Great Experience for Your Kids."[6]

If winning is what everyone so desperately wants, how can it be that we are losing this battle and failing our children so badly? Surveys and studies like the ones above can paint an ugly portrait. But the real-life snapshots of repugnant behavior by adults and their poorly raised children fill page after page of a scrapbook so hideous much of society dares not open it up. Take a moment to flip through the following edition of that scrapbook: a collection of the unthinkable acts against sports officials during the one-year period beginning in February 2003 and ending in February 2004 (reprinted from the National Association of Sports Officials' Web site):

- *Pennsylvania (basketball):* A parent body-slammed a high school referee after he ordered the man's wife out of the gym for allegedly yelling obscenities during a basketball game (Feb. 6, 2004).
- *Kentucky (basketball):* During a fifth-grade Little League game, one player's father (and a teacher for the school district) physically

confronted the game official during halftime after the official ejected several players for fighting (Jan. 2004).

- *New Jersey (soccer):* A 50-year-old referee was slugged in the head and neck after ejecting a Clayton High School player who had received a yellow card earlier in the game for incidental cursing and was later given a red-yellow card for taunting.

- *New Jersey (baseball):* A 39-year-old man was indicted by a grand jury and charged with assault at a youth sports event for allegedly bumping and then punching the umpire during an argument (Oct. 2003). He could face up to 18 months in prison and $10,000 in fines.

- *Illinois (football):* A 43-year-old man was charged with two counts of aggravated battery and one count of battery after allegedly charging onto the field and attempting to choke a game official (Sept. 2003).

- *Kentucky (baseball):* A father of a T-ball player was briefly jailed after an outburst against an umpire during a game involving five- and six-year-olds. The accused threatened to beat the umpire moments before walking onto the field and starting a fight. A girl who was playing in the game suffered a minor injury when she was struck in the face during the scuffle (July 2003).

- *Illinois (softball):* An irate father headbutted the umpire in a confrontation following the game. The mother had earlier been ejected for berating the umpire (July 2003).

- *Oklahoma (basketball):* Five players and a spectator were charged with beating a referee following a rec-league game. All six allegedly struck the referee on the head several times, pushed him to the ground and kicked him about the head and body "with force and violence" police records report (June 2003).

- *Oklahoma (baseball):* A high school coach allegedly attacked the umpire in the umpires' room following a game. The ump suffered a bruised lip, knot over his left eye, and a sore right shoulder. The coach resigned his coaching position with the school (July 2003).

- *Ohio (soccer):* A Major League Soccer coach was fined for entering the Referee Secure Area, which is against league rules (April 2003).

- *International (soccer):* A Brazilian soccer player sat out three matches for the national team because he hit a referee (March 2003).

- *Hawaii (soccer):* A referee was pushed to the ground by a high school player following a state quarterfinal game. The coach of the team was banned for five years from participation in any state sports event and the team is on "conduct probation" after the discovery of "overwhelming evidence" of other acts of poor sportsmanship by the team during the season. The coach was then fired (Feb. 2003).

- *Illinois (baseball):* A fan at a major-league ballpark attacked an umpire, trying to wrestle him to the ground. He was charged with felony aggravated battery and misdemeanor criminal trespass, the bail was set at $250,000, and if convicted, the fan faces two to five years in prison (April 2003).

- *Maryland (hockey):* Fans of the losing home team during an NHL playoff game littered the ice with bottles and other debris after the final goal was scored (April 2003).

- *New York (hockey):* A linesman trying to break up a fight between two players during a junior varsity high school hockey game was pulled backward by his uniform and knocked to the ice, where he hit his head. The man was arrested and charged with third-degree assault with intent to injure and third-degree attempted assault (March 2003).

- *Iowa (basketball):* The parent of a high school player forced his way into the referee locker room, upset about a call at the end of the game, and assaulted a referee who suffered injuries to his right arm and face. The man was charged with assault with injury, a serious misdemeanor (March 2003).

- *Texas (basketball):* An NBA player was suspended for one game for bumping a referee (Feb. 2003).[7]

Sports officials who used to plan which restaurants to frequent after games now have plans to cover their injuries in case they are attacked. Instead of lobbying to change rules to improve their games, they lobby state and national legislators to change laws increasing penalties for those who physically assault them. Instead of enjoying the surroundings of a newly built arena or smaller venue, they anxiously ask about evacuation plans in case there is a problem with irate fans. It is disappointing that a majority of states still do not have laws providing stiffer penalties for fans who physically confront officials.

USA Today columnist Christine Brennan, appearing on *CNN Live This Morning* on June 8, 2001, said, "My goodness, now there are 16 states in the country that have laws that prohibit assaulting . . . a sports official by a parent or a kid. So you know, obviously I think we're headed probably to 50 out of 50 states on something like that." But more than three years later, there are only 17 states with such laws on the books, and only two more states had legislation pending at the time this book was written. It is no wonder that little has changed in the way of curbing violence at youth sporting events when lawmakers have failed to change their thinking on how important this issue is.

The list of violent acts above is not a comprehensive one. Doug Abrams, a law professor at the University of Missouri, tracks news stories about rage-related incidents at youth sports events, and he suspects there are dozens more, if not hundreds, for every one reported.[8] And these reports involve only acts of violence that warranted suspensions, fines, or criminal prosecution. There are, no doubt, numerous cases that were not reported to NASO and perhaps hundreds of incidents of extreme verbal abuse or less severe physical contact that were not meant to inflict physical harm but were enough to rattle already wary game officials. Florida State Representative Eleanor Sobel (D-Hollywood) is cosponsoring a bill that would upgrade the maximum penalty for assaulting a sports official to three years in prison and/or a $10,000 fine because officials are often in positions of authority and are responsible for controlling unstable situations, much like peace officers. "That's the only way you can stop this," Sobel told the Florida *Sun-Sentinel*. "Otherwise you won't have sports officials." Sobel recognizes that there is a nationwide shortage of officials, especially at the youth sports level where often there is no presence of police or security.[9] Just as disconcerting is the impact this violent behavior has on the many children who are either participants or spectators at these events. There are several potential outcomes:

- Children with their own volatile emotions may join the verbal or physical abuse.
- Children, and everyone in attendance, may store the memory of this incident and use it as a license to act similarly in future incidents.

- Adults who commit acts of violence send a confusing signal that may lead kids to believe violence is an acceptable measure in resolving conflict.
- If kids do recognize that the behavior by adults is wrong, their level of respect for the parent or coach decreases, a trend that is eroding the credibility of authority figures (see chapter 14, "Who's in Charge? Administration Is Part of the Problem").
- Children become frustrated at seeing the anger and violence, and they grow disinterested in participating in sports. Most studies of sports participation patterns conclude that close to 70 percent of kids who play youth sports quit by their freshman year of high school, many because bad sportsmanship makes for bad experiences.

The travesty is that society's administration of youth sports is failing so severely that an overwhelming majority of children—64 percent, by the NFL/PTA survey's count—are dissatisfied with playing in organized leagues. But why must this fact dissolve from our minds so easily, disappearing from most reader's radar screens by the start of the next chapter? Yet this has been the trend with this crisis—it's not a crisis until the next published report tells us it is. Society needs to wake up—and not simply by realizing the problem exists but by combining efforts to stamp out a perfectly understood problem. Perhaps the simplicity of the situation causes a lack of concern for how damaging it is. Despite a decade of hearing about the deterioration of the core values that should be associated with youth sports—the importance of sharing; playing fair; getting along with, respecting, and forgiving others; and teamwork—the problem has not only persisted, but it has grown into a monster that 64 percent of kids want to run away from. Adults can typically soothe a child's discomfort, but not when they are the cause of it.

SIX UNACCEPTABLE MISTAKES

There are at least six unacceptable mistakes committed by parents and coaches who use inappropriately aggressive approaches to youth sports, thereby eroding the pleasure of sports for kids and fans.

1. Pushing Kids Too Hard

When adults lose perspective for what youth sports are supposed to be about—kids having fun, learning life skills, coping with losing while aiming to improve and succeed, etc.—those who are most hurt by this are the kids themselves. There are many levels of pushing. No parental debacle has been more publicized than that of Marv Marinovich, whose son Todd was being prepared for his athletic career from the day he was born. Following is a summary of the Marinovich story taken from a Louisiana sports-writing award-winning special report in the *Shreveport Times* entitled, "Building the Perfect Athlete":

> Instead of commercial baby food, Todd ate frozen raw kidney chunks for the right vitamins and minerals. According to *The Los Angeles Times*, refined sugar, animal fats, nitrites, coloring agents and white cake flour were not allowed in Todd's diet. If a classmate's birthday party featured a cake with some of those ingredients, Todd had to abstain.
>
> After Todd failed to hustle to dad's satisfaction during a youth basketball game, Marv forced him to run eight miles alongside his car on the way home. The boy worked out 365 days a year, including holidays, and underwent a series of esoteric tests and drills to sharpen his vision, improve his eye-hand coordination and cut down on his reaction time.
>
> When Todd arrived at USC in 1989 as a record-setting quarterback, most of the country knew him only as the boy whose father wouldn't let him eat a Big Mac. He was tagged with the nickname "Robo QB."
>
> Less than three years later, an arrest and jail time earned him a new, startlingly telling moniker: "Marijuana-vich."
>
> Todd played two seasons in college, two in the NFL. This spring (1999), six years after the Raiders cut him, he tried out with the Seattle Seahawks. He didn't make the team.
>
> Marv denies he tried to build the perfect athlete. Few people, he says, talk about the math homework and violin lessons and museum trips.
>
> "We set out to produce a healthy, balanced child," he says.
>
> But sports psychologists say his methods are chillingly out of balance.[10]

Marinovich represents an extremist in terms of pushing a child to succeed in sports—literally from infancy—instead of encouraging that child to enjoy youth sports and choose his own level of participation based on his wishes. But just because other parents are not as fanatical—even psychotic—as Marinovich, does not earn them a pass for their actions. Take, for example, the actions of Randy Bowers of

Shreveport, Louisiana, as told by Brian McCallum of the *Shreveport Times* in 2002:

> Years before his sons Chris and Chase were old enough to play high school football, Randy sought the advice of a nutritionist on how to help his boys get bigger and stronger. At first, he made shakes consisting of milk, powdered milk and a banana every night. Since then, the family has moved on to sports supplements containing protein and creatine.
>
> "It was pretty unscientific at the beginning," the elder Bowers said. "It kind of made them sick to their stomach until their bodies began to get used to it."
>
> As for those who wondered whether Randy was pushing his kids to do something they didn't want to do, he had a simple answer.
>
> "My response was always that it didn't matter if they like it; they're going to take it," he said. "There was no controversy in it because it was all just stuff from the refrigerator."[11]

Parents should always be in control of their children, but they must also police themselves very strictly to ensure that they are not pushing or even leading a young athlete in a direction that brings more satisfaction to the adult than to the child.

2. Putting Too Much Emphasis on Winning

Most parents do not come close to the extreme methods Marinovich's father used to prepare his son for competition. In fact, a majority of parents are not involved enough in their child's practice time and development, limiting their responsibility to driving to and from practices. But when game time arrives, parents far too often become overzealous cheerleaders and overenthusiastic sports experts. A list of the "Top 10 Things Parents Don't Get About Kids and Sports," a compilation of actual quotes from kids compiled and printed in the September 1996 issue of *Sports Illustrated for Kids* (see sidebar 11.1), revealed what kids feel about such parents. Common complaints included:

- Parents coaching them, perhaps for the first time all week, during car rides to games or practice.
- Parents who try to pump kids up before games.
- Parents who become instant experts on the sport.

Sidebar 11.1: Top 10 Things Parents Don't Get About Kids and Sports

Reprinted with permission from Sports Illustrated for Kids:

You may not want to hear this, but most kids have a lot to say about their parents' involvement in their sports lives, especially what they don't like about it. Here is our Top 10 list of kids' advice for parents, gleaned from comments by S.I. FOR KIDS readers.[1]

10—During car rides to games or practice, kids don't want you to tell them how to do this or that. "I am not stupid," said one 12-year-old. "I know how to play the sport I play."

9—Kids can get psyched for a game without your help. "I hate when parents say, 'Are you ready? We're going to win,' like they're playing," said one kid.

8—It's your duty as a parent to sit quietly and watch your kids do wonderful things. Kids get bummed out when you miss games or yak it up too much with friends in the stands. "We're sweating and playing the game, and they're busy socializing," complained one girl.

7—If you don't know what you're talking about, kids don't want you to talk. Typical comments: "Parents think they know the rules, but they don't." "My mom asks annoying questions." And "I hate when my mom tells me to do things even when she doesn't know the first thing about sports."

6—Even if you do know what you're talking about, kids don't want you to talk (unless you're the coach). "I hate when parents tell us to do the exact opposite of what the coaches say," said one child. Added another: "If your parent isn't the coach, he or she shouldn't try to be one."

5—Kids wish you would practice what you preach about sportsmanship. "My mom always wants me to be a 'good sport,' but a lot of the time she blames the loss on the ref," claimed one kid. "Arguing with the refs is not only embarrassing, but it takes up time," said another.

4—Kids often can't hear you yelling when they're concentrating on the game. Sometimes, they can. Either way, they don't like it. "Parents yell advice you don't hear because you're so into playing the game. Afterward they say, 'Why didn't you listen to me?'" complained one child. Said others: "I feel embarrassed when my parents yell so loud that the whole town can hear," and "They yell and scream and look like dorks."

3—After they lose, kids don't want to be told it doesn't matter. Typical reactions: "I hate when we get knocked out of the playoffs and my parents say, 'You'll get them next time!'" and "When parents try to cheer you up after a loss, all they do is remind you of the score."

2—After they lose, kids don't want to be told that it does matter. "Parents take losses harder than we do," wrote one boy. Advised one girl: "You win some, you lose some, no big deal! Get over it!"

1—Kids just want to have fun. Parents just don't get this, kids say. Many kids say they would *rather play on a losing team* than sit on the bench on a winning one. Some would like to skip practice once in a while. "The thing that bugs me the most is that my parents take it too seriously," summed up one child. "They act like it's school."

- Parents who don't practice what they preach about sportsmanship.
- Parents who yell—criticism or advice—in the middle of the action.
- Parents who take losses harder than kids do.
- Parents who take the games too seriously when kids just want to have fun.

With all of this working against their enjoyment of the game—before, during, and after—it's no wonder kids are quitting sports. Fred Engh, founder and president of the National Alliance for Youth Sports, says the pressure that coaches and parents put on players is not worth it. "The travel teams, the all-stars, the championships—they're what the parents want. But children under the age of 10 don't necessarily want competition. What they want is to have fun."[12]

As with many problems in society, the combination of powerful media messages and parents' failure to help children understand these messages can be a major contributor to this growing crisis. Mike Legarza, a former small-college all-American basketball player with 18 years of college coaching experience on the West Coast, was working as a senior trainer from the acclaimed Positive Coaching Alliance at Stanford University to conduct clinics across the country aimed at "transforming youth sports so sports can transform youth." In a speech to parents in Mandeville, Louisiana, in 2002, he said: "The media tells you that if you're not No. 1, you're nothing. As a result, kids don't want to disappoint the coach or their parents. They're afraid to make mistakes, of looking stupid or incompetent, like they don't know what they're doing. And all the joy that used to be in youth sports can be destroyed."[13]

Sidebar 11.2: Commentary: It's Inexcusable When a Youth Coach Breaks Rules, Our Trust

Editor's note: The following commentary by John McCloskey was originally published on August 28, 2002, in the Shreveport Times, *where he was the sports editor in charge of an award-winning project entitled "Winning at All Costs."*[1]

My wife could see it on my face and hear it in my voice during a 10 p.m. dinner out last week.

The grind. The deadlines. The boss.

We've all felt it. She sensed it. And she had the perfect remedy.

"What's the *best* thing that happened to you today?" she asked.

And one thing immediately came to my weary mind.

Before a single word of this special series on winning at all costs had ever appeared in print, we received a phone call from a faithful reader who happened to catch an advertisement in the lower-right-hand corner on the very last page of the sports section.

It was an ad from our marketing department, perfectly designed to promote our eight-month investigation into this subject. The ad read: Whatever happened to "it's not whether you win or lose; it's how you play the game?"

Do we go to extremes to win at all costs?

What are the costs ethically and morally?

What is the message we are sending to our children?

This reader's story was of a football team of 9-year-olds whose coach broke the rules in order to win.

The rules of this league state each team must play all of its 9-year-old players for at least half of the game. These are 9-year-olds who eat lunch on a colored tray, get excited to dress up for Halloween and are not yet embarrassed to hang out with their parents in public.

They might, however, be embarrassed someday of the coach who kept the starters in the game long enough to secure an unbeaten season. Too bad he didn't realize how badly he was losing.

Losing because the opponents who played their not-so-good reserves were cheated.

Losing because his players couldn't possibly feel like winners if they knew their coach was cheating.

And losing because those players on his team who were not as good as the others didn't get the one thing in life 9-year-olds who join fun football leagues should get to do—play the game.

For some kids it's not about who scores or who wins. It's about wearing your jersey on the day of the game. It's about running through the banner the cheerleaders are holding. It's about trying your best and having fun.

Some of these less talented kids won't get to play on a team when the rules aren't so friendly. This is their only shot.

So was the best thing that happened to me last week this sad story? You bet. We can only hope more of you call or write us to tell us your examples of winning at all costs.

The purpose of this four-day series is to help everyone—including us—remember that winning isn't the most important thing.

You see we're in the business to win, too. We try to win more readers, advertising dollars and awards. Sometimes we miss what's important.

We invest a lot of time researching how many readers follow stories if we continue them on inside pages. We tell ourselves, "the best teams will get the best ink because more fans follow winners." And sometimes we give our readers what they want instead of what they need.

The coach of the 9-year-old team wants to see his name alongside his kids' names in this section. What he needs—and what his players and their families need—is to understand how much harm he is doing. He needs to be stripped of the privilege of being a leader, a role model, an adult respected by his 9-year-old team.

Is your child, your coach or your team cheating? If you suspect it, investigate it. And then tell us about it. Because while we are in the business to sell newspapers, some of us, including everyone who contributed to this project, care about the kids playing the games we cover every day.

Telling us a sad story might just be the best thing that happens to us all day.

3. Losing Control of Emotions and Accosting Officials, Opponents, and Players

Most of the research done in this particular area by news organizations has relied on shock value to gain the attention of readers and viewers. The truth of the matter is that some incidents are shocking, to say the least, such as the three examples used by the *Palm Beach Post* in a 2002 article on sportsmanship:

- In August 2000, more than a dozen parents and coaches were involved in a brawl over an umpire's call in a Miami T-ball game *for four- and five-year-olds*!

- In 1999 in Allentown, Pennsylvania, a former police officer was convicted of assault after offering $2 to a 10-year-old pitcher to bean a batter.
- And in 2002, a Massachusetts father of a 12-year-old hockey player was convicted of involuntary manslaughter for beating a coach to death after they argued at their sons' practice.[14]

But, as has already been mentioned, hearing these stories does not seem to affect a public that believes these incidents are so few that they do not warrant our concern. The following statistics, however, should clarify the myth that this brutish, shocking behavior is isolated:

- "An informal survey of youngsters by the Minnesota Amateur Sports Commission found 45 percent saying they had been called names, yelled at, or insulted while playing. An additional 18 percent said they had been hit, kicked, or slapped while participating."[15]
- According to a 2001 study published in *Sports Illustrated For Kids*, 74 percent of the more than 3,000 youngsters who responded said they had seen out-of-control adults at their games.[16]
- A survey in South Florida in 1999 of 500 adults found 82 percent saying parents were too aggressive in youth sports, and 56 percent said they had personally witnessed overly aggressive behavior.[17]

These events happen everywhere, in everyone's hometown. Whether you hear about it depends on the severity of the transgression and the local media's decision on where the story is presented among a lengthy list of daily or weekly news priorities. The founder and publisher of *Referee* magazine and the president of the National Association of Sports Officials, Barry Mano, has invaluable insight and intelligent analysis as to why parents lose control so often at events that are, in theory, geared toward recreation, relaxation, and enjoyment:

> One of the reasons you do what you do as a sports fan is because you feel fewer restraints than you do in your normal life.... [Fans] come [to games] to get away from restraint and what do they get confronted with? Somebody with a plastic whistle who when they blow it, the world stops. They give you something you didn't want to hear.[18]

Or the opposing team gives you something you didn't want to see. Or the opposing coach . . . or your coach . . . or someone on your team . . . or your own child. It's all about what we want, and when we don't get it, we can become furious. It's purely selfish behavior. Anyone who exhibits this behavior, who claims to be looking out for the "victimized" children of a rotten call, a questionable strategy, or a team member's consistently bad play, is missing a very crucial piece of evidence: According to the National Alliance for Youth Sports, 78 percent of children (and up to as much as 90 percent in other studies) would much rather play on a losing team than warm the bench for one that wins. The rotten calls and mistakes are not a big deal to most kids in youth sports. And for those kids who do get upset by these events (an increasing number as they become older), there are parents and coaches who have taken the time to stress sportsmanship over success and who should have no problem correcting their child's attitude. But again, parents with poor attitudes create an overwhelming majority of these problems by losing proper perspective, losing their tempers, and losing control of their actions.

4. Ignoring Serious Injuries

An informal survey of youngsters by the Minnesota Amateur Sports Commission found that 22 percent said they had been pressured to play while injured.[19] Professional athletes are often pressured by their coaches—Cowboys' Bill Parcells is a prominent example—to play hurt, and youth coaches are applying similar pressures. And just as pros are rushing back from these injuries, coaches are asking kids to do the same. Here are four areas of primary concern in terms of youth sports injuries:

Concussions

Although it was discussed in detail in chapter 10, the fact that a majority of concussions go undetected should cause great concern for any youth football coach who witnesses a player on the field absorb or dish out a severe helmet-to-helmet hit. Players who are struck in the head via other collisions—with a player's knee or the ground—should also be given special attention to prevent a second, potentially deadly collision in the same game. A key point to remember is that a player who suffers such an injury may not be able to communicate his injury. The tougher the player, the more dangerous the situation, because a player who can "take a hit" might hop up after a collision and still be in a complete daze. If he can find the huddle, the sideline, or the position on the field that he needs to be in on the next play, others may not recognize he has been severely injured. Therefore, coaches must be alert and prepared to take major hits seriously.

Overuse/Year-Round Participation

Athletes specializing in a sport that requires year-round participation, or athletes in more than one sport who are using the same repetitive motions, may be more susceptible to injury, especially at the youth level. Proper rest, stretching, and warm-up techniques may sound like simple solutions, but they are not being properly managed by coaches according to most studies on youth sports injuries:

- About one in three children, ages 5 to 14, who play organized sports will be injured at some point while participating in individual and team competition, according to a survey released this month by the National Safe Kids Campaign, a Washington, D.C.–based nonprofit group dedicated to preventing childhood injury.[20]
- Dr. Len Remia at the Cleveland Clinic Hospital says teenage pitchers are undergoing elbow reconstruction surgery four times as often now as they were five years ago. "If a kid has pain, and it's not going away, it's not normal."[21]
- The *Physician and Sportsmedicine* journal estimated that 30 percent to 50 percent (3.6 million to 6 million) of youth sports injuries are related to overuse, which has replaced traumatic injuries as the most common reasons children visit doctors with a sports injury.[22]
- The Consumer Product Safety Commission reports that roughly 4 million kids between ages 5 and 16 suffer sports-related injuries each year that require a visit to the doctor's office. Other groups estimate that as many as 8 million more kids just shrug it off and play hurt. Those numbers are about double of what they were 10 years ago, according to the commission.[23]
- Each year, an estimated 50,000 athletes, the majority of whom are between the ages of 15 and 25, tear their anterior cruciate knee

ligament. Girls are more susceptible than boys to the injury, and with more of them playing competitive basketball and soccer, the numbers have gone up.[24]

Premature Return to Competition

Athletes who do sit out do not want to sit out for long. When winning is placed above an athlete's health—especially in youth sports where bodies are still developing, are less mature, and are therefore more fragile—the premature return to the athletic field after an injury can do permanent damage. The *Los Angeles Times* reported in May of 2004 that organized sports have a 20 percent re-injury rate, according to the National Youth Sports Safety Foundation, a nonprofit organization based in Boston that tracks youth injuries in sports. Kids often attempt to come back before rehabilitation because of external pressures focusing on personal character or team needs.[25]

Weight Training

The debate as to when a child can safely begin strength training using weights can seem as heated as an emotional contest between crosstown rivals. But, as with the sporting events, cooler heads and common sense should prevail. Carl Dubois' reporting in the *Shreveport Times* in 1999 summarizes this issue by imploring parents and coaches to use caution in allowing children to lift too much weight too early:

> Josh Smith, a fitness trainer who specializes in youth strength training for the Cooper Institute of Aerobic Studies in Dallas, says children can lift weights before their growth plates are set.
>
> "You go to an orthopedic surgeon who will take an X-ray of the knees, look at the joint and can tell if a person has some growing left to do," Smith says. "You can lift if you haven't stopped growing but you have to be extremely careful."
>
> Kyle Pierce, an adjunct instructor at LSUS, has a doctorate in exercise science from Auburn University. He's a director and coach for the USA Weightlifting Development Center at LSUS, a joint venture of the university, the Shreveport Regional Sports Authority and USA Weightlifting.
>
> He believes children can start early to make the most of the body type they have.

"You can always do some sort of strength training," Pierce says. "A baby pulls himself out of a playpen or crib. That takes strength. Some parents are always against lifting weights or strength training, but no parent stops a kid from taking the groceries in or carrying a heavy bag of fertilizer, even though the bag might weigh more than the weights they'd be using."

Pierce says 11 years old is usually the ideal age to begin formalized weight training—under strict supervision by a qualified coach.

As for worries about a child's growth plates being a determiner of when and how much to lift, Pierce says there's a lot of misinformation being sold as expert advice.

"I always ask for physicians to show me the literature on that," he says. "It's just not in the literature. Growth plate damage can occur in youth football and basketball. There are fewer injuries in weight lifting than those, because it's supervised much better."

But Dr. Jim Brown, an Atlanta-based expert on youth sports and sports medicine, says it's difficult to know exactly where to draw the line about strength training and enhancing body type.

"You can't take little kids and put them in a research program," Brown says. "There are ethical considerations and laws to prevent that, so a lot of doctors make their best educated guess based on their training and what they see with their patients."

Dr. William S. Bundrick, a sports medicine specialist who works with the Shreveport Captains and Louisiana Tech athletes, says the "growth centers" aren't hindered unless children try to lift more weight than they should.

"The ones who try to 'max out' at a high weight, to see how much they can lift one time, they're the ones at risk," Bundrick says.[26]

5. Pushing Athletes Too Early

Georgia Tech sports medicine expert Dr. Jim Brown, in his book *Sports Talent: How to Identify and Develop Outstanding Athletes*, writes: "Does a child have to be a star at 8 to be a star at 18? No. Earlier is not necessarily better in terms of sports-specific training. There is plenty of evidence to show that the real athletes kick in at age 13 or 14. . . . I am alarmed that kids start playing organized sports at 5, 6, 7 years old because I think they are missing the kind of backyard neighborhood experiences that do a lot toward building sports skills and social skills such as settling arguments in an unstructured way."[27]

6. Mistaking a Child's Age for Their Preparedness to Compete

This is very different from number 5 because often we equate a child's age to his or her readiness to participate in certain levels of sport. Former Buffalo and Penn State University standout Mike McBath was an undersized 150 pounds as a senior in high school, bulked up in college, and became big enough to compete in professional football. "Just because kids are the same chronological age, they're not always the same physiological age," McBath says. "I have a 15-year-old son and I run into this a lot—parents who are expecting all the players at a certain age to be on a level playing field and it just doesn't happen like that. Parents can't expect their undersized kid to compete against someone who develops early. At the same time, kids who are late bloomers should not be counted out. My situation is proof of that."[28]

> As youngsters learn the intricacies of a sport, they must contend with growing bodies that can leave their coordination wobbly at times. And young athletes are often grouped by age, not by height and weight, resulting in opponents who are the same age, but vastly different in size. Particularly in contact sports such as football, the mismatches can lead to injury.[29]

All of the "problems" above also have their exceptions:

- Some kids need and benefit from being pushed harder than others.
- There is great value in teaching youngsters the importance of setting goals, working hard to obtain them, and always aiming to succeed, not fail.
- Emotions can be good in sports. Being fired up is not a bad thing in many situations.
- Growing tougher by overcoming minor injuries helps build character and can increase the effort and dedication of teammates.
- Returning to the playing field as soon as safely permitted can ignite a team and can earn the respect of others for an athlete.
- Athletes who truly have fun competing at an early age should not be deprived of competition if they are physically and mentally ready to participate.
- There is a great lesson to be learned by the youngster who is able to overcome physical limitations and succeed despite being smaller than other competitors, if it is safe for that child to compete.

The key is that these exceptions remain just that—exceptions and not the rule. Too often the problems in youth sports are not viewed as problems but as rites of passage.

- Iron sharpens iron, but an eight-year-old need not become a chiseled weapon in a Little League war.
- As Vince Lombardi has said, and is misquoted 99 percent of the time: "Winning is not a sometime thing; it's an all the time thing. You don't win once in a while; you don't do things right once in a while; you do them right all the time. Winning is a habit. Unfortunately, so is losing." He was right, but he was talking to grown men playing professional football, so surely Lombardi's important lesson can wait until after the Pop Warner season ends (and Lombardi never said winning is the only thing).
- Young athletes often have fond memories of the coaches who spit fire when motivating a team to win. But consider how effective a team of nine-year-olds can be while walking around with wide eyes and gaping mouths, having just received an emotional charge to dive into battle.
- Overcoming injury, age, inexperience, or size is something a youngster can and should be proud of, but "safety first" should be a commonsense rule and not a worn-out cliché. There's a reason why a 70-pound seventh-grader is not asked to lock horns with a heavyweight.
- Above all, the line separating fun from fanatical should be reserved for elite athletes at the professional level. And youth sports coaches and parents should not seek to find elite athletes because they are too far from reaching that level. If they are truly great, they will succeed without being molded into the perfect athlete. Ask Marv Marinovich.

This chapter's intent was not to fill page after page with examples and personal testimonies of past and present problems. In fact, much of this type of writing was purposefully left out because the point is to move forward in a meaningful, organized, and hopeful direction by providing expert opinions for why and how these problems exist and persist. Chapters 16 and 17 will focus on solutions to ethical and moral problems in all of sports, including the ability that leagues, coaches, and parents have in solving these problems in youth sports.

There are countless resources (many of which are listed in sidebar 16.1) from which to construct a quality plan to maintain a healthy sporting environment—from selecting players to practicing to playing for championships. It is not enough, however, to have an organized plan. Nor is it sufficient to leave the administration of this system to coaches who have been trained or certified. The evidence is clear: knowing the right thing to do is not enough. Parents may know right from wrong, but they are blinded by their obsession to force success upon their children. Penalties must be harsh for breaking sportsmanship codes. It is our belief that, while each state, county, and city will have its own rules, a national organization is needed to carry out the uniform penalties when these rules are broken. Several of these organizations or alliances exist, but a uniform code of ethics and a structured system might enable more leagues to benefit. Too often a youth can be banned from one league only to begin playing in another league across the river. More needs to be done at the legislative level to ensure that enough pressure is being placed on leagues to take note of a person's background before taking their registration fee. Future generations of parents will raise children based on the environment they are observing today. Sadly, an entire generation seems to have slipped out of the grasp of the current inconsistent system. Many reckless parents and coaches are leading young athletes, and there is little or no sign of improvement in sportsmanship or morality. The improvement must start—in a meaningful way—right now.

12

Winning at All Costs:
What We're Driven to Do and Why

If sport and life are inseparable, and if the major problems with organized sports today reflect the struggles of a society faced with a daily battle between good and evil, how are we to solve the ills that stain the purity of sports when society cannot even agree on what is good and what is evil? We can start by taking what we all agree is wrong—performance-enhancing drugs, violent and poor sportsmanship, and purposeful, premeditated cheating—and increase by tenfold the penalties for breaking the rules. But therein lies the biggest problem facing sports today. It isn't the steroids, the attacks on referees, or the use of ineligible players that corrupts competition so much; it is, instead, the fact that those who possess the power to punish are themselves choosing to push the envelope between what is right and what makes them rich. Take steroids as an example: Fans want bigger, faster, and stronger stars, and leagues always want more fans, so rules against performance-enhancing drugs have been slow to come by, slow to become stringent, and soft when it comes to the penalty phase. The line between good and evil is disappearing (see chapter 14, "Who's In Charge? Administration Is Part of the Problem").

The dilemmas sports face today do not come as a surprise to Michael Josephson, who founded the The Joseph & Edna Josephson Institute of Ethics, "a public-benefit, nonpartisan, nonprofit membership organization with a goal to improve the ethical quality of society by advocating principled reasoning and ethical decision making." The Josephson Institute is a leader in teaching organizations of all sizes and statures—from big businesses to little leagues—the obvious but oft-forgotten ethical foundation upon which all true successes must be built. Josephson has a clear perspective on good versus evil.

The world is always filled with Darth Vaders and Luke Skywalkers—the dark side of the force and the light side of the force. At various times in our society one side seems more dominant. Right now we are, in my mind, way too skewed toward the dark side. There is an expediency mentality that is perpetuated by shows like *Survivor, Temptation Island, The Apprentice,* shows that are blatantly and openly celebrating manipulation and deception and winning at any costs. But those people pay a very high price. And for whatever reason, people who are controlling these television reality shows are not concerned with that.[1]

D. Stanley Eitzen, author of a 1995 thesis for the annual Angelo State University Symposium on American Values, entitled "Ethical Dilemmas in American Sport," does a good job summarizing *"The Winner-Take-All Society . . .* we heap incredible rewards on winners and barely reward others . . . winning supersedes all other considerations . . . moral values have become confused with the bottom line." Eitzen's thesis is, "American values are responsible for many of the ethical problems found in sport. We glorify winners and forget losers." This sounds simple enough, but Eitzen more than proves his point by connecting good with evil—"strategy" with "cheating"— and by thoroughly describing and specifying normative cheating and normative violence:

> Getting such a competitive edge unfairly is viewed by many in sports as "strategy" rather than cheating. In some sports, illegal acts are accepted as part of the game. . . . The forms of normative cheating are . . . more widespread than commonly thought, and they clearly violate ethical principles. In basketball, for example, it is common for a player to pretend to be fouled in order to receive an undeserved free throw and give the opponent an undeserved foul. In football, players are sometimes coached to use illegal techniques to hold or trip opponents without detection. The practice is common in baseball for the home team to "doctor" its field to suit its strengths and minimize the strengths of a particular opponent. . . . Home teams have been known to gain an edge by increasing the heat by several degrees from normal in the visitors' dressing room to make the athletes sluggish. (Several college football programs paint the visiting locker room pink, a color said to make players less aggressive). . . . "Normative cheating" acts to achieve unfair advantages that are accepted as part of the game. The culture of most sports is to get a competitive advantage over the opponent even if it means taking an unfair advantage. When this occurs, I argue, then sport is sending a message—winning is more important than being fair. In this way, sport is a microcosm of society where the bottom line is more important than how you got there.[2]

Eitzen also successfully defends the theory that athletics hinders, not helps, moral development:

> A widely held assumption . . . is that sport is a primary vehicle by which youth are socialized to adopt the values and morals of society. The irony is, however, that sport does not enhance positive character traits. Philosopher Charles Banham has said, ". . . [sport] encourages selfishness, envy, conceit, hostility, and bad temper. Far from ventilating the mind, it stifles it. Good sportsmanship may be a product of sport, but so is bad sportsmanship." . . . It is not surprising that research reveals consistently that sport stifles moral reasoning and moral development. . . . Physical educators Sharon Stoll and Jennifer Beller (found):
>
> 1. Athletes score lower than their non-athlete peers on moral development.
> 2. Male athletes score lower than female athletes in moral development.
> 3. Moral reasoning scores for athletic populations steadily decline from the ninth grade through university age, whereas scores for non-athletes tend to increase. "While sport does build character if defined as loyalty, dedication, sacrifice, and teamwork, it does not build moral character in the sense of honesty, responsibility, and justice."[3]

A final important note Eitzen makes solidifies the connection between poor moral judgment on and off the playing field. This link shows that there is little to no separation between the actions of athletes and nonathletes.

> Moral development theorists agree that the fundamental structure of moral reasoning remains relatively stable from situation to situation. Thus, when coaches and athletes—in their zeal to succeed—corrupt the ideals of sportspersonship and fair play, they are likely to employ or condone similar tactics outside sport.[4]

Many others agree with this thinking:

- Barry Mano, president of the National Association of Sports Officials: "Sports is life with the volume turned up. So to some measure, we shouldn't be surprised by the characterization [of sports mirroring life]. We should be disappointed, but not surprised."[5]
- David Callahan, author of *The Cheating Culture: Why More Americans Are Doing Wrong to Get Ahead*: "There's a new social Darwinism in that the rewards have become so large for the people

at the top that the incentives to do anything to get there become greater and greater."

- Sociologist Harry Edwards: "Any time you find society in crisis, athletes get drawn into it." Edwards has long argued that sports have a profound impact on the larger culture and that a serious problem arises when people lose their role models. "We're being stripped of our heroes, of our Horatio Algers. Then we become in danger of believing in no one and nothing. Losing faith in everything is a very dangerous thing to happen to the world's only superpower that's used to thinking of itself as having higher moral authority."[6]

- Jack Marshall, president of ProEthics, a Virginia-based ethics training and consulting firm: "That's why the Iraqi prison scandal has been so damaging. It undermines our whole foundation of belief. And baseball is supposed to be about apple pie, motherhood, the great American way. If it becomes about cheating, it loses what makes it so valuable to our society. . . . The sports story just contributes to the general feeling that nobody is playing by the rules. The public can get to the point where it says, 'I've been a real sap. Nobody embraces any real values, and I might as well cheat just like everybody else.' "[7]

- Brenda Light Bredemeier, a psychologist who codirects the University of Notre Dame's Mendelson Center for Sports, Character and Community: "First of all, there's no question that within sports is the great opportunity to teach moral values. [Within sports], the greatest predictor of moral behavior is the child's perception of how his or her coach and peers define success. That becomes the norm for the child. And athletes take that norm off the playing field and out onto the street."[8]

- Charles Yesalis, Penn State University professor, author, and steroids expert: "There is so much money involved. . . . We are so appearance-oriented. We live in a society [without regard for] ethics. Kids went through eight years of Bill Clinton having sex in the White House. Patrick Moynihan said it nicely: 'We down-define deviance so low that there ain't nothin' wrong anymore!' We have some journalists who fabricate stories. We have some professors who fabricate research. We have some corporate officials who behave in the most egregious manner. How many other types of entertainers besides athletes, whether they be singers or actors or actresses, use drugs."[9]

- Michael Josephson, Josephson Institute of Ethics: "Good decision-making always has ethics as a ground rule, but people in the business world aren't always interested in ethics; they're interested in getting a job done, and they're willing to consider ethics. Our approach [in helping organizations better understand the importance of ethics] is that a good decision is both good and ethical. You can't call it a good decision if it doesn't work, if it doesn't accomplish a goal. What our mission statement means is we must begin to ingrain into decision-makers—whether they are at corporate level . . . military . . . law enforcement or kids—is that decisions need to be guided by moral principles as well as pragmatic considerations. Clearly in society, people are going to be looking at the decisions made by Enron, WorldCom, Arthur Anderson, Adelphia, or for that matter the Catholic Church and its decision to cover up and repress the information about sexual abuse. All of those decisions were not only unethical but were quite self-destructive and societally destructive.

  Everybody wants to be in some sense successful. You want a book that's read. A preacher wants to reach people's lives. So, effectiveness is a critical aspect of people's motivation. Unfortunately, in modern times the ethical dimension has become less and less relevant to decision-makers. So, young people are deciding to cheat on exams at a huge rate, in respect to 74 percent overall who cheated on exams last year—and these are the ones who admit it—without conscience, because all they focused on was effectiveness and accomplishing goals."[10]

Academic fraud that is regularly committed in pursuit of "accomplishing goals" is, perhaps, the most telling sign that society's acceptance with cheating—a steady slide into the pit of normative cheating—will not be correcting itself. And it will not be corrected without an enormous effort on behalf of everyone, beginning with parents, along with major responsibilities falling on guidance counselors, teachers, principals, education boards, college recruiters, advisors, professors, and even legislators. The epidemic is especially concerning at the collegiate level, where keeping players eligible ap-

Sidebar 12.1: Commentary:
Winning at All Costs Is a Big Loss in Game of Life
By James D. Nickel[1]

I used to be a student-athlete. I have known the exhilaration of sinking a basket with no time left and putting the game into OT, of scorching the nets for 30-plus points, of competing on championship teams.

Those wonderful times are part of a season of opportunity long past. I've got "salt and pepper" hair now and according to the ancient writings, gray locks equal wisdom (in my case, I think it is wisdom learned through hard knocks and not necessarily wise choices).

I love sport—everything about it—the competition, the strategy, the heroics, the statistics. But I am concerned about where sport is going.

Like most, I am concerned about the excess money, the corruption in some places, the cheating (especially in the academic arena). Sport to some has become the absolute grid through which everything in life is to be interpreted. When sport becomes *the* grid, when winning at all costs becomes *summum bonum* (the highest good), then the outcome of such a fallacious commitment is not winning, but losing.

History teaches us many lessons. In sports history, once every generation or so, a student athlete comes along who blazes a trail of principled instruction. One such athlete was Eric Liddell (1902–1945) of Edinburgh University, nicknamed the "Flying Scotsman" for his swift feet on the running track.

To Liddell, his running was an extension of his governing life principle. This standard can be reflected in a verse from the Old Testament (I Samuel 2:30), ". . . them that honor Me I will honor, and they that despise Me shall be lightly esteemed."

Liddell was no pushover; he ran to win. He would often quip to news reporters that he "hated to lose." In the 1924 Summer Olympics (in Paris, France), he was a member of the Great Britain team and he was slated to run the premier race of the Games, the 100 meters. When he discovered that the heats for this race were to be run on Sunday, he refused to run based upon his principle of honoring God. He would not surrender this principle for any price whether it be the glory of a "blue ribbon," country or King.

Although he did not run the 100 meters, another race just "happened" to appear on his radar. That race was the 400 meters, a distance that turned out to be a "natural" for Liddell's stride. He won by 5 meters and set a world record (47.6 seconds). Shortly after the Paris Olympiad, Liddell graduated (BSc in Pure Science) and sailed for China as a missionary. In 1945, he died in a Japanese internment camp in occupied China.

Liddell perceived his running through a grid greater than sport or himself. As he confessed, "God made me for a purpose, for China. But He also made me fast and when I run I feel His pleasure."

He ultimately competed for a gold medal that was "not corruptible, but incorruptible." The wisdom lesson to be dispensed is this: If one wants to truly compete and love sport, then one must view sport through a grid that is greater than the temporality of any human glory (whether it be money won, trophies received, or simply winning at all costs).

To do otherwise is to lose in the game of life.

pears to be a purposeful sham organized by the athletic departments themselves. This unimaginable quest to win has in recent years undermined the core of institutions like Minnesota, New Mexico State, California, Marshall, Southern California, Fresno State, St. Bonaventure, Georgia, Fairfield, Missouri, Baylor, and more. These instances will be addressed in detail in chapter 13 since the undeniably wrong cheating originates from those who are supposed to in charge. It is yet another example of morality's decline, which is leading to the disassembling of the education system's ethical framework. It is an enemy of the state that is eroding this country. And, not surprisingly, it coincides with a decline in religious values. Between 1993 and 2002, the number of people who said they had no religion rose from 9 percent to nearly 14 percent, according to a study by the National Opinion Research Center at the University of Chicago.

The case of Saratoga High School (California) illustrates how cheating has become routine in America. During the 2003–2004 school year, the top-ranked public school was involved in a highly publicized cheating scandal initially uncovered when a student who had obtained a copy of an advanced-placement history exam in advance of the test was turned in by classmates who caught him reviewing the exam in the school library. His was just one of several incidents of cheating revealed by the school's subsequent investigation. As the San Jose *Mercury News* deduced during weeks of interviews with dozens of students, teachers, parents, and administrators, "a school like Saratoga may have an especially tough time combating cheating, because it can't change significantly one of the root causes: its high-achieving, pressure-packed culture."

- "You always have the feeling you have to get ahead because every-one else is," one student at Saratoga said.
- "The parents do play a role, creating the mindset that without a good college, your job is going to be working at Target," said an-other.
- "Pressure is pushing kids to the limit," said the father of a student suspended for accepting a stolen English test.[11]

Justifying the cheating as necessary or minimizing cheating for any number of unacceptable reasons is bad enough, but finding blame in America's intense pressure to be the best is pathetic. What's more, this is not a new phenomenon. Competition has always existed and it should never cease to. There is nothing wrong with separating the best from the rest—in or out of sports—as long as it is done within the obvious boundaries of ethics and morality. The world should de-termine who is rewarded the best positions in the workforce and be-yond by the credentials and accomplishments of its people—not politics, wealth, connections, or race. So pressure and competition should not equate to a justification of any kind for cheating. Yet somehow, this type of dishonesty is a growing problem and threatens to become normative cheating, if it has not already crossed into that territory.

The Saratoga student who obtained the stolen copy of the test at-tempted to deflect some blame and reduce the severity of the offense by claiming that he had not asked for the stolen test and had studied the night before. "I don't consider it an extreme form of cheating," he said. It is yet another example of how the mind-set in America and elsewhere today is that some dishonesty, when combined with some good, honest, well-intentioned hard work, is acceptable to override feelings of guilt. When confronted with the evidence, not many peo-ple—unless, perhaps, they are arguing in a court of law with hopes of receiving a reduced sentence—will deny that their actions are wrong. Cheaters who are caught often 'fess up, as was the case at Saratoga High School, but it is their lack of guilt that led them to cheating in the first place, and this attitudinal flaw intensifies the problem. Was Martha Stewart wrongfully singled out and punished too harshly for her questionable actions? Perhaps, but it is the fact that she did not 'fess up—devoting her time to explaining how she became a victim instead of accepting any responsibility—that is the reason her company laid off hundreds of employees, lost millions in profits, and went from being one the strongest brand names to ranking lower than Enron.

"Today is a shameful day, a shameful day for me and my family and for my beloved company and for its employees and partners," she told the judge. "What was a small personal matter became over the last two years an almost fatal circus event of unprecedented proportions. I'm very sorry it has come to this." What it came to is not just a five-year prison sentence for her and big losses for her company; the impact stretched much further. "It has cost us [taxpayers] probably $5 million to prosecute her. Plus, 200 people, many high-level, have been laid off in her company," veteran entertainment industry analyst and media investor Hal Vogel says. "On top of that," he added, K-mart's sales of Stewart's household brands suffered drastically, and "investors and pension funds, such as large state funds for teachers and nurses, may have sustained losses in the billions of dollars."[12] Stewart said she was sorry that others had been hurt by the scandal, but her insistence to this day that she was not guilty and that her selling of the stock after receiving inside information, "a small personal matter," is simply wrong. It's the quintessential example of ethics being minimized and justified both internally and externally with the same fervor. It does not matter whether she feels the crime should go unpunished because of her enormous power or because the magnitude of her offense is so insignificant. For whatever reason, she believes some cheating is acceptable—again, normative—and she's not alone. National surveys show cheating is widespread and growing in America's high schools. The San Jose *Mercury News'* reporting on the Saratoga cheating scandal offers evidence of this:

In December, the *Saratoga [High School] Falcon*, the student newspaper, ran six stories examining plagiarism and other cheating on campus. In one story, staff writers Shenje Hshieh and Lauren Sun quoted an unnamed junior: "I really don't like cheating. But sometimes there's so much to do and so little time to do everything. Usually I end up either not finishing my homework or not being able to study for tests. I can't afford to let my grades drop, so I just end up cheating on the homework or tests." Teachers struggle with such attitudes. Three years ago, in response to an amnesty offer, 27 of 31 students in one of Kerry Mohnike's English classes admitted to completing an assignment on *The Great Gatsby* by plagiarizing from an online study guide. All but two of the 27 told Mohnike that they didn't have the time to do the work themselves.[13]

Without enough time to do the work, these students took "shortcuts." This is the word the United States Anti-Doping Agency chose to use in each of six public service announcements (PSAs) on its Web site in 2004 featuring Olympic athletes promoting clean competition. Track cyclist Giddeon Massie's brief video ends, almost as an afterthought, with this statement: "Taking shortcuts and stuff, that's not going to get you anywhere." But how true is this? Shortcuts such as steroids actually work. Their success and popularity are their greatest danger. Believing otherwise, or pretending that kids will buy this, seems ineffective. Shot-put thrower John Godina looks at it from a different perspective. He knows trying to scare people away from using performance-enhancing drugs won't work either. "Kids are educated viewers," Godina says. "They're going to catch on if you try to intimidate them. Kids know it's their choice. If they see you trying to be too tough, they won't take you seriously." Godina, in his announcement, explains that, "By taking shortcuts, you're going to build an inadequacy in yourself and a feeling that you cheated yourself." As we have learned from other doping experts, some athletes will cheat no matter what. Education, including PSAs featuring model athletes, is aimed at reaching anyone who has yet to make up his or her mind. Cheaters don't care about inadequacy. In fact, they almost appear to believe you have no right to question their adequacy when they are accused of doping. Perhaps they have to convince themselves that cheating is OK in order to defend themselves. Tim Montgomery told a grand jury that he used steroids, which is rather shocking having heard his vehement public denial of doping. He must have known the truth would come out eventually, but he was aggressive and arrogant, perhaps as an overcompensation for his inadequacy.

Just like the line between good and evil, the one separating feeling inadequate and seeking improvement is wearing thin from being crossed frequently. Bulking up with weight training and supplements can be a legitimate path to success. But the mentality of those who seek and usually find rapid gains in size and strength is dangerous because there is a sense of always needing more, which we have already discovered can lead to the well-traveled bridge to steroids. Several examples taken from the *Shreveport Times'* national award-winning series in 2002, entitled "Winning at All Costs," bear this out:

- A 110-pound Haughton High School (Louisiana) sophomore receiver and defensive back in 2001 used weight training and nutritional supplementation to gain 50 pounds in the summer before his junior season. "I was little," he said. "I wouldn't be playing football right now if I wasn't taking anything. I'd just be serving water. I've worked hard this past year, but I wouldn't weigh as much [without supplements]."[14]

- Another player from Airline High School (Louisiana) grew from a 150-pound cornerback his freshman year to a 210-pound linebacker, his goal by the 2002 season. Airline strength coach Gary Smith says, "You can take away the supplements and he'd still be pretty strong." But now that he's on the smaller side as linebacker at a Division I-AA school, the temptation to juice will be stronger than ever.[15]

- Haughton baseball coach Glenn Maynor said the number of kids putting in the time in the weight room has skyrocketed since he graduated from high school in 1989. His team now starts in the fall, lifting weights three days a week. "It's made a great difference in our program," he said. "We hit more home runs, and singles in the gap turn into doubles in the gap. Pitchers get more velocity, and it makes you faster."

- Bucs' third baseman Seth Holloway, who will be the second-year starter at quarterback in the fall, said the weight room is catching on with all ages. "Used to be there was nobody working out. Now you have kids that are going to be in the eighth grade coming up there," he said. "That's why they open it in the morning and the evening. It's amazing."[16] But the power of incentives and the pressure created by more competition is also amazing.

After high school, the incentives and pressures become significantly greater. Bossier City sports psychologist Edd Wilbanks told the *Shreveport Times* in 1999 that "90 percent of high school sports participants are just that—participants. Only 10 percent are real athletes." In college, he says, the ratio reverses. Ninety percent of those on college teams are bona fide athletes.[17] That being so, the discovery in 2004 that the University of Colorado was one of many football programs to lure recruits with alcohol and sex was not a surprise to many who have long known of the violations regularly being committed by schools in search of star athletes. Former Miami and NFL defensive lineman Dan Sileo told the *Calgary Herald* he was drunk during his visits to Miami, Minnesota, Ohio State, Pittsburgh, and Maryland in the early 1980s. "I don't remember a recruiting trip I didn't get drunk on," Sileo said. "No strip clubs, but there were always plenty of girls. At Ohio State, I got so drunk I fell down 25 steps at a bar called the Mine Shaft and the coaches thought it was cool. It's all about showing the kid a good time."[18] Jim Fitzpatrick, who played at Illinois State from 1977 to 1981 and later with the Tampa Bay Bandits of the United States Football League, added: "I went on recruiting trips. I was given money to treat recruits to a great time, including all the beer or booze they can drink, all the food they can eat and, last but not least, all the girls they could get. Some of the stories were so bad they can't be repeated. It's been going on for decades. Unfortunately, with the moral decline of our country, so goes the expectations of what defines a great time. With all the XXX-rated films on Showtime and HBO, the profanity on every network, how can anyone expect a teenager to stop in his tracks after everybody else says it's OK?"[19] In a FOX Sports television special (*Beyond the Glory, Season 4*) that aired on April 4, 2004, Pro Football Hall of Fame and Dallas Cowboys running back Tony Dorsett said, "I had everything imaginable offered to me. I'll never forget this one university [offering] me so much I said, 'There is no way you can do all of that for me.' . . . [and then a] very prominent coach coming to me and opening up an envelope full of money—I mean just *full* of it."[20]

The most recent recruiting lowlights:

• *Colorado University, 2004:* Three women are suing the program after claiming they were raped during or just after a December 2001 off-campus party for football players and recruits. Katie Hnida, a former place-kicker for the university, told *Sports Illustrated*'s Rick Reilly that she was raped and endured a year of sexual harassment by many of her teammates.[21] Also, a former athletics department employee said she had been raped by a university football player in September of 2001, but that Mr. Barnett had promised to back the player "100 percent." Boulder Police investigated a total of seven claims of sexual assault at the university since 1997.[22]

- *University of Miami, 2004:* Willie Williams, the team's top recruit this year, has been arrested 11 times since 1999—a record school officials said they were unaware of when he signed a national letter of intent.

Sports Illustrated's story on the Colorado scandal detailed similar incidents at other major universities, fueling speculation that the occurrences were the norm and not exceptions:

- *Michigan, 1996:* Five basketball players entertaining high school star Mateen Cleaves with strippers and alcohol at a party in a Detroit hotel were involved in a car accident when their SUV rolled over. Then-Michigan president James Duderstadt personally apologized to Cleaves' parents. Cleaves chose to play at Michigan State and led them to a national championship.
- *Florida, 2000:* While on a recruiting trip to Gainesville, offensive-line prospect Jason Respert of Warner Robins, Georgia, was arrested and charged with burglary and attempted sexual battery for an incident that occurred after he'd been drinking in a bar with a fellow recruit and a Florida Gators player. Respert plead to lesser charges of criminal trespassing and simple battery. He is now a junior at Tennessee.
- *Alabama, 2002:* The NCAA banned the Crimson Tide team from postseason play for two years for violations that include players inviting strippers on campus to entertain visiting high school recruits from 1997 to 1999.
- *Oregon, 2002:* During his recruiting visit to Eugene, blue-chip running back Lynell Hamilton of Stockton, California, was taken to parties where, he says, he was offered alcohol, marijuana, and sex. Hamilton is turned off by the experience, telling the *Stockton Record*, "Oregon was my number one choice, but they blew it for both of us." He signed with San Diego State and rushed for 1,087 yards as a freshman in 2003.[23]
- *Alabama State, 2003:* After an in-house investigation, fired football coach L. C. Cole exposed that he allegedly paid strippers to entertain recruits.

- *Minnesota, 2003:* Several Gophers players took top offensive line recruit Lydon Murtha of Hutchinson, Minnesota, to a strip club during a December campus visit. Murtha later rescinded his verbal commitment to Minnesota and signed with Nebraska, though he told the Minneapolis *Star-Tribune* that the club visit had nothing to do with his decision. Other 2004 recruits later said that they too were taken to the establishment on their visits and supplied with alcohol. The university is investigating the charges.

- *Brigham Young University, 2004:* Provo, Utah, police probed allegations that a sex crime occurred at a late-night party for Cougars recruits in January at a house shared by three football players. Investigators found no basis for criminal charges but turned up evidence of other recent football parties that included sexual advances and alcohol. Consuming alcohol and engaging in nonmarital or extramarital sex violate the school's honor code, and university officials are investigating. (Running back Reynaldo Brathwaite has since been expelled, and cornerbacks James Allen and Shannon Benton and defensive tackle C. J. Ah You were suspended.)

- *Colorado State and others, 2004:* Steve Lower, owner of Denver-based Hardbodies Entertainment, told the *Rocky Mountain News* that his company, which has branches in Houston and Las Vegas, had sent strippers to entertain recruits at parties at Colorado State, Houston, Northern Colorado, Rice, and the University of Nevada at Las Vegas, in addition to Colorado. Officials at all the schools denied knowledge of such activity. Rice president Malcolm Gillis made the following university statement: "I can't believe any of our athletes are that stupid."[24]

(See chapter 14, "Who's in Charge? Administration Is Part of the Problem," for a look at more than two dozen incidents of academic fraud or other extra benefits from 2002–2004.)

While recruiting scandals would appear to be limited to the college level, where the rules allow recruiting, many sports fans know recruiting has also occurred to some degree in high school. Some lowlights from across the country:

- *California:* Santa Fe Christian football player Chase McBride, a senior in 2001, said his school "has started putting more emphasis on really building up the sports programs."[25] The school has hired former NFL quarterback Brian Sipe as football coach, and despite just 280 students, the school's athletes reached No. 1 in the state in its division and sent four athletes to Division I-A. Former major league pitcher Rick Aguilera is an assistant baseball coach.

- *Colorado:* The *Denver Post* reported that about 2,600 students changed high schools without changing their home address last year.
- *Florida:* In Orlando, iconic football coach Bill Gierke left Dr. Phillips High School for Edgewater High School. Edgewater received an influx of talented players, who exploited loopholes in the state's transfer laws. Following this situation, Orange County Public Schools instituted a new transfer policy, making transfers ineligible for high school sports for one calendar year.
- *Georgia:* EastCobbbaseball.com is an independent traveling summer baseball team based out of Marietta that brings in players from several high schools throughout the area. It is alleged that members of the team actively recruit other student-athletes to come play at their high schools.
- *Illinois:* The Quincy High School boys basketball team, one of the top teams in the nation, faced an investigation by the Illinois High School Association (IHSA) for allegations the team recruited foreign exchange students, for example Dejan Dokovic and Kristjan Makke. The IHSA ended its investigation in July, closing the matter. "While it is apparent a violation of the IHSA recruiting bylaw may have occurred, we are closing out the investigation with no action being taken by the IHSA office," IHSA Executive Director Martin Hickman said.[26]
- *Indiana:* School superintendent Dan Tanoos has told the school board he plans to form a committee to look into athletic transfers—both within and outside the district—after Terre Haute South lost two tall male basketball players to Lawrence North in three years. The two are archrivals in the Metropolitan Interscholastic Conference.
- *Maine:* The Maine Principals Association began a preliminary investigation in 2002 into the growing problem of Maine students transferring from one school to another for athletic purposes only.
- *Mississippi:* The Mississippi High School Activities Association forced West Lauderdale High School, a powerhouse in Mississippi

baseball and the 2001 defending Class 3A state champion, to forfeit six Division 5-3A wins for allegedly using an ineligible player, a junior pitcher whose residence was determined to be in the South Lauderdale district. The forfeits caused the team to miss the playoffs and ended the school's streak of 19 consecutive district-division championships.

- *Missouri:* Hickman High School near Columbia was ruled ineligible for the Class 4A baseball playoffs for allegedly using a player who lived out of district two years ago. The violation cost the school its first district baseball title in 10 years.

- *Nebraska:* The Nebraska School Activities Association passed a rule in 2002 forcing kids to sit out one semester after transferring. Previously, athletes were allowed to play immediately, and private schools had been accused of abusing the policy.

- *Nevada:* In an effort to cut down on the numbers of athletes who transfer from school to school purely for athletic reasons, the State of Nevada passed a "one free transfer" rule last summer. The rule allowed nonvarsity athletes to make one move to another school without penalty during their high school careers.

- *New Jersey:* The New Jersey State Interscholastic Athletic Association (NJSIAA), the state body governing high school athletics, ruled two ice hockey players ineligible for playing at a school outside their own district and town. The ruling confirmed rumors that perennial state power Brick High used illegal players.

- *North Carolina:* R. J. Reynolds High in Winston-Salem built a high school basketball power by taking advantage of an open selection process to attract top athletes.

- *Ohio:* Moeller High School's high-profile football program was reported to the Ohio High School Athletic Association (OHSAA) by private rival Catholic and other area schools for sending out a pamphlet to public school students inviting students to a recruiting meeting. It was also alleged that coach Bob Crable recruited players at a Pee Wee football practice, which was deemed to be against the "spirit" of OHSAA bylaws.

- *South Dakota:* In September 1993, the South Dakota High School Activities Association claimed basketball coach John Jordan had arranged for three black youths from New York City to come live with him on the Pine Ridge Indian reservation and attend his school.

- *Tennessee:* Brentwood Academy, a private school with a powerful football program, appealed a ruling by the Tennessee Secondary School Athletic Association (TSSAA), which found the school's coaches had recruited four middle school athletes away from Nashville public schools. The school said prohibiting a private school from talking to athletes at another school infringed on its First Amendment rights.
- *Virginia:* Transfers play immediately. No waiting, no questions.
- *Wisconsin:* In 1998 two-time individual state wrestling champion Jereme Maye took advantage of the state's open enrollment law to transfer from Crivitz to rival Coleman, a state wrestling power, to get better coaching and win a team title.[27]

With a pair of powerhouses in its back yard—a public school girls basketball team that had won six of eight state championships[28] and a private school football team that won eight of 10 state titles[29]—the *Shreveport Times* devoted part of its 2002 investigative series, entitled "Winning at All Costs," to the topic of high school recruiting. The challenge of limiting this practice falls upon a Louisiana High School Sports Athletic Association (LHSAA) that is grossly understaffed for what is demanded of it. Many states have no rules limiting recruiting, while others have no ability to enforce the restrictions that are in place. In any case, the example set by coaches and parents who actively recruit kids from outside their district for the purpose of competing in athletics is another incidence of normative cheating, one that administrators admit is difficult to control.

LHSAA assistant commissioner Mac Chauvin has been involved in his organization's investigation of recruiting violations for 20 years. He said adults who try to bypass the rulebook to recruit the best players are hurting kids. "They're teaching the kid to lie and cheat," Chauvin said. "That's the bottom line, circumventing the rules. I just think it's a poor example for high school kids."

His boss, commissioner Tommy Henry, said his office is not staffed to investigate every allegation, and every time he thinks the LHSAA has a handle on the problem, someone finds another way to get around the rules.

"The snake will grow a lot of heads," he said. "It goes back to this: our association is set up on the integrity of the school—the principal, athletic director and coaching staff. . . . The right thing to do is to abide by the rules. If we can't trust our principals, then who can we trust?"[30]

Since it is obvious that no one can be trusted in sports—parents, principals, or priests included—winning at all costs has become synonymous with the survival of the fittest. What might have been viewed as extreme in the past is standard today. Doing whatever it takes has taken almost everything over. Some other examples:

- *Faust's (Olympic) Gold:* The Olympics, the ancient tradition that for so long has symbolized all that is pure and good about amateur athletics, succumbed long ago to the business side of competition in the mega-marketed and media-driven modern world. If you want to bring home the big prize at today's Games, you better have your Visa card. For the United States Olympic Committee (USOC), there was no shame in shelling out more than $40 million over four years leading up to the Salt Lake City Olympics to finance its eight winter sports' national governing bodies. (Never mind the fact that even landing these Games would not have been possible without the infamous bribes that, when discovered, helped break a long-standing unethical tradition of cheating to win the right to be the host.) The extra spending—common for a host country—was more than twice what the USOC had spent on the previous Winter Olympics in Nagano, Japan.
  - The return on the investment: a record 34 medals, far exceeding their once-ambitious goal of 20.
  - The ratio of dollars to medals: $1.2 million for every one.
  - The big picture: The number of medals was 5.5 times their dismal six-medal showing just 14 years earlier in Calgary, a performance that led to the formation of a special panel to revive the U.S. Winter Olympic team. Chaired by big-spending, win-at-*any*-cost New York Yankees owner George Steinbrenner, this commission reported that the United States' sole Olympic mission should be winning medals, which would come at a price. A big part of the $40 million price—$18 million—went to the PODIUM program, designed in part by Jim Page, the managing

Sidebar 12.2: A Senior Season Lost at a Burger King: LHSAA Rules Move, Loophole Improper
By Brian McCallum, Reprinted with permission from the *Shreveport Times*[1]

Carlos Harris lost his senior season in a Burger King.

Most of the decisions that followed a chance meeting between his dad and a crosstown coach in a fast food joint would eventually cost him the rest of his high school basketball career.

The details of the story can be as difficult to follow as they were for Harris to accept.

There was a move from one school to another, bypassing a third. A legal separation. A controversial ruling on a man's job status. And charges that one school was out to get a former coach who had already taken away his son.

Those involved admit the motives were all about basketball. The price was the loss of one athlete's most important season.

"[Basketball is] very important," Harris says. "I've been playing since I was little—real little. It's all I like to do, pretty much."

As it turns out it was important for officials at Bossier High—where Harris had played for three years—to keep the younger Harris from playing for the Lions, a top rival in a tight district.

A CHANCE MEETING

It began in July of 2001. Carl Harris, Carlos' dad, found himself in line at Burger King standing next to Booker T. Washington boys basketball coach Bobby Joe Rusley. The two knew each other through coaching circles, and Rusley knew that Carl was interested in coaching at the high school level.

When Carl mentioned he would be retiring from the Air Force within two months, there was a job offer. Carl says then-Evangel coach Todd Foster had previously offered him a job but that he decided not to pull Carlos out of Bossier High for his senior season.

He changed his mind for the opportunity to work with the Lions.

"The timing was right for me. That's why I went ahead and accepted the job after I talked to my wife," Carl says. "We still hadn't mentioned it to my son. It was just my wife and I talking, and I wasn't going to accept it if he didn't come along with me."

Carl says Rusley told him at the time of the job offer that Carlos' decision on where to play would be "up to you and your son," but Carl never doubted he would want Carlos to follow him to BTW.

"In my heart, [it was] automatic, because what father wouldn't want their son to be [playing for him]," Carl says. "He thought about it and he said, 'Yeah dad, if you're going to be over at Booker T., I want to be, too.'"

The move itself involved three schools. While Carl was in the Air Force, the Harrises lived in the Bossier district. The family bought a house in the Parkway district upon his retirement, but it was BTW where the two wanted to end up.

Three schools competing in the same basketball district.

It meant an LHSAA ruling on Carlos' eligibility, and Carl wanted to test the waters before putting his son's career in jeopardy. Carl Pierson, a friend of the Harris family and the Caddo athletic director, made a call to the LHSAA and talked to assistant commissioner Mac Chauvin.

Carl Harris' version of the conversation is that Chauvin gave the tentative green light to the switch.

"[Chauvin said] 'Yeah coach, we've never turned down a father-son coaching combination. As long as he coaches there, he'll be eligible to play,'" Harris says.

Chauvin doesn't remember the specific conversation, but he says callers often provide only some of the facts with those requests. He said Carlos was ruled ineligible because his dad "did not meet the rule of the full-time teacher [at BTW]."

Carl is a full-time employee with the Caddo school system as security co-ordinator at West Shreveport Elementary and he coaches in the afternoons at BTW. He is certified through the state as a coach.

A CONTROVERSIAL RULING

Tommy Henry denied immediate eligibility for Carlos in BTW's initial request, so the school appealed. Pierson believes Henry—who once coached at Bossier—made the decision based on Bossier's alleged antipathy toward its former coach.

"That's what it was, and it was almost admitted," Pierson says. "I don't personally remember any situation where the LHSAA has not given credence to a son playing for his dad. It ought to be a courtesy."

The only thing Henry thought "ought" to be done according to Pierson is monitor the actions of Rusley. Pierson says Henry was friendly and told him "everything will be all right" before the appeal hearing in Baton Rouge.

In the meeting, Pierson says it was a different story as Henry "was jumping around" and argued that "we can't keep doing this for the same school."

Pierson claims he was told afterward by Henry, "you need to watch Bobby Joe Rusley."

Carl was in despair after the committee denied the appeal, so the group returned to Shreveport and began "scouring the books trying to see if there's a loophole somewhere to get him eligible, because it just wasn't right."

A FAMILY SPLIT

The only chance for Carlos Harris to play for the Lions was to live in the BTW district, so he and his dad moved into the house of another family member via a change in family status.

Carl and Gloria Harris decided to separate.

"To be honest, we were trying to get him eligible to play," Carl says. "We felt like we were wronged. We were frustrated with the whole system. I wouldn't have done this to be one of those parents to try to circumvent the system. My son would have been just fine at Bossier High. I just wanted to get at Tommy Henry, and I wanted my son to play."

He did. For six games Carlos wore the uniform of the Lions, but when he led his team to the championship of the Bossier tournament, the report of his performance drew the attention of a visitor to town.

"I read in the paper where he scored so many points, and I wondered how can this be," Henry said. "They should have gotten a ruling on that."

If they had, BTW officials would have learned that Carlos was required to sit out 45 days from the official custody ruling which allowed Carl to move him to the new district. By playing before that time, an LHSAA rule was broken. It was part of a ruling which included two other athletes and cost the school 18 victories while ending Carlos' career.

It was a shocking decision to Carlos, who said Rusley had promised to "get it fixed."

"I was under the impression that he knew what to do or whatever. He went through the same situation with his son, and they let his son play."

Either of the principals at Bossier or Parkway could have written a letter of support for the Harris move and possibly influenced the appeals committee enough to change the outcome according to Henry.

Neither did.

"[Bossier principal Bud] Dean said he would not write the letter," Carl Harris remembers. "He said he's a Bearkat and he was with his coaches. Coach [Ronnie Howell] told him he didn't want him to write the letter. . . . If it took him writing the letter for my son to play and compete against his school, then he wouldn't do it."

Dean and Howell, who says he expected Carl to be his starting point guard after starting for 32 games as a junior, agree that it was Dean's decision to not write the letter.

Dean based his decision on how Carl's addition to the Lions would affect Bossier's place in the District 1-4A standings.

"That was simply it," Dean says. "That was the whole thing."

Parkway principal Joe Huffman says he felt like a middle man in a conflict between BTW and Bossier, so he wrote a letter saying only that he would be able to live with the decision of the committee.

It was not the recommendation the Harrises wanted, and Pierson believes it was not Huffman's choice.

"I really think—and I don't know; this would be speculation on my part—that . . . it was a collective decision. I don't think the guy at Parkway was free to make the decision that he would have made."

It is Pierson's theory that the two principals and Henry agreed to prevent Carlos from playing for the Lions. Dean denies that, saying that he and Huffman "never spoke about it."

"I was not told to do anything by anybody," Huffman says. "Mr. Dean, obviously, and his coach were upset. . . . I simply called Mr. Dean to say, 'Did you have the young man over there for three years?' "

A PLAYER TORN

For his part, Carlos says he had doubts about leaving Bossier after playing there for three seasons, but he decided to move for one reason. He is adamant that it had nothing to do with winning.

"I play to win, but that's not the reason that I transferred. I transferred because my dad was coaching over there. I didn't transfer to go beat Bossier."

The Harrises simply wanted father and son to play together, and months after the school year ended Gloria Harris still found it difficult to talk about.

"They didn't punish Bobby Joe. They punished my child and my family," she said. "My child cried every night to sleep, and when you see your baby cry himself to sleep, you have to cry, too."

Carlos remembers the sadness around his family's house, and his life lesson is "how different people can act and how people have power over certain situations."

Does he think BTW opponents are right when they accuse Rusley of hiring Carl to get Carlos' services?

"Sometimes. Like when I used to go to Bossier I would see coach Rusley and since he got the coaching job at BT he always came up to me and said he wanted me to come over there and play for him because he liked me as a freshman. . . . So I know he always wanted me to play for him."

For six games, he did.

A FUTURE UNCLEAR

Carlos doesn't regret leaving Bossier, but he does think the suspension hurt his chances at a college scholarship.

"I know since I was going to be the only senior on the [Bossier] team, I was going to have all the senior leadership and the ball was going to be in my hands most of the time," he says. "So I knew if I played good and we were winning I'd have a chance to play on the next level in college."

Carlos still played AAU ball during the summer, so he has had looks from college coaches and has had discussions with a junior college coach in Oklahoma. Playing again has also brightened his outlook a good bit.

But there's still that missing senior year. He says even if he were to go on and win championships at the collegiate and national level, he will never forget what happened to him in the most important season of his basketball life.

"All the other years it matters, but not like your senior year because it's your last year of high school and you really want to play good your last year. That hurt real bad."

director of sports performance services for the USOC. "We knew that our success would be measured by the number of medals we won," Page said. "So we developed the PODIUM program, which stands for Partnering Olympic Dreams Into Utah Medals. We analyzed the sports where we had the best chance to win."[31] And those sports—and the athletes determined to be within striking range of medaling, received funds that allowed them to train full time. If you were an athlete in a sport where the competition was too great and you were likely not going to medal, you did not qualify for money from the PODIUM program.

- *It pays to win:* Since 2002, high school sports coaches in Louisiana have earned bonuses, such as $250 for making the playoffs, $500 for winning a district title, and $1,000 for a state championship. The added incentives have not come without additional worries for coaches, like Woodlawn's Mike Green, who are concerned the new system might tempt some coaches to break rules in order to win and earn the extra money. "It worries me a little bit because you get a reward for getting into the playoffs," Green said. "Any coach wants to be rewarded, but I'm just afraid that maybe down the line some recruiting will increase."[32] Val McGyvers, an assistant professor of psychology with the University of Louisiana-Lafayette whose primary research interest is in achievement motivation, says, "Any time you increase external motivation you're going to increase the proportion of illegitimate shortcuts that are taken. Now you're going to see a situation where the coaches are going for the money. That means they will put an enormous amount of pressure on their athletes because the athletes are the ones getting them the money."[33]

- *Tough road to the top:* The *Shreveport Times* reported in 2002 that, while the NCAA has rules regulating the number of hours a student-athlete can be required to attend practice sessions, no such limitations are in place to protect athletes from extended travel required to compete in contests. "I speak from my heart when I say that if the WAC doesn't go to divisional play, then I won't coach in this league long," legendary Louisiana Tech Lady Techsters coach Leon Barmore said in 2002. "Where have we lost track of the student-athlete? This league is very close to taking the student off that phrase."[34] Barmore, sometimes known to pass on the long conference trips to Hawaii, retired a short time later for many reasons, but the extensive travel was certainly among them. Former Louisiana Tech basketball player Marco Cole discovered how being an athlete hurt his standing as a student. By missing the first seven days of the winter quarter during a lengthy road trip, he was forced to drop an English class that kept him from graduating on time in May. "I didn't think it was fair. I missed several 100-point quizzes and the professor wouldn't let me make them up."[35] Jane Jankowski, an NCAA public relations representative, said student-athlete welfare is one of the basic premises of the NCAA, but "if you're looking for a rule that says a student-athlete cannot be away from class more than 'x' hours, you're not going to find that rule."[36]

13

Recurrent Unexplained
Deaths in Sports

Julian Bailes, M.D.

There is no question that the incidence of illicit drug use in modern Western society has markedly increased in the years following World War II, especially since the 1960s. The accessibility and acceptance of numerous street drugs has also permeated athletics. While amphetamines were already popular for athletes, and their use was well documented even at the NFL level in the 1960s and beyond, the emergence of cocaine was rapid and pervasive. As a recreational drug, cocaine became one of the most widely abused illicit substances, and its abuse by athletes was no exception. At the same time, anabolic steroid use continued to grow in many sports. G. I. Wadler and B. Hainline, in their book *Drugs and the Athlete*, documented eleven athletes during the 1980s whose deaths were contributed to or caused by the use of PEDs such as cocaine, steroids, amphetamines, and narcotics. During that same decade, they reported nearly 200 high-profile amateur and professional athletes who had major news media coverage for similar drug use, including that of drug-masking agents.[1] In addition, as always, alcohol use continued to be a problem for numerous athletes.

Although this behavior in large part reflects the attitudes and practices of society, it also introduces a certain acceptance of either recreational drug use or of the winning-at-all-costs attitude. The latter evokes, at least, a tacit acceptance of a recognized and appreciated benefit of players getting bigger, stronger, and faster, as well as hitting the ball farther and other feats, with the ends justifying the means. Athletes came to be pressured to push the limits of training and performance and were enabled, just as are many people who abuse street drugs, by their trainers, coaches, federations, governments, and other entities. This has led to an apparent increasing desire to experiment with and consume a multitude of PEDs for competitive sports.

The emergence and evolution of various herbs, medications, and newly synthesized "designer" drugs in sports is now understood. From ancient athletes and warriors to today's aspiring and elite competitors, there has been a great tendency to seek perceived advantage by utilizing foreign substances for performance improvement. In modern times, however, the question has arisen as to whether there are more powerful, alluring, and ultimately dangerous drugs available to the athlete, and what the consequences of this practice are. It has been suggested that numerous deaths have been caused by this lifestyle, yet that fact is not fully appreciated or feared by those most at risk. There is a constant reminder of the ancient Olympic motto of *citius*, *altius*, and *fortius*: faster, higher, and stronger.

The 1987 death of the famous German heptathlete Birgit Dressel was felt throughout the sports world, as it was widely reported that she had been an eager consumer of multiple PEDs, having been injected at least four hundred times with various substances. It has been noted that her father felt that she was a victim of the pharmaceutical industry.[2] Her case also emphasized not only the role of the industry but also that of often numerous enablers for aspiring or elite athletes, including their coaches, trainers, and physicians. Hundreds of European amateur and professional competitive cyclists have purportedly died from drug use, overdose, or secondary formation of malignant tumors.[3] There is the ever-present temptation to tamper with human physiology, to push the barriers of athletic achievement as well as the pressures, pain, and emotional toll which all competitive players endure. While most of the side effects of PEDs do not lead to premature death, there is also the constant specter of real and proven adverse events or damage to critical organs, which may become lethal.

Several unexpected and shocking deaths in recent years have led to an interest in the further examination of the causes and types of demise in otherwise presumed young, healthy athletes. These fatalities have occurred unexpectedly in elite athletes involved in soccer, cycling, American football, track and field, and wrestling.[4] While a certain number of spontaneous deaths happen each year, primarily as a result of undiagnosed cardiac conditions, as detailed in chapter 9, the incidence in these sports is greater than the natural history based on the exposed population. That is, the deaths are excessive from what would be predicted by statistical models for these athletes, and therefore beg the question of how and why there are so many. Perhaps there is a common thread to their training habits, athletic lifestyles, and causes of death.[5] In addition, these were all non-traumatic deaths that were otherwise listed as death from "natural causes."

In a seven-year period, 65 wrestlers died unexpectedly in the prime of their lives from various causes and at a much higher rate than would be expected in that age group. During this period, it has been estimated that only three died from traumatic injury in the ring.[6] Although several died from suicide, among various other theories it has been suggested that they experienced some form of side effects from abuse of PEDs, particularly the anabolic agents and especially steroids. One of the most likely possibilities is that some of the premature deaths were caused or contributed to by the known steroid effects on the heart. The $500 million wrestling industry had previously tried to regulate substance abuse through steroid testing; however this was abandoned by professional wrestling in the late 1990s. Professional wrestling does not ban or test for PEDs, including anabolic steroids, in its athletes, and their use has become ingrained and accepted. This phenomenon has been well detailed in an article by Jon Swartz in *USA Today*.[7] The use of PEDs is not the only possible association, as a career with the lifestyle of the professional athlete, in this case a professional wrestler, is apparently contributory. The psychological pressures of innumerable expectations and of winning may have taken an unmistakable toll.[8] Many had discussed the multiple injuries they constantly received that required the use of painkillers, including narcotics, which may have led to a cycle of dependency and abuse. The deaths of several professional wrestlers have been attributed to an overdose of narcotics as well as other substances, including cocaine.

Olympic gold medalist Florence Griffith Joyner died at age 42 amidst rampant but unproven speculations of an early steroid-associated demise.[9] In addition to wrestling, the deaths of ten European cyclists occurred in a six-month period and were reported as sudden deaths, believed to be heart related.[10] Jean Paul Escande, former head of the French National Doping Commission, stated that he was "appalled by the explanations for these sudden deaths" in the March 2004 edition of *Le Monde* magazine. These unexpected deaths included those of cyclists Marco Pantani and Fabrice Salanson and footballers Marc-Vivien Foe (Cameroon) and Miklos Feher (Hungary), all of whom were discovered deceased without having suffered a traumatic event. These elite athletes, which include six cyclists, have been alleged as victims of doping and suffering lethal cardiac or other effects.[11] One suspected cause is the use of the blood doping agent EPO, which causes a rise in the erythrocytes, or red blood cells, within the bloodstream. This attempt at increasing oxygen-carrying capacity may also have a major untoward effect by creating a hyperviscosity or sludging of the blood, which may lead to the formation of clotting within the blood. This may lead to clots within such major organs as the brain (stroke), heart (heart attack), lung (pulmonary embolism), or lower extremity blood clots, which may travel to other parts of the body.

Several recent, highly publicized fatalities in organized sports have prompted great concern regarding a perceived increased incidence of death due to heatstroke and has led us to review and analyze the available data concerning this phenomenon. While there is an inherent risk of death as a result of head and cerebrospinal injuries or cardiac-rhythm disturbance, we wish to emphasize the recent trend toward a growing number of deaths that are a result of heat-related illness. This small but important increase in the years after the deregulation of dietary supplements has occurred despite what we think is adequate and effective knowledge of the clinical science of dehydration and its treatment by physicians, athletic trainers, coaches, and players.[12] This increase in heat-related fatalities transpired while the number of direct injury-related football deaths had generally remained level. Although we also acknowledge that numerous factors may be operative in causing non-traumatic deaths in athletes, the use of dietary supplements, among other variables, should be considered causative or contributory during training in extreme heat conditions. In addition to the multitude of anabolic agents widely purported to be used by many athletes, the amphetamines, such as ephedrine, appear to be prime candidates for contributing factors to the deaths of these otherwise healthy individuals. The deaths in recent years of

Korey Stringer of the Minnesota Vikings, Rashedi Wheeler of North-western University, Steve Bechler of the Baltimore Orioles, and others have been attributed to the use of PEDs, particularly those containing ephedrine.[13]

Do these deaths mean that there is a modern and current trend toward higher fatalities in our elite athletes, or merely that they reflect the expected mortality in this age group, which is being noticed due to better reporting and dissemination of the news? Certainly today's athletes push themselves to further goals and limits and are often willing to accept any risk for the pursuit of excellence and accomplishment. The breakdown of human performance barriers has often meant that the human body's normal physiology must be exceeded, and that for this result many have been willing to turn to exogenous substances. The resultant culture has evolved to include an Internet- and computer-savvy generation of athletes who have free access to information and guidebooks on do-it-yourself doping, black-market drug dealing, newly emerging "designer" drugs, and an ever-increasing pressure to achieve. Financial and marketing possibilities are at an unprecedented high for those who are successful at many amateur, Olympic, and professional sports. It remains to be seen whether the deaths discussed above are merely coincidental; however, a preponderance of evidence seems to suggest that recent deaths indicate that the modern elite athletic lifestyle has real and lethal risks. By continuing to monitor and observe these occurrences and by questioning their cause, we may make a difference in preventing unnecessary sports fatalities in the future.

Hoberman, in his book *Mortal Engines*, discusses the phenomenon of the transformation of athletics, as science and sport have combined to create a new meaning for the term sportsmanship. This fusion has led to the disappearance of self-restraint, resulting in a crisis of both conduct and identity. In the former, behavior may occur that knows no ethical boundaries as long as the desired result occurs in competition. The crisis of identity implies that this person possesses a character with which no one can any longer identify, which will resort to any means to transform itself both physiologically and psychologically with drugs.[14] A century ago, medical experts warned of athletes attempting to exceed the physiological boundaries of the human body by building large muscles, overtraining, overexerting, and racing against time. We have come to accept that many of man's apparent physical obstacles can be overcome, but where should we draw the line in terms of reaching for outside or exogenous support?

Is there a common thread in the deaths of these elite and dedicated athletes? Does dietary supplementation or the use, in one form or another, of various PEDs lead to a lifestyle that includes not only extreme training but also doping to increase athletic productivity? If discussed with athletic trainers today, they will state that at high levels, including elite and professional athletes, consumption of a multitude of available substances, some legal and some prohibited, is one of the greatest potential risks they fear for their athletes. At the same time, many will suggest that what is consumed is ultimately the athlete's responsibility, which has certainly been the premise of drug-testing programs. As discussed earlier, there are innumerable combinations of drugs, hormones, and blood doping that exist to provide the athlete or aspiring athlete with temptation to circumvent the rules in order to win or gain some advantage.

Today's athletes are not only at risk for their current behavior, but future athletes and athletic generations will also continue to suffer through the possibility of sudden and non-traumatic death. In addition, new and emerging methods will exist which will make this problem not only more pervasive but also more unpredictable, undetectable, and lethal. Will the technology be available and will the potential for gene doping allure the competitive athlete preparing for the 2008 Olympics, as some have suggested? What role do the federations, professional organizations and teams, and the administrators and leaders play in sanctioning and allowing such behavior to be perpetuated and condoned? Is there going to be one sport, athlete, or federation leader who assumes a forward role in prevention or change of these attitudes and behaviors? The answers to these and other questions will in great part determine the progress or regression made in many sports in the upcoming years.

14

Who's in Charge?
Administration Is Part of the Problem

No one in sport or society can deny a natural need for order and authority. As it relates to society, the laws of the land—in the United States and around the world—are maintained to ensure the survival of future peaceful generations. Sports rulebooks are similarly set up to preserve the peace, fairness, and enjoyment of the game. One of the earliest rulebooks that commands us to obey authority figures is the Bible. One interpretation of the instructions to "honor thy father and thy mother" is not limited to our parents but to all of our superiors. One of the most important figures of the Protestant Reformation, Frenchman John Calvin, wrote: "We should reverence them whom God has exalted to any authority over us, and should render them honor, obedience, and gratitude."[1] Regardless of your religious beliefs, logic dictates that we must honor and respect those who have earned their positions of authority. It is a foundation on which order is built. Unfortunately, there are far too many weeds and cracks in this foundation today. An increasing number of kids do not respect the rules, the officials, the history, or the integrity of the games they play. While their actions cannot be entirely linked to those of their mediated peers in the spotlight of professional sports, it is impossible not to compare a tantrum on the playground to that of poor sportsmanship by grown men on television each week. Part of baseball's tradition allows managers to protest instantly the call of an umpire. It is an unwritten rule that such protests—in baseball and other sports—can interrupt the game, without consequence in most cases. But this was never intended to give irate athletes a right to spit on, head butt, or otherwise disrespect, belittle, or harm the authority figure charged with maintaining the order, safety, and integrity of the game and all of its participants. The plight of the referee is further addressed in chapter 15 ("Struggle for Sportsmanship: Through a Ref's Eagle Eyes").

Officials are not the only ones who fail to receive the respect they did in the past. Head coaches, who often make less money than their players, are in a battle to regain respect that has been steadily disappearing. Never mind the tremendous win-now pressure from ownership that keeps quality head coaches spending more time clearing out offices than night crews spend cleaning them. Coaches at all levels today are finding themselves expendable. *Sports Illustrated* chronicled the modern professional coach's plight in August of 2004:

- *NFL:* 16 of 32 teams changed coaches from 2002 to 2004, most notably the 49ers' Steve Mariucci, who was fired for "what was perceived as a passive approach." He was 57–39 and went to the playoffs four times in six years. Also, Tony Dungy was fired after leading the Bucs to the playoffs in four of his final five years in Tampa.
- *Major League Baseball:* 21 of 30 teams changed managers from 2002 to 2004, most notably the Giants' Dusty Baker, who led his club to within one win of the World Series. Baker, a three-time National League Manager of the Year left "over differences with ownership." Also, Grady Little was fired by the Red Sox after leading them to within five outs of the World Series.
- *NHL:* 20 of 30 teams changed coaches from 2002 to 2004, most notably Joel Quenneville, whose Blues were 29-23-7-2 during the 2001–2002 season. He was 307-209-77 in seven-plus seasons with St. Louis and never finished below .500. Also, Jacques Martin was fired by the Senators with a 341-255-96 record in eight seasons with the club.
- *NBA:* 21 of 29 teams changed coaches from 2002–2004 (and 17 of 29 changed from the end of the 2002–2003 season to the end of the 2003–2004 season), most notably Rick Carlilse, who won 50 games in each of his two seasons in Detroit. Also, Byron Scott was fired the season after he took the Nets to back-to-back NBA Finals appearances.[2]

NBA coach George Karl told *Sports Illustrated,* "One of the real pillars of the game is being destroyed. Coaches are the leaders and teachers, and when their authority is undermined, it's bad for sports.

It's gotten way out of control."[3] San Jose Sharks coach Ron Wilson was in the overwhelming majority of coaches interviewed by *Sports Illustrated* who believe, as we have stated, that the nation's overall moral decline is resulting in a loss of respect for all coaches: "Why don't teachers get respect anymore? If you can answer that question, then it answers the question about coaches. Where has personal accountability gone in a lot of our society?"[4] Finally, South Carolina basketball coach Dave Odom told *Sports Illustrated*, "People look at the coaching profession as something less than honorable."[5]

The lack of respect is not limited to professional coaches. Rick Wolff, the chairman of the Center for Sports Parenting (www.sportsparenting.org) and author of 17 books, including *Coaching Kids for Dummies* (IDG, 2000) and *Good Sports: The Concerned Parent's Guide to Competitive Sports* (Dell, 1993), wrote a bimonthly column in *Sports Illustrated* in 2004 entitled "Parents' Guide To Youth Sports."[6] In the August 2nd edition entitled "Losing the Leadership of Our Classic Coaches," Wolff describes how youth coaches are joining youth umpires and sports participants in quitting early amid increasing pressure and depressingly poor sportsmanship from parents. "With heavy parental involvement and interference today," Wolff writes, "many influential coaches who once played such important roles in the community are driven to give it up, citing the stress and pressures of the job."[7]

Despite these very real pressures, professional coaches are still incredibly well paid. The median salary for NBA and NFL coaches is about $3 million. The best NFL assistants make more than $1 million a year. Top college football and basketball coaches are not far behind. And while big paychecks bring huge expectations, what is certainly expected out of a leader of young men is character. Too often in recent years this has been sorely lacking among so many college coaches, which can only further damage the diminishing honor today's coaches are clinging to. The worst and most recent examples (2003–2004) include:

- *Alabama's Mike Price:* He was fired only months after being hired after he was seen drinking heavily at a topless bar while representing the school at a golfing weekend in Florida. He was later alleged to have had sex with topless dancers in his hotel room.

- *Baylor's Dave Bliss:* He resigned as basketball coach for having made improper tuition payments to player Patrick Dennehy. A week later, secret tape recordings revealed that Bliss tried to cover up the payments by portraying Dennehy, who was murdered, as a drug dealer.
- *Fresno State's Jerry Tarkanian:* He retired but not before his basketball program was found guilty of committing academic fraud and providing improper financial aid and benefits to players.
- *Georgia's Jim Harrick and Jim Harrick Jr.:* Head coach Jim Harrick resigned and assistant Jim Harrick Jr. was fired following accusations of academic fraud and improper player benefits.
- *Iowa State's Larry Eustachy:* He was paid ($960,000) to resign as basketball coach after photographs were taken of him drinking at a party with Missouri students after an ISU road game. Not altogether surprising, four players were suspended after they were arrested and charged with drunk driving and marijuana possession.
- *Washington's Rick Neuheisel:* He was fired for gambling in off-campus pools on the NCAA basketball tournament, profiting by more than $5,000. He also lied about his gambling and kept secret a job interview with the San Francisco 49ers.

Three coaches with questionable pasts (Tarkanian, Harrick Sr., and Neuheisel all had been linked to improprieties at their previous employers) and three incidents of completely bizarre behavior (Price, Bliss, and Eustachy implicated in plots involving sex, lies, and photographs, respectively) are just the tip of the trash heap. So-called leaders have been involved in an unacceptably high number of NCAA violations, with academic fraud being the most disturbing. When Minnesota's basketball program was placed on four years' probation in 2000 and forfeited six seasons' worth of victories, including a 1997 Final Four appearance, many thought the severe punishment, which included the firing of coach Clem Haskins, would significantly impact academic fraud in collegiate athletics. They were wrong. What follows is a list of other noteworthy major infraction cases featuring academic fraud since 2000, according to an NCAA database:

- *New Mexico State, June 2001:* The men's basketball team was placed on four years' probation after an assistant men's basketball coach was found to have helped arrange fraudulent correspondence courses for two junior college transfers.

- *Southern California, August 2001:* The football and women's swimming and diving teams were placed on two years' probation after employees of an academic service office wrote papers for three student-athletes.
- *Marshall, December 2001:* The football team was placed on four years' probation after an assistant professor in the physical education department provided copies of a final exam to players in advance of testing.
- *California, June 2002:* The football team was placed on five years' probation after a professor awarded credit to two players who had not attended a sufficient number of classes or completed a sufficient amount of coursework.[8]
- *St. Bonaventure, 2003:* School president Robert Wickenheiser resigned after it was learned that he improperly declared junior-college transfer Jamil Terrell eligible to play basketball when Terrell had not met NCAA transfer requirements.

Incidents of academic fraud or other extra benefits that were either ruled to be in violation of NCAA rules or were still under investigation by the NCAA since 2002 include the following:

- *Missouri, 2004:* Men's basketball team is hit with 57 NCAA violations, including paying a player (who was later imprisoned for violating parole by physically assaulting his girlfriend) $250 and making excessive phone calls to recruits.
- *Duke, 2002:* Star point guard Chris Duhon's mother moved to North Carolina, landed a job that was never posted at a company owned by a Duke booster, was paid more than the position's standard despite questionable qualifications, and received a big raise within months. Another former star's father, Carlos Boozer Sr., landed a $40,000 (according to Boozer) administrative assistant position at a pharmaceutical company run by a friend of Duke coach Mike Krzyzewski.
- *Louisiana-Lafayette, 2000–2003:* Though two investigations failed to uncover violations, the New Orleans *Times-Picayune* reported that the address of men's head basketball coach Jessie Evens was used as the official address listed for a basketball player's resi-

dence and for the registration of a 1996 Cadillac of the same player's girlfriend. The woman also owned a Cadillac Escalade that was driven by the player.

- *Ohio State, 1998–2002:* Coach Jim O'Brien was fired for paying $6,000 to a recruit who never played for the Buckeyes. The violation came out of a lawsuit against two Ohio State boosters who allegedly arranged and paid for another player to live with a woman who now claims she was not compensated per an oral agreement with the boosters.

- *Ohio State, 2003:* Star running back Maurice Clarett was suspended for multiple games (he left the school before serving the suspension) for receiving improper benefits, among them the use of a car by a Columbus, Ohio, dealership.

- *LSU, 2002–2003:* LSU admitted violating NCAA rules dealing with improper aid offered to students by tutors at the academic center, including helping one football player write and type a term paper, typing papers for other players, and giving a prospective player free tutoring before he enrolled at LSU. The NCAA added a sixth violation (a tutor underlined key passages in a textbook available to all student-athletes) but did not increase self-imposed penalties (i.e., forfeiting two football scholarships in 2005 and four on-campus official visits in 2004).

- *Auburn, 2004:* The NCAA put Auburn's men's basketball program on probation for two years after an AAU coach, acting as a representative of Auburn, arranged to wire $3,125 for one player and to buy a 1996 Dodge Stratus for another.

- *LaSalle, 2003–2004:* The school fired its men's and women's basketball coaches—Billy Hahn and John Miller—for failing to report the rape of a female basketball player. The woman claims the coaches discouraged her from going to police. The coaches say she told them not to speak about the allegation made against a member of the men's team in 2003.

- *Villanova, 2001–2003:* The men's basketball program was put on probation for two years for numerous small infractions that the coaches insisted were unintentional, inadvertent, and provided a minimal recruiting advantage.

- *Oregon, 2003:* The football program was placed on two years' probation after an assistant coach instructed a recruit to date his letter of intent (as well as the forged signature of his father) a day earlier to meet a national deadline.

- *Arkansas, 2003:* The football team and men's basketball team lost scholarships and were placed on three years' probation for infractions that included athletes being overpaid at a booster-owned business in Dallas during the 1990s.
- *Cal State Northridge, 2003:* The men's basketball team lost one scholarship and was placed on three years' probation by the NCAA for academic fraud for the late addition of two classes and fraudulent grades for a player.
- *Gardner-Webb, 2000–2002:* The school was placed on three years' probation by the NCAA for grade-tampering arranged by since-fired school president Christopher White, who approved the removal of an "F" from a basketball player's grade-point-average calculation.
- *Arkansas, 1994–2000:* After some 20 Razorback football and basketball players were paid for work they did not do, the school was put on three years' probation, lost 10 football scholarships in the period 2001–2006, and was limited to 50 expense-paid visits in 2003–2004. Also, Arkansas was required to develop and implement a comprehensive educational program on NCAA legislation and compliance rules.
- *Salem State College, 2000–2004:* The school was placed on two years' probation by the NCAA, and its men's soccer program was barred from postseason play and all off-campus recruiting activities for the 2003–2004 season because of $11,900 in loans given to a soccer player via two men's soccer coaches in 2000.
- *Fairfield, 2003–2004:* An NCAA investigation of former men's basketball coach Tim O'Toole's program neared completion in the summer of 2004, concentrating on allegations by former players of academic fraud, a falsified drug test, and cash handouts.
- *Iona, 2003–2004:* An NCAA investigation of the men's basketball program was still in progress in the summer of 2004. The school violated NCAA rules by hosting prospective student-athletes at postgame booster-club receptions.
- *Mississippi State, 2003–2004:* The school admitted that a football booster arranged a part-time job for a recruit, another booster loaned a player $750 for tires for his pickup, and the school paid

three recruits nearly $400 for automobile expenses they didn't incur.

- *NCAA, 2003–2004:* Fourteen of the 56 Division I-A football teams playing in bowl games this year graduated less than 40 percent of their players, according to a study by the Institute for Diversity and Ethics in Sport. Moreover, half of bowl teams graduated less than 40 percent of their African American players.[9]
- According to NCAA statistics, 25 percent of the NCAA's "major infraction cases" since 2000 have involved academic fraud, up from 11 percent during the 1980s.[10]

Coaches who pretend the problem is not potentially calamitous despite mountains of evidence are a very big part of the problem:

- *Florida State coach Leonard Hamilton's perception:* "I don't mean to diminish what has happened over the past year, but the way I see it, we had a few unfortunate situations [at Arkansas, Auburn, Baylor, Cal State Northridge, Duke, Fairfield, Fresno State, Gardner-Webb, Georgia, Iona, Iowa State, LaSalle, Louisiana-Lafayette, Missouri, New Mexico State, Ohio State, St. Bonaventure, and Villanova over a three-year span] in succession and people started to paint us with a wide brush, when in reality, 95 percent of coaches already have programs to govern themselves from an ethical standpoint."[11]
- *The reality:* The wounds of one year bleed into the next. No fewer than 20 independent examples (at least 15 in basketball alone) of extra benefits violations within a three-year span does not constitute a "few unfortunate situations." Most cases were irrefutable instances of unethical violations—several were abominable—and that number does not even include the extremely suspicious occurrences at Duke (Duhon and Boozer) and Louisiana-Lafayette.
- *Duke coach Mike Krzyzewski's perception:* "It's not a statement that everyone's doing it bad. It's a statement that obviously there were a couple of pronounced episodes in violation of an ethical code."[12]
- *The reality:* There were a couple *dozen* incidents, not a "couple."
- *Michigan State coach Tom Izzo's perception:* "I am all for us taking more measures to better ensure that we can police ourselves. But I do have a problem with three or four out of 320 or so Divi-

Who's in Charge? Administration Is Part of the Problem

235

sion I programs having some difficulties, and all of a sudden there's this need to sound the alarm like we're in a crisis situation. That still means that 98 percent of the programs are doing what they can to try and stay out of trouble. Our image has to be perfect in some people's minds, and that's impossible. There are so many middlemen involved in the recruiting process now that it's unrealistic to think you can wave a magic wand and suddenly clean up everything."[13]

- *The reality*: Again, there were 23 or 24 "difficulties," not 3 or 4. And none of them involved middlemen, unless these characters also have titles such as coach, athletic director, and president.

Hamilton's "programs to govern themselves from an ethical standpoint," Krzyzewski's "ethical code," and Izzo's absurd assertion that 98 percent of schools are "doing what they can to try and stay out of trouble" all sound very similar. They are theories that fail to materialize in the new billion-dollar business of college sports. As has been proven by today's incredibly flawed drug-testing programs, only a small percentage of cheaters are actually caught. The same holds true when it comes to academic fraud and improper benefits to college athletes. The *Atlanta Journal-Constitution* provided the proof of this in pointing out the number of allegations made against schools by former players who leave after a falling out. Without their need to seek revenge, the following violations would never have been discovered.

- *Tony Cole, Georgia:* He was kicked off the Georgia basketball team in 2002 after being accused of aggravated assault with intent to rape. Cole accused assistant coach Jim Harrick Jr. of paying for phone and hotel bills and giving him an "A" in a class he never attended.
- *Gene Jelks, Alabama:* He received $24,400 in loans from football boosters and never repaid them. He eventually went public with his information, including audio tapes of an assistant coach promising that he would be taken care of financially. The NCAA's investigation, which included looking into charges that defensive back Antonio Langham was allowed to play in 11 games in 1993 despite signing with an agent, resulted in Alabama's being banned from a bowl game in 1995, losing 13 scholarships, and forfeiting eight

victories from 1993. In addition, athletics director Hootie Ingram was forced to resign.

- *Eric Ramsey, Auburn:* He received cash and other benefits totaling at least $4,000 from a football booster. He also got monthly payments from an Auburn administrative assistant and an unsecured bank loan of more than $9,000 approved by a booster. Ramsey secretly taped coach Pat Dye and others involved. Dye resigned in 1992, and in August of 1993, Auburn received a one-year ban on television appearances, a two-year ban on postseason play, and lost 11 scholarships in each of the next three recruiting classes.
- *Hart Lee Dykes, Oklahoma State:* This wide receiver got an ample array of extra benefits during the late 1980s. Dykes was given immunity in exchange for information about violations involving Oklahoma State, Illinois, Texas A&M, and Oklahoma. Oklahoma State was dealt a two-year TV ban, a three-year bowl ban, and the loss of 15 scholarships.
- *Lester Earl, LSU:* The 6-foot-8 basketball star was dismissed for violating team rules in January 1997. He transferred to Kansas, but on his way out of town Earl testified to the NCAA, saying he had received $6,000 from an LSU assistant and another $4,000 from a booster. The NCAA cleared the LSU assistant, but not the booster, and LSU lost six scholarships over three years. Coach Dale Brown retired at the end of the 1997 season.[14]

Players who receive benefits and remain happy at their given schools do not bite the hand that feeds them money, cars, grades, or girls. Simply having a self-governing program does not ensure that the program will be properly administered. There are many other cases in which the NCAA's understaffed infractions committee is unable to find enough evidence to satisfactorily prove wrongdoing. This means the dismal ethics report card of college athletics is likely even worse than it appears. No one knows this reality better than Linda Bensel-Meyers, a faculty member at Tennessee for 17 years before being forced to resign after receiving death threats and enduring break-ins for her role in sparking an NCAA investigation into the Volunteer athletic department. The accusations didn't stick and Bensel-Meyers, who claims Tennessee became very good at being very bad, didn't stick around long after the case was closed. She told the *San Antonio*

Who's in Charge? Administration Is Part of the Problem

237

Express-News that there is a simple explanation as to why such academic fraud cases are so prevalent today. "The faculty no longer has a voice on campuses structured under a corporate system where athletics are big business. I see more and more universities willing to do whatever it takes to maintain successful athletic programs. And the public is willing to accept it. People want to believe there's nothing wrong."[15] While the NCAA might not have proven her words to be true in Knoxville, there are plenty of others who say her thinking is right on.

Highly successful former Virginia basketball coach and athletic director Terry Holland told the Knight Commission, a group charged with reforming collegiate athletics, "the forces driving intercollegiate athletics today are compromising these outstanding individuals (those who oversee college athletics) at an alarming and increasing rate. How else can one explain the growing litany of outrageous (and irresponsible) behaviors of athletes, coaches, athletic administrators, governing board members and college presidents?" Holland, who resigned from a consulting position at Virginia in 2004, has not retired from the fight against the assault on college academics by collegiate athletics. In his report to the Knight Commission, Holland quotes "two (anonymous) outstanding professors who have taught at four different Division IA institutions in power conferences." Their stark positions mirror Bensel-Meyers' assertion of a system-wide lack of control:[16]

1. "In my opinion, college presidents, independently or on NCAA boards, will never solve the problem. They are part of the problem. It is all about money and keeping their jobs. In a sense, they are more guilty than anyone because they should know better, and they let it happen, even encouraged it.

   "The simple truth is that many college athletes should not be in college, and many others have no real reason or opportunity to behave like students once they get here. The problem is decades old, but it is now worse because of the money and TV. I believe that the only potential solution is a faculty revolt across universities, but apathy runs deep and who would organize it."

2. "It seems to me that, whether they want to be or not, Brand and the other presidents are prisoners of this huge cash generating co-

lossus. No one can convince me that they care one whit about the academic achievements of athletes and I don't see them backing any reform that represents any risk to them personally.

"The saddest thing to me is that fans, like me and my faculty friends, accept this situation. No one believes that the majority of basketball and football players are qualified to be students and everyone knows that their sports take all of their time and leaves very little for academics. What you propose makes so much sense and I believe anyone who is honest would agree. But I think there will be a thousand reasons for doing nothing."[17]

Doing nothing apparently has been the preferred action by athletic programs across the country—football in particular—when it comes to recruiting violations. Tony Dorsett's claim in the previous chapter of being offered "everything imaginable" by schools interested in signing him might have left a lot to the imagination a year or two ago if not for the sex scandal that wallopped Colorado football and helped reveal nearly a dozen similar cases—some that had never before been reported. It was truly a cross-section of the nation's colleges and universities—from the usual suspects (Florida and Miami) to private schools whose administrations were appalled (BYU and Rice), from proven powerhouses (Alabama and Michigan) to lesser-known lightweights (Alabama State and Northern Colorado). In every case, nothing much had ever been done by coaches to curb potentially fatal results of unsupervised and underage partying during recruiting trips. Michigan president James Duderstadt told the *New York Times* that he had personally apologized to the parents of Mateen Cleaves following his near-disastrous visit to Ann Arbor. "I had to meet with the parents of Mateen and explain to them how a university allowed their high school son to end up in such dire circumstances (in a one-car roll-over accident coming back to campus from a party with strippers in a Detroit hotel)," Duderstadt said. "That is not a conversation any parent should ever have to hear, not from a university."[18] Obviously Michigan did not go out of its way to bring attention to the 1996 incident, but the fact that these types of parties persist gives some indication of the level of concern coaches and administers have always shown to these recruiting tools and rites of passage. Eight years after Cleaves' crash, it has taken an eight-member panel, appointed by uni-

Who's in Charge? Administration Is Part of the Problem

239

versity regents of the State of Colorado to review CU's policies, months to learn that the school's administrators did not have enough control over the athletic department, and head football coach Gary Barnett did not have the proper control over his program. "There hasn't been a clear line of accountability, and that has to be addressed," CU consultant John DiBiaggio told the *Denver Post.* "The public is saying, 'Some of these things apparently have been going on for a long period of time, and there hasn't been an adequate response.' That's very clear."[19] To the NCAA's credit, doing nothing is now far from acceptable. The steps taken by the NCAA in response to these recruiting scandals were swift, significant, and smart. The fact that such changes are so late in coming is reason to believe there is much work to be done to clean up college sports, but, as will be detailed in chapter 17, the NCAA did very well in moving toward that goal.

Plenty remains unsolved for the NCAA and other organizations whose coaches are either not properly respected or do not deserve to be respected. Academics crusader Terry Holland is not nearly as nice with his criticisms. "We have to acknowledge the system is failing rapidly because we have some incredibly intelligent people doing some incredibly stupid things at every level, including our presidents," Holland says. "Those who won't admit that are absolutely crazy."[20] Holland is not alone in recognizing the enormity of the circumstances. William C. Friday, president of the University of North Carolina system from 1957 to 1986 and chairman of the Knight Commission says, "What is happening here is an illustration of the pressure to win, the pressure of money in college sports. It's not a happy scene. We've turned college sports into a religion in the United States, and that pressure, coupled with the insatiable appetite of commercial interests (are) beyond a president's ability to control."[21] Whereas presidents at Colorado, Baylor, and many more respected institutions may have stumbled into trouble after discovering they had exhibited too little authority over their athletic programs, there are several examples of presidents being directly involved in the improprieties that plague college sports:

- *Georgia:* President Michael F. Adams personally selected Jim Harrick Sr. as the men's basketball coach, despite knowing that Harrick lied about an expense report at UCLA, which led to his firing. A sexual harassment suit against Harrick's staff as well as minor NCAA violations committed during his tenure at Rhode Island had not been made public when he was hired at Georgia. "We had discussed how important doing the right thing was at the University of Georgia, and I think everybody had good faith that that would be taken seriously," Adams told the *Chronicle of Higher Education.*[22]

- *Fresno State:* President John D. Welty hired popular Fresno State alumnus Jerry Tarkanian, despite the fact that his previous two programs were punished for NCAA violations (Long Beach State and UNLV). Tarkanian retired before Fresno State also went on probation, lost scholarships, and forfeited victories for violations that included academic fraud, a lack of institutional control, and players competing while ineligible. "In hindsight," Welty said, "maybe it wasn't the best decision."[23]

- *St. Bonaventure:* President Robert J. Wickenheiser was forced to resign after admitting he ordered subordinates to circumvent the school's policies to allow an ineligible player to play. "Throughout this process, I made a series of well-intentioned decisions based on a series of assumptions and interpretations," he said in a written statement. "The NCAA has come to a conclusion different from the one I reached."[24]

- *Gardner-Webb:* President Christopher White resigned after allowing a star basketball player to continue playing even though the president knew he was ineligible. "I am sorry that what I did two years ago out of fairness to a student has led to such turmoil and controversy," White said in a statement.[25]

These examples are extreme cases and are certainly the exception. But they are also the only well-publicized examples of university presidents playing a major role in compounding the ethical problems colleges face. Many other questionable hires slip by unnoticed. And moral breakdowns by people in other administrative positions also receive less attention. But if a president can lower his standards or drop his guard (whichever story you believe), corruption can exist at any level and at any school. It is, as Holland and others complain, an environment that does not necessitate change for the good, and therefore changes are slow to come about. The status quo will remain because of the "unbridled commercialism and competition that threatens the academic integrity of every Division I campus," Holland says.[26] It may sound dire, because it is. So too is the impact of a crumbling academic base on the student-athletes. There are no limitations in place to protect athletes from extended travel required to compete in contests. The NCAA has and always will be concerned about its players, but not enough to override the television schedules or the huge contracts that come with them. Thus, the overall time burden of competing in college does not afford most athletes the ability to obtain a quality education. Even the best students struggle to keep up, let alone the majority of collegiate athletes who consider schoolwork secondary to their task on the field. It's no wonder athletes see academics as secondary.

- Some kids are told they won't have to go to class.
- Look at how many incidents are reflected on these pages; papers are written for athletes, grades are manipulated, classes are taught by coaches and are drastically dumbed down.
- Parents approve of holding children back in school for the sole purpose of allowing them to mature physically in order to better prepare them for the chance of a college scholarship. This has proven to stunt social and academic development, and it lowers expectations for students who are repeating coursework that no longer challenges them. There are always exceptions, but the message being sent is not correct.

From presidents to parents, those in charge are failing to fulfill their obligation to instill character and ethics into the children and young athletes they supervise. Until this tragedy is attacked, there is little hope, because those who are capable of implementing solutions are still such a major part of the problem.

As discussed in detail in chapters 3 and 4, professional sports authorities have often been more a part of the problem than of the solution. One overwhelming example comes from Cincinnati Reds catcher Johnny Bench, who in his autobiography, *Catch You Later*, wrote: "[Amphetamines] were misused, and not just by pitchers, and for that I blame the trainers who dispensed them as much as the players who took them. In the pros, you look for any leg up, and a lot of guys, especially pitchers facing a tough start, thought daps and dexys were that edge."[27]

15

Struggling for Sportsmanship: Through a Ref's Eagle Eyes

In this chapter, we present an interview with Barry Mano, president of the National Association of Sports Officials.[1] The founder and publisher of *Referee* magazine and the National Association of Sports Officials (NASO), Barry Mano is a retired 23-year basketball official who worked nine seasons at the NCAA men's Division I level. He is a renowned public speaker and administrator and a member of the NASO-initiated Officiating Development Alliance.

Q&A WITH BARRY MANO

Question: Sports seems to mirror society in its growing disregard for authority and morality. What are your thoughts on this connection?
Answer: Sports is life with the volume turned up. So to some measure, we shouldn't be surprised by the characterization [of sports mirroring life]. We should be disappointed, but not surprised, because that's kind of the crucible of emotions acting out; the loss of restraint in your daily life. One of the reasons you do what you do as a sports fan is because you feel fewer restraints than you do in your normal life. And to some measure that might be why some people lash out so virulently against sports officials as authority figures, because [fans] come [to games] to get away from restraint and what do they get confronted with? Somebody with a plastic whistle who when they blow it, the world stops. They give you something you didn't want to hear. You see this at the youth level, particularly with parents. The frustrations of the day well up and assault them again during this leisure-time activity. That's where we see our biggest problems.

The difficulty of each passing generation is that people have not been accepting decisions [from authority figures]. If when you're being raised, you are always [responding to a parent's orders by] asking, "Why?" and your parents keep giving you reasons why, over and over, it carries over to the classroom and it carries over to the basketball floor. So you make a call on a kid, the reaction is, "Why?" They want an explanation and you're put into the situation where the answer is, "It's that way because I called it." It's much more challenging today than it was 20 years ago. People were much more accepting of a decision. There wasn't constant review of that decision—and I don't mean in a technical sense such as videotape. Today, it's like this with everything. How many hearings do you see on TV with politicians grilling people. It's constant daily fare now. Every decision-making level gets hauled in to sit in front of somebody. It's a different world. We are swept up in that and as officials, we have to hang on mightily. I'm not saying we're not wrong; we do make mistakes. But I think what's important is that we as society continue to accept the premise that when an official makes a call—right or wrong—it is the call.

Q: It appears the situation is getting worse when it should be getting better. What's your perspective?

A: We now have liability insurance—$3 million for each of our 16,000 members. We have assault protection insurance; and we're getting ready to initiate game-call insurance to protect our members and pay for legal defense. The day will come when we get hauled into court over a decision we make that say pulls a high school team out of a tournament, which means the college scouts don't get to see a kid and the parents lodge a lawsuit because of loss out of economic potential. It's already happened, but it was summarily dismissed because the courts have yet to rule against us. The courts are very assiduous in saying we are not going to get involved in the decision-making process of sports officials.

Sport is part of the culture, of the society. Those major forces have to be dealt with and made manifest in the sports world. The interesting question for me is can you uncover certain values that are coming the other way. Are sports creating a certain culture, certain values and habits, etc., that then drive their way back into the larger culture. That to me is a fascinating question. Because there's so much media focused on sports and on every little thing that happens. And does that drive itself back into society's daily culture. It's like the lyrics of some rap music; people are asking if these lyrics are basically anti-feminine. Are they driving certain behaviors in larger society. You can ask the same question about sports. Is it OK to use corked bats and pump up on steroids? If it's OK there, how big a step is it stealing stuff from your office when you go home at night?

NASO held a national summit in August of 2004 in Washington D.C. The theme of the event was, "The Official's Role in Promoting Sportsmanship." As officials we are changing the focus a bit. We want to talk about what is our role in sportsmanship; what exactly are we doing to make it better and in what ways are we making it worse right now. That's really not a focus in other sports summits.

Nobody has a real body of information. All we can say is from what we've been witnessing in the last 10 years is that there are more physical assaults against officials than ever before. More are being reported so there are more today than ever before. Absolutely, there is no doubt about it, that physical assaults against officials have been on the rise. Obviously it's bad enough that 18 states have passed legislation to increase the penalty for physically assaulting a sports official. That in itself tells you that people out there in the larger society realize there is a serious problem.

Q: *So what's taking the other states so long to pass their own similar form of legislation?*

A: When you do this sort of thing, you are defining yourself as a protected class like teachers, public transportation drivers, police. Some politicians say, "An assault is an assault—why should it be different than against somebody on the street?" They don't look upon officials as a protected class. We make the case that our role in sports and therefore in society is much more significant than somebody walking down the street. That type of protection and recognition is important.

If you've ever been at a sporting event when an official is assaulted, it's a pretty horrible thing. One of two things can happen. One, is that the crowd just moans because they know they're witnessing something that's just terrible. It would be like in court if someone started beating on the judge we would be just outraged. If you saw that on TV you'd probably stand up and scream. It's the same way in sports. The other action that can happen [when a sports official is attacked] is people cheering. In either case it's pretty grim, so a lot of people are fighting and scratching to stop this. Many organizations—from the NCAA to youth groups—are struggling mightily to get this thing turned around because it's a cancer in sports. From our standpoint, we're having a harder and harder time recruiting people to officiate. There's a shortage of bodies. We're not able to keep up, to replenish, to get people into the lower levels where there is either no compensation or very minimal monetary compensation. So we're constantly struggling to get new officials, and to retain them.

Every meeting we're ever in, recruiting and retaining officials is one of the top topics. In youth sports, unfortunately, the top topic is pedophilia. Beyond that, the topic of how you find people to become officials is the No. 1 problem. If people finally say we're not going to referee, what are you going to do? Have parents referee the games? They're even less skillful, there are liability issues.

Q: So what are the possible solutions?

A: Some things we can do is not pour gasoline on the fire. When you're an official, I don't care if it's a soccer pitch, a football field, baseball diamond or a basketball court, there are little kindling fires on all of those at all times. As a referee we can either pour gasoline on those fires or we can pour water on them. In the old days when my dad refereed—in the olden days—he could turn around say to someone: "Shut up and sit down!" You can't do that today. We are a different society. It's just not permitted to say, "Shut up. I don't want to hear it anymore!" You have to have a whole new, unique set of skills in dealing with people from a position of leadership to be able to reach the goal of good, effective game management. The kindling fires I'm talking about have to do with things like two players jabbing each other and trash-talking running up and down the floor and you know this stuff is going on and you're doing nothing about it. That's pouring gasoline.

Part of the challenge in D.C. [was] to do some self-inspection to see if what we're doing is making things worse; how we go about conducting ourselves. It takes a good bit of restraint to be a referee when someone's chewing on you like crazy. You might want to have a strong verbal reaction to that but we're not permitted to do that, by not putting ourselves in positions we can't extricate ourselves from.

Another problem an official can have is not enforcing the rules. There are many rules on unsportsmanlike behavior and many times we pass on them. We use warnings. We try to be good game managers; try to be good guys; try to get along with people and make it all come together when in fact we should be enforcing the rules. We have to step up with respect to that issue. And we can never say, "People are going to get angry if we enforce this rule." We referees have gone too far in using warnings. And if you look around at society, you see it everyday. You're at the airport and a kid starts acting up and his mother says, "Johnny stop doing that." He keeps it up and she says, what? "Johnny, I told you to stop doing that." Then she tells him for the fifth time, "If I've got to tell you one more time . . ." That's what we've become [as a society]. We've devalued our words. The kid's not stupid. The kid knows mom's going to do this five times, so he's going to push her through the first four. This plays out in sports. It plays out in respect to how officials interact with players.

Q: *What positives have you witnessed that give you reason to believe society is working toward solutions?*

A: Obviously there is positive news in my mind in that consciousness has been raised. Hey, we really have a problem here. Look at the NFL. They saw this as a problem, with players running onto the field and stomping on the Dallas Cowboys' star; all the doggy dancing and all that. It reflected poorly on the sport and people were not happy with that behavior. Finally the NFL came out with some strict penalties and even produced a video that was presented at one of our [NASO] conferences, showing kinds of behavior that officials were going to flag. You had Terell Owens and the next guy and the next guy and by the time you've seen 10 of them you're ready to throw up. My point in this whole anecdote is this: That effort got started by the veteran NFL players. The NFLPA [players association] threw their hands up because they couldn't get the young bucks to listen to them that doing this stuff was not good. They went to the league and they jointly came up with the ruling, the video, and that got circulated to every team. I find it interesting that the players themselves took this action. If the fans want more of that stuff, then shame on the fans. It's disrespecting the other players. If people think putting cell phones in goal posts [Joe Horn, New Orleans Saints] is cute, then it's a sad commentary of what we're expecting from sports. It's turning it into the WWE football league. We, the fans, are the consumers of sports. And consumers rule in a market economy. Fans tell us very clearly what they want; what they're willing to pay for. I think the league showed great leadership there. We're supposed to be talking about football, not about in-your-face stuff. There's a lot of pressure put on referees to stop this unsportsmanlike behavior. The league wanted it stopped. And they're doing it. You're seeing it in the NBA and in baseball and certainly in the high schools. There's a strong movement toward getting this thing turned back around to the level that people find acceptable.

Q: Are officials better trained to handle the problems?

A: We used to have a saying: "It's nothing until I call it." That was the arrogance of being a ref. Today, it's still nothing until I call it but, boy oh boy, your instincts are so different. The conversations we have now in pre-game meetings, a lot of it has to do with security. We used to go in and talk about a few rules and then we talked about where we were going to get some beers after the game. Today you go to the big venues and you want to meet the head security guys. You want to know who's going to be where; who's taking us on the floor. Where are the security people going to be when we're coming off the floor. When we have trouble with the fans, where do we turn to get it stopped. In the old days you'd have refs go into the stands to get rid of people. It's very different today, but that's another very positive outcome. We've had to go "back to school" to learn these skills and to be much more aware of how we treat people with our language, how we look at people, all of these things.

There is a men's recreation league in Chicago, and they're doing radio advertisements to get people to play in the league. One of the main things they say is that they have hired the best officials. They're making a point of this to say they are better trained so they're going to make the games safer and more fun, etc. I think that's a neat, positive outcome. There the market's working right? People want good officials and they're willing to pay for it. A lot of these leagues are brutal and a lot of it's because the officiating is not good.

Q: What's important for parents to know or work on?

A: Their acceptance that there are going to be incorrect calls in games, and we have to accept that. Some of them might be terrible calls, for whatever reasons: the ref didn't see it or the ref's not good. Frankly, it's not important. What's important is to understand that sports at that level is an educational experience. Part of that education is to know you are going to get incorrect calls. It happens. Sport is supposed to train us. That's the most important lesson of all.

Number two is to continue to be a role model, regardless of how agitated or unhappy you are. Be a role model in public places.

And number three, when you're going home with the kids, make sure you don't permit the kid to offload responsibility to the officials for something that did or did not happen. That to me is unacceptable. Most importantly, we're not going to sit here and shift the responsibility. And if a kid says, "But dad . . ." I don't want to hear that. That doesn't teach anything except a lack of responsibility. We're big on that in this society. We believe that somebody else is at fault. We are unable today to accept the smallest bit of injustice. We say, "This stinks. I don't deserve this."

Q: What do coaches need to work on?

A: [Coaches] must be role models, too. They are so important in this because they have an overreaching influence on the kids. We have to be sure to understand the old phrase "sports is an extension of the classroom." Would you permit a teacher to act the way some coaches act during youth games?

Q: What do athletes need to work on?

A: As far as athletes go, sportsmanship is such a character builder. Officials can see kids who are destined to be great people. When they are blatantly the recipient of an incorrect call, but they handle it correctly—and they may say something; they may ask the ref about the call in a polite way and the ref may say, "I blew that call," but we move on. When I see kids do this, that's character. That's refreshing. Referees can't see everything. If I make an incorrect call and say A touched the ball last so it's B's ball and I later know that by the way player A reacts that I've made the wrong call, I'm still giving the ball to B. You don't have all the info all the time. I missed that call but by rule, [if another official didn't see the play] I cannot change the call.

A perfect example happened at a Braves–Rockies game [in April of 2004]. A player reached into foul ground, caught a fly ball, and a fan snatched it out of his glove when he opened it up. It happened in a matter of seconds, but the rule is that you have to do something positive with the ball—for example take it out of your mitt as if to throw it.

The rule exists so that when a catcher catches a ball and it gets knocked out of his glove by a base runner, it's not an out. Or if an outfielder makes a catch running full speed into a wall and hits the wall two or three strides later and the ball pops out, it's not an out. People don't know that rule. The manager didn't know that rule and he argued so much that he got thrown out of the game. The umpire got the call dead right in a very tense situation because he knew that rule. It's a lousy deal. I don't disagree, but it's a rule and it's there for a good reason. . . . My point is there are intricacies of the rules that players don't always know. A good rule of thumb is for players to give referees the benefit of the doubt. Because we study the rules and kids and coaches don't.

Q: What responsibility does the media have in promoting sportsmanship and supporting officials?

A: It's not so much for our cause [as officials] but for the cause of sports. They [the media] need to be better. I understand you don't have lot of time and having a little bit of controversy is good, but the fact is that the media is perpetrating so much bad information that reflects poorly on officials. You should have heard these two announcers on the Rockies game. I mean they went off on the ump. I mean, big time. Fact is, the umps were correct. That's why the NFL has set up live feeds into 240 Park Avenue, into the 15th floor. Director of Officiating Mike Pereira and others are watching these games. Let's say we had a situation like this baseball play in the NFL, Mike would actually call over to the [network satellite] truck. And he'd tell them, "Hey would you tell John Madden upstairs that here's the ruling, the ruling is correct." It's so they can tell the fans. We need much more of that because the media has a tremendous impact on how we perceive sports and what sports officials do. We just get killed by the media, because they don't have the knowledge.

One of the problems [the media face] is the gag rule. We can't talk to you. I would like to see that changed. At the same time, when you do that then we officials have to have some training in dealing with [the media] because [they] are notorious about taking stuff out of context, about hearing what [they] want to hear. We have no guarantee that [the media] will actually listen to and hear us. It's a very challenging thing. The pro leagues today will bring the media together ahead of time, they'll bring them to camps and other places, we'll have media at our [national convention] in Washington D.C. just trying to instill in them the need for more of this. There are some broadcasters who will not correct themselves on the air [even if they are given a correct ruling]. They won't admit they're wrong. Others will do that. I think it would be great information. What's the big deal.

Q: What help can the government provide?
A: We need to be a protected class [by law]. We need to get all the protection offered to teachers, police, fire people. Our role in sports is tantamount to that. Just like judges. Having that heightened class distinction is very positive. Other than that we don't need help, we just need to do our jobs, enforce the rules.

16

Solutions: Winning without Losing Perspective

Individual commitment to a group effort—that is what makes a team work, a company work, a society work, a civilization work.

—Vince Lombardi

The contents of this book may cause many to wonder if individuals can ever correct the piles of problems plaguing sports today. Lombardi, if he were alive today, would say they are right and wrong. For a sports book wrought with adversity, such as this one, a reminder of the importance of teamwork is a must before solutions can be sought. Unfortunately, America's culture—especially considering the sad, deteriorating state of the family—encourages an individualistic approach that builds more obstacles than bridges. Fortunately, sports will always have the power to bring people together—all races, all religions, and all social classes for all time. The bond of a sports fan and his or her favorite team is rarely broken (even for a Cubs fan). If only the energy from individuals who pour their hearts into one winning season could be duplicated and put toward winning a much more important fight. The pages ahead are filled with solutions that individually will do little but collectively can begin to beat back the immoral and dishonorable behavior in sports and beyond. It is up to our readers to recognize their roles on this team—to lead, contribute, or perhaps to simply show support or show restraint from putting too great an emphasis on winning.

SOLUTIONS IN SCIENCE

The prevention of catastrophe in athletic events has numerous aspects. The strategies include such areas as rules, laws, and other legislation that impact various areas of each sport; protective equipment design and manufacture; and proper coaching and training. The hope for prevention of deaths and serious injury in sports follows one of several pathways. We know that certain catastrophic injuries and deaths are going to follow predictable patterns and may not be amenable to education programs, changes in participation, or the rules of the sport or activity, and inexorably will continue to occur. The education of the athlete and all others involved in sports is paramount for increased understanding and safety. Later in the chapter we focus upon those programs and policies that have been shown to be advantageous to accomplish improvement in athletics. First, however, we will consider possible solutions for avoiding some particular risks in both recreational and organized sports.

The most common reason for sudden death in athletes from a non-traumatic cause is a cardiac event. The potential for unsuspected cardiac conditions is present in every person, and thus every athlete. In young and highly conditioned athletes, it is always difficult to determine beforehand if a life-threatening cardiac abnormality exists primarily because it is not apparent by taking a medical history (the person has no heart symptoms) or by performing a routine, preseason physical examination. In fact, sophisticated heart tests are often necessary to detect such a problem as an irregular heartbeat, a heart valve abnormality, or a blockage in a coronary artery, but these tests are not infallible in determining their presence. Several recommendations have been made by authorities in this area. In general, any athlete who suffers chest pain or unexpected shortness of breath with exertion, has a heart murmur, passes out, or experiences other unexplained symptoms should be evaluated by his or her physician and possibly by a cardiologist. Any potentially serious medical condition that can impact the athlete, such as asthma, should be thoroughly evaluated prior to participation.

Another example of a non-traumatic death in sports is heatstroke, and its prevention is possible through proper fluid replacement and practice regimens, by avoiding extreme environmental training sessions, and by banning the use of PEDs or exogenous substances. The period required for heat acclimation is approximately two weeks. During this time, numerous physiological responses are occurring in the body to help it adapt to the new environmental stress. These responses include a reduction in loss of electrolytes through the urine, retention of fluids to expand blood plasma volume, a reduction in heart rate, and an increased sweat rate, among others. It is important to provide the body with enough time to adequately readjust to the heat-stressed environment, and this is the single and most sensible factor for athletes and coaches to consider in their training.[1] New portable cooling devices that lower body temperature by drawing heat away through application of a specially devised glove and a cooling vest are examples of high-technology solutions for avoiding heat-related illness in athletes, but thus far these tools have not been universally adopted.[2] A very effective initial treatment for someone who may be suffering from heat-related illness is immediate immersion into an ice bath, followed by medical attention if appropriate.

Motorized sporting activities such as snowmobile and ATV riding, bicycling, snow skiing, and others are prime areas for prevention strategies. In essentially every sporting activity in which head injury is a possibility, helmet use remains the single best prevention mechanism that can be implemented. Numerous studies have shown that protection of the head and face affords the greatest benefit against impact and penetration injuries. In ATV accidents, our research has confirmed that helmet use would likely prevent at least 50 percent of serious or fatal injuries. In addition, the concomitant use of alcohol was seen in nearly one-half of serious or fatal ATV mishaps, and the strict prohibition of alcohol use while operating any recreational motorized equipment would result in a marked reduction in the number and seriousness of these accidents. Legislation to implement several laws concerning the operation and operating conditions of ATVs, including those to protect young riders, is paramount in improving their safety record.

No type of central nervous system lesion lends itself as well to prevention as does the diving injury. Although such programs as "Think First" have had a dramatic impact on reducing the incidence of diving injuries in some regions of the United States, traditionally diving accidents have persisted in spite of previous public warnings. Public service announcements and cervical spine injury prevention programs remain a top priority. The seasonal nature of diving accidents justifies the continued need for public awareness during summer months. The cost to society, in terms of human suffering and financial burden, is incalculable. The retrieval mechanism of a person with a known or suspected spinal cord diving injury should follow established guidelines, with careful maintenance of a neutral anatomic position until spinal injury has been ruled out. When an in-water diving injury is suspected, the victim may be floated supine in the water with assistance until professional help arrives. It is calculated that when diving from deck level or higher, it takes almost double the individual's height in water depth to allow complete deceleration of the body. Above ground, shallow swimming pools are notoriously dangerous for diving. The causative role of alcohol use in these injuries also deserves emphasis. Similar to the warnings the public receives concerning the dangers of drinking and driving, they should also be made aware of the risk of drinking and diving.

Our research has shown that boxers who fight for prolonged periods, and who have absorbed multiple, unblocked, or unparried blows to the head, sustain the greatest risk of fatal outcome, particularly in bouts which have gone the distance or lasted into the late rounds. In these instances it is believed that there are a threshold number of punches that may be landed to the cranium before the chances of irreversible brain injury are increased, and death usually results from widespread and untreatable brain swelling. Future improvements may result if a system of scoring and continuing a boxing match would depend not only on the usual requirement that a boxer be able to defend himself while mounting some offensive movements, but also that he may be disqualified if he absorbs a specified number of unblocked head shots during the course of the fight. Other methods that objectify the impacts incurred during a match may be helpful in the future, such as the use of an accelerometer, which is a device for measuring the force imparted to the head.

The evolution in our thought concerning prevention, either primarily through equipment and rule changes or via improved clinical management, is important in understanding the current recommended treatment of athletes with concussions. At the same time, the United States' legal system has evolved in the past two decades to allow a much more liberal interpretation of laws regarding assumption of risk; negligence on behalf of coaches, athletic trainers, and team physicians; and product liability for protective equipment or its fitting and other aspects of sports-related injury. For instance, the number of

U.S. helmet manufacturers has fallen dramatically in the last few years as liability insurance rates have simultaneously soared.

The ability to intervene on behalf of prevention in an athletic contest is necessarily limited by the regulations as well as by the nature of the events of contact sports. Therefore, efforts to lessen the incidence of serious injury or concussion have focused on the protective equipment and playing rules as they are formulated and enforced. The playing surface, although the source of study and efforts for improvement, has been primarily correlated with major joint and soft tissue injuries. A previous study has shown that regardless of the type of playing surface, whether grass or artificial turf, there was no difference in terms of the incidence of concussion. Many sports are played on a hard surface, such as the ground or ice, and this is unlikely to be modified in the future.

The implementation of helmet use has become more widespread than ever before and is now commonplace not only in organized sports, such as ice hockey, but also in equestrian sports, bicycling, and other endeavors. The purpose of a helmet in general is twofold: (1) it has a hard outer shell that serves to spread the force of impact over a large surface area, preventing scalp injuries such as lacerations; and (2) it contains an inner lining, often with an advantageous web or suspension design, to help dissipate the kinetic energy of the acceleration forces by an energy-absorptive mechanism. Current helmet designs have limitations in terms of size, appearance, weight, materials, and other engineering factors, in addition to being subjected to numerous medical and legal influences of product liability.

In all helmeted sports, we have seen a marked reduction in the incidence of head and facial injuries. Proper equipment, and its correct fitting, should be an integral part of every sport that utilizes such equipment, particularly the contact sports. Studies of fatal pole-vaulting accidents have confirmed that the majority of deaths are caused by improper landing techniques, specifically when the vaulter lands outside of the pit. This can and should be corrected by the enlargement of the pit, with greater protective padding, along with proper coaching to instruct the athlete of the potential for injury in this manner.

The importance of proper conditioning and training is emphasized in order to help contact sports athletes to best sustain the energy forces to which they are subjected. This has been especially true for avoidance of cervical spine injuries, as it has been shown that the neck musculature can be developed for effective injury prevention strategy. Overall, optimal strength and conditioning are paramount for proper coaching and playing. The attention to rules and their enforcement by game officials is of great importance to help prevent injuries to the central nervous system, as the effects of "spearing" in football have been demonstrated to increase the risk of such catastrophic injuries.

It is worth mentioning that basic, sensible, nutritional guidelines will ensure an athlete has the necessary fuel to maintain an active year-round competitive sports schedule. This fact is applicable to all athletes but can be especially important to parents who do not want their children taking any supplements. As 2004 U.S. Olympic triple jumper Kenta Bell says, and medical experts agree, eating a well-rounded diet that includes vegetables of all colors is a great way to get the right amount of vitamins, minerals, and antioxidants. Bell suggests that athletes refrain from using any protein supplements, but instead "eat a couple chicken breasts" to get the same amount of protein. Bell, however, does use creatine safely (avoiding unnecessary "loading" and taking the recommended dosage). Leslie Bonci, director of sports nutrition at the University of Pittsburgh Medical Center, and Julie Hartley, clinical/wellness dietitian at Willis-Knighton Health System in Shreveport, Louisianna, agree that using food rather than supplements for energy is a recommended option to ensure the best overall health. "I tell athletes the fuel going into their body—whether it's from pasta or fruit—is really what is sustaining them over their athletic endeavors, not the supplements," Bonci says. "Even though eating a bagel doesn't sound nearly as sexy as taking a Ginseng, it does go much further."[3] Adds Hartley: "The food pyramid most people are familiar with is basically an accurate guideline. . . . Proteins definitely have a place, but a good ratio for an active child is that at least 60 percent of their diet come from carbohydrates."[4] It is true that some supplements are safe and even beneficial, but as Bell reminds us, "one in five supplements contain banned substances." Their exact contents are often unknown, and long-term health effects are still not completely understood. A safe bet is to eat right, and there is a buffet of resources available to parents, coaches, and athletes interested in monitoring this basic but vital area.

SOLUTIONS IN YOUTH SPORTS

As the authors of this book, we would like to encourage the collaborative efforts of the many organizations and individuals working toward the betterment of young athletes. The Joseph and Edna Josephson Institute of Ethics, the Citizenship Through Sport Alliance, the National Association of Youth Sports, Adolescents Training and Learning to Avoid Steroids, and other successful organizations are leaders in this charge already. As the World Anti-Doping Agency hoped to unify policy and support to eradicate doping in all sports, our hope is for as many youth coaches, leagues, and schools as possible to sign on with one alliance, or at least follow an approved code of ethics in which all participants vow to institute practices of outstanding sportsmanship and citizenship. At the risk of oversimplifying an enormous task, we are all fighting the same battle; joining forces seems to be a sure-fire way to succeed in small and grand ways.

Before individuals can commit to the group effort, those in charge must make the team's goals and guidelines clear. For those involved in youth sports, the most important goal should be enabling children to have fun again. If this is a goal on which we all can agree, there must be a way to agree on the steps we can take to work toward that end. John Leavens, the executive director of the Citizenship Through Sports Alliance (CTSA), wants this to be a reality. A coalition of the largest professional, amateur, and Olympic sports organizations in the nation, CTSA is one of many similar groups across the country that is doing tremendous work. But as Leavens points out, with millions of children competing in youth sports, no one organization can effectively reach every community. "We understand there are a number of youth sports organizations out there. We're interested in finding unifying seeds, fundamental enduring values that ought to be standard for all of these organizations. And we want to measure if we're making progress. We know there are problems in youth sports but what is not known is how extensive those problems are.

"Our three major areas of focus include this idea of creating a collaboration [of groups]—a clearinghouse for organizations across the country interested in Citizenship Through Sports Alliance's programs. No. 2, we want to increase public awareness of our programs. And No. 3, we're searching for a means to measure progress over time."[5]

Sidebar 16.1: Tips for Coaches, Parents, and Players

FOR COACHES:

Scott B. Lancaster, NFL Youth Development senior director, offers seven principles for coaches to achieve success in youth sports from his book *Fair Play: Making Organized Sports a Great Experience for Your Kids:*[1]

- *Make It Fun.*
- *Limit Standing Around.*
- *Everyone Plays.*
- *Teach Every Position to Every Participant.*
- *Emphasize the Fundamentals.*
- *Incorporate a Progression of Skill Development for Every Participant.*
- *Yell Encouragement, Whisper Constructive Criticism.*

FOR PARENTS:

Darrell J. Burnett, sports psychologist, on what parents should not do, taken from his *Playbook for Kids*, a free pamphlet produced by Gatorade:[2]

- *Don't yell out instructions*: During the game, I'm trying to concentrate on what the coach says and working on what I've been practicing. It's easier for me to do my best if you save instructions and reminders for practice or just before the game.
- *Don't put down the officials*: This embarrasses me, and I sometimes wonder whether the official is going to be tougher on me because my parents yell.
- *Don't yell at me in public.* It will just make things worse because I'll be upset, embarrassed or worried that you're going to yell at me the next time I do something wrong.
- *Don't yell at the coach*: When you yell about who gets to play what position, it just stirs things up and takes away from the fun.
- *Don't put down my teammates*: Don't make put-down remarks about any of my teammates who make mistakes. It takes away from our team spirit.
- *Don't put down the other team*: When you do this, you're not giving us a very good example of sportsmanship, so we get mixed messages about being good sports.
- *Don't lose your cool*: I love to see you excited about the game, but there's no reason to get so upset that you lose your temper. It's our game, and all the attention is supposed to be on us.

- *Don't lecture me about mistakes after the game*: Those rides home in the car after the game are not a good time for lectures about how I messed up. I already feel bad. We can talk later, but please stay calm and don't forget to mention the things I did well during the game.
- *Don't forget how to laugh and have fun*: Sometimes it's hard for me to relax and have fun during the game when I look over and see you so tense and worried.
- *Don't forget that it's just a game*: Odds are, I'm not going to make a career out of playing sports. I know I may get upset if we lose, but I also know that I'm usually feeling better after we go get a pizza. I need to be reminded sometimes that it's just a game.

Ian Tofler, a psychiatrist at LSU, on suggestions for parents hoping to avoid trying to live vicariously through their children's sports activities:[3]

- Balance your child's total development needs with sports goals.
- Reclaim "decision authority" for the child's welfare. The child should not be allowed to say, "This is my decision."
- Monitor your own motivation by asking, "How will this affect my child?" and "Am I doing this for myself or for my child?"
- More questions for parents to ask themselves:
  - What is my background or agenda in this sport?
  - What are the child's physical limitations?
  - What are the potential physical or emotional risks?
  - Are the financial requirements unreasonable?
  - Does this affect other important aspects of life?
  - Is this child emotionally ready?
  - What do our friends say about my involvement?
  - Do my emotions get out of control?
  - How does this affect the rest of my family?

FOR PLAYERS:

Dr. Burnett, on the characteristics of good players:[4]
Good players will . . .

- Follow the rules.
- Avoid arguments (stay focused on the game).
- Share in responsibilities of the game (be a team player).
- Give everyone a chance to play.
- Play fair (no cheating, no drugs to enhance your performance, etc.).
- Follow the directions of the coach.

- Respect the efforts of the other team (know that they are trying hard to win, too).
- Encourage their teammates.
- Accept the calls of the game officials (without complaining or arguing).
- End the game smoothly (without pouting, threatening or ugly behavior).

BOOKS ON YOUTH SPORTS AND SPORTSMANSHIP:

- *Kids & Sports: Everything You and Your Child Need to Know About Sports, Physical Activity, Nutrition, and Good Health—A Doctor's Guide for Parents and Coaches,* Eric Small, M.D.
- *Sports and Children,* K. M. Chan
- *Good Sports,* Rick Wolff
- *Positive Coaching,* J. M. Thompson
- *Goal: The Ultimate Goal for Soccer Moms and Dads,* Gloria Auverbuch, Michael Hammond
- *Children and Youth In Sport,* F. L. Smoll and R. E. Smith
- *Sport Parent,* T. Hanlon
- *Moms and Dads, Kids and Sports,* P. McInally
- *Parenting Your Super Star,* R. J. Rotella and L. K. Buncker
- *Sport For Children and Youth,* M. R. Weiss and D. Gould
- *Coaching Mental Excellence,* R. Vernacchia, R. McGuire, and D. Cook
- *Strength Training for Young Athletes,* W. J. Kraemer and S. J. Fleck
- *The Cheers and the Tears: A Healthy Alternative to the Dark Side of Youth Sports Today,* Shane Murphy

WEB SITES WITH TIPS ON SPORTSMANSHIP/FAIR COMPETITION:

www.charactercounts.org/sports/sportslinks.htm—Links to dozens of sports organizations and sportsmanship-centered sites, including many of those below

www.josephsoninstitute.org—The parent organization for Character Counts

www.sportsmanship.org—Citizenship Through Sports Alliance

www.nays.org—National Alliance for Youth Sports has developed a parental-sportsmanship course that includes a handbook, a video, and an ethical code

www.decatursports.com/articles/NYSCA—National Youth Sports Coaches Association code of ethics for coaches, players, and parents www.momsteam.com—Site founded by youth sports expert Brooke de Lench

www.kid-e-sport.com—Kid-e-sport offers helpful advice from the experts at the National Alliance for Youth Sports, aimed at children up to age 13 and their parents

www.cmonmom.com—C'mon Mom! lets soccer moms get in the game

www.sportsparents.com and www.sikids.com—Sports Illustrated for Kids

www.internationalsport.com—Institute for International Sport

www.naso.org—National Association of Sports Officials

www.tandl.vt.edu/rstratto/CYS/index.html—Coaching Youth Sports newsletter

www.nfhs.org—National Federation of State High School Association

www.positivecoach.org—Positive Coaching Alliance character-building programs

www.fairplaytoday.com—A youth program of the NFL

www.djburnett.com—Sports psychologist Dr. Burnett's official Web site

www.youth-sports.com—a Web site offering articles and advice on youth sports topics

www.kidsource.com—Education and healthcare information

http://ed-web3.educ.msu.edu/ysi/—Institute for the Study of Youth Sports

www.pecentral.com—Site for Health and Physical Education teachers

www.naysi.com—North American Youth Sports Institute

www.healthycompetition.org—Blue Cross Blue Shield Association educational Web site on performance-enhancing drugs

www.usantidoping.org/athletes/ambassadors.aspx—U.S. Anti-Doping Agency Athletes Ambassadors program

www.steroidabuse.org—National Institute on Drug Abuse

www.1.ncaa.org/membership/ed_outreach/health-safety/drug_ed_progs/index—NCAA: Alcohol, Tobacco, and Other Drug Education Programs and Grants

www.monitoringthefuture.org—University of Michigan's Monitoring the Future survey

WEB SITES WITH INFORMATION ABOUT SUPPLEMENTS:

www.consumerreports.org/co/supplements and www.consumersunion.org—Consumer Reports

www.fda.gov—U.S. Food and Drug Administration

www.mskcc.org/aboutherbs—Memorial Sloan-Kettering Cancer Center

One powerful partner of the Citizenship Through Sports Alliance is the Josephson Institute for Ethics. The Institute's creator, Michael Josephson, agrees that coming together as a team is essential. "Collaboration is the whole theory of character counseling and our Gold Medal Standards for youth sports. [Participants in this program include] the president of Little League Baseball, the executive director of American Youth Soccer Organization, the U.S. Olympic Committee's representative for volleyball. You do have to collaborate. Sport is a context in which ethics and character can and should be taught. The problem with sports is that they do have a built-in proficiency, especially since they rely so much on volunteers and parents to run them. . . . There are more than 500 organizations now that are a part of the Character Counts coalition. . . . One of the fundamental principles is concert in action, collaboration, not to reinvent wheel, but to take organizations like the YMCA that has always been character oriented and team up with them to help them be more proficient. It allows there to be this notion of we're all in this together."[6]

Collaborating and/or unifying the many youth sports associations in the United States would have immediate positive effects.

Protecting Referees

Beginning with the fundamental need for authority to be established, respected, and protected, youth leagues that join forces would have one very loud voice in support of increasing the number of states to pass bills calling for stiffer penalties for a physical assault on a sports official (currently 16 states do, with a 17th pending). This is an absolute necessity because of the facts discussed in chapter 11, "Caring For Youth Sports":

- "Little League Syndrome" or "Sports Rage" incidents are on the rise.
- Incidents of violence at youth sports events tripled from 1998 to 2002.
- Measuring the law's effects is difficult, but it is logical to assume the law is a deterrent.

Protecting Children's Health

As has also been described in chapter 11, injuries among youths are increasing, many from overuse by kids who play the same sport and make the same physical motions in hopes of honing skills enough to compete at elite levels when they get older.

Common examples include:

- "Little League Elbow" (repeated stress on the elbow from overhand throwing).
- Osgood-Schlatter's Disease (swelling and tenderness just below the knee, usually occurring during growth spurts or in sports that involve a lot of running and jumping).
- Torn anterior cruciate ligaments (an estimated 50,000 occur each year, the majority to people between the ages of 15 and 25, with girls being more susceptible, especially since more are playing basketball and soccer).[7]

Potential solutions include:

- Mastering the mechanics of pitching through instruction.
- Warming up, gradually building endurance, and limiting the number of pitches thrown per week.[8]
- Youth sports coaches can employ more stretches and injury-prevention techniques to their practices each season.
- Everyone can watch for signs of overuse and fatigue.
- More and more careful evaluations (seeking a physician's opinion for serious or lingering injuries, or those requiring medications).
- Refusing to allow children to compete when injured.
- Encouraging young athletes to try other sports and activities to allow off-seasons as a time for rest and recovery.[9]

Educating Adults

Sportsmanship needs to be reviewed or even relearned. Leagues that currently do not require such education can benefit from joining forces with organizations that have effective plans in place to eliminate the consistent, damaging mistakes adults make in overseeing youth sports.

From chapter 11, those common mistakes and their results include:

- Pushing kids too much
- Emphasizing winning too much
- Losing control of emotions

- Ignoring injuries (concussions, overuse/repetitive motion injuries, returning to play too early, weight training, etc.)
- Pushing athletes too early
- Mistaking a child's chronological age as an indicator that they are physically ready to participate in a certain sport or at a certain level
- *The overwhelming result*: Kids are noticing the poor behavior by adults and are not having fun.

The two primary parts of this education process—the policy and the punishment—should and can be taken from a collaboration of organizations that specialize in building character in youth sports:

1. *The Policy:* Not all parents who want their children to be the best are out of control, but even some parents who think they are doing a good job can benefit from understanding a simple formula that can be used to ensure parents are not losing perspective: Having fun should always be more important than being No. 1. Teaching kids life skills should be a secondary priority, including encouraging them to improve while maintaining a good attitude. Winning can be a part of the formula, but its importance should be minimized.

2. *The Punishment:* In a *Sports Illustrated for Kids* poll of 3,000 child athletes, more than a third said adults who can't control their tempers should be banned from games.[10] Since we have not yet learned that unsportsmanlike conduct by adults makes for an unenjoyable time for kids, perhaps it's time to listen to the children who believe the punishment for adults who get out of line needs to be much more severe. Standards that have been adopted and that are working across the country can be implemented and enforced more easily if there is a central clearinghouse that requires leagues to adhere to the rules. Setting stiff penalties everywhere gives this action the teeth it needs.

Success Stories

The following are some success stories from those communities that have organized policies or philosophies on sportsmanship (the list is by no means comprehensive as there are many programs not listed that are as or more deserving of credit for their efforts):

- *Mandeville, Louisiana:* Prior to the start of the 2002 fall basketball season, recreation supervisors and advisory board members at Pelican Park hired Mike Legarza, a senior trainer from the acclaimed Positive Coaching Alliance at Stanford University, to conduct a series of clinics aimed at "transforming youth sports so sports can transform youth." One piece of invaluable advice from Legarza can serve as a talking point and should be memorized by all coaches, parents, and league administers: Coaches, players, and their parents should "redefine [a] winner" as someone who makes maximum effort, continues to learn and improve, and refuses to let mistakes—or a fear of mistakes—stop them, regardless of the game's outcome.[11]
- *Nationwide:* Scott Lancaster is the senior director of NFL Youth Football Development and author of *Fair Play: Making Organized Sports a Great Experience for Your Kids.* His program includes such components as eliminating the scoreboard, removing coaches from the sidelines, and recruiting parents to help teach skills. The focus, he said, can then be not on winning and losing but on making sure that every child learns from the experience and has a good time in the process.[12]
- *Washington, D.C.:* John McCarthy, a former minor-league pitcher, teaches baseball to kids at his Home Run Baseball camp and to disadvantaged kids at an inner-city elementary school. He emphasizes basic skills and qualities such as concentration, persistence, generosity, humor, improvement, teamwork, hustle, and perseverance. McCarthy encourages coaches, parents, and teammates to cheer, but only to encourage and praise, not criticize.[13]
- *Bossier City, Louisiana:* Robert Reynolds, head umpire for Dixie baseball and a member of the National Association of Sports Officials, is listening more to parents and coaches with complaints instead of quickly jumping into arguments. "It's preventing anything before it even starts," Reynolds says. "Games are at more of a faster pace and with that emotions are up." Also, Bossier City Parks and Recreation Coordinator Bob Carter follows a sportsmanship program established by the National Alliance of Youth Sports. It became mandatory for coaches in 2002. "Summer ball is going on right now and you'd think there was a party over there

every night," Carter said. "They love it. There's no cuss words. The umpire's always right. It's really refreshing."[14]

- *Jupiter, Florida*: The Jupiter-Tequesta Athletic Association, the originator of the NAYS system now used nationwide, has seen a similar effect among its parents and coaches. Tempers flared less often, coaches could coach, officials could officiate, and kids could just play. "When we first introduced the program, we did get a lot of coverage from the media as you can imagine," JTAA Director Don Fradley said. "All of the parents were positive in getting certified. It had a huge impact on our organization. Parents seemed to have more manners and they were very conscientious of how they were behaving."[15]
- *South Dakota Cooperative Extension Youth Development/4H*: This organization is fighting poor sportsmanship by promoting two meaningful resources:
  1. *Putting Youth Back into Sports*: A program developed by Dr. Ann Michelle Daniels, South Dakota State University, and Dr. Danny Perkins, Penn State University, which provides a research-based curriculum to address the developmental attributes and needs of each age. Topics include:
     - Community Youth Development and Sports
     - Child and Youth Development Competencies
     - Differences between Female and Male Athletes
     - Understanding What Youth Want from Sports
     - Cooperation versus Competition
     - Parents and Youth Sports
     - Coach: Building a Positive Relationship with Parents
     - Coach: Building a Positive Relationship with Youth
  2. *Pursuing Victory with Honor*: A part of the Josephson Institute of Ethics' Character Counts! program, which is a campaign to help coaches and other adults equip youth with values to meet life's challenges on and off the field, the curriculum includes:
     - Child-Centered Developmental Objectives
     - State Mission and Objectives
     - Provide a Safe Environment
     - Consider Social, Emotional, and Physical Developmental States

- ○ Educate Coaches to Achieve Program Objectives
- ○ Train Officials to Achieve Program Objectives
- ○ Educate Parents to Play a Constructive Role in the Pursuit of Program Objectives
- ○ Evaluate Program Effectiveness Annually

Benefits to Parents

Aside from gaining valuable information about how to help children enjoy youth sports, parents from across the country who are involved in a collaborative sportsmanship effort can borrow valuable information from other parents with experiences in similar past situations. This can include helpful background information about a particular sport, tips or advice, and even encouragement. Parents can also benefit simply by being involved more positively in their child's sports choices, something a mandatory introductory education program would facilitate. Some of these benefits include:

- Almost 70 percent of parents with children playing sports reported

Sidebar 16.2: Teaching Sportsmanship Tips

Here are five things parents can do to show children (and other parents) how to be "a good sport." The advice comes from Shane Murphy, Ph.D., a sports psychologist in Trumbull, Connecticut, and author of *The Cheers and the Tears: A Healthy Alternative to the Dark Side of Youth Sports Today*, and Brooke de Lench, publisher and founder of MomsTeam.com, a 2002 International Institute of Sports Ethics Fellow, a member of the Board of Advisors for the Institute for Preventive Sports Medicine and the Board of Directors for the Matthew Colby Head Injury Foundation, and the executive director of Teams of Angels, which works to prevent sports injuries to children. The complete article can be found on momsteam.com:[1]

1. *Cheer for all the children, even those on the other team.*
2. *Thank the officials.*
3. *Talk to parents of the other team: they're not the enemy.*
4. *Be a parent, not a coach: resist the urge to critique.*
5. *Stay physically active.*

better relationships with their children, according to the National Alliance for Youth Sports' Start Smart program.

- 95 percent of these parents said they learned new ways to help their children develop sports skills.
- 74 percent of parents experienced an increase in awareness of their child's physical capabilities.
- 67 percent of parents say they are more likely to be involved in their child's sports experiences.
- Parents of at-risk families reported more positive parenting attitudes and behavior as well as more positive parent-child relationships.[16]

Some additional information that could be a part of such an education program that would benefit parents includes:

- The National Center for Educational Statistics reports less than 1 percent of children playing organized sports will receive any type of college scholarship.
- "I always recommend to parents that for kids between the ages of 3–8, let them try everything," says Chris Hirsch, co-owner of Jill's Gymnastics in Shreveport, Louisiana. "They'll find the sport that they like."[17]
- Parents can do research on leagues, coaches, administrators, the condition of facilities, etc. Search for coaches who are concerned about your child's learning and growth, not just about winning.[18]
- Bill Cushing, a coach and regional youth sports director in the Albany, New York, area, told *USA Today*, "I'm very concerned that at even younger ages than ever before, our children are learning how the rules do not really matter unless you get caught breaking them, and if you do, the penalties are not really bad." He suggests parents take a more aggressive approach to solving these problems, such as forming a group to bring complaints against coaches, parents, or entire leagues that are not adhering to the adopted code of ethics.[19]

Benefits to Children

Aside from safety concerns, a healthy sports program can positively impact a child's well being in many ways. For the reasons below, among others, efforts should be made to reverse the number of youth sports participants who drop out of athletics by the time they reach their freshman year of high school (estimated to be around 70 percent). Benefits to children, compiled by David Carmichael of the Sport Alliance of Ontario, include:

- Physical activity during the high school years reduces delinquent and criminal behavior.
- Sports are a positive influence for students overcoming high school drug abuse in terms of responsibility, self-esteem, and discipline.
- Girls who are involved in sports are 92 percent less likely to use drugs and 80 percent less likely to have an unwanted pregnancy than girls who are not involved in sports.
- Sports and other activities were reported to significantly decrease vandalism and antisocial behavior in a pilot project for economically disadvantaged children in a public housing complex.[20] Additionally:
- "We know from a lot of research that kids who participate in sports tend to do better academically," says Mark Goldstein, a psychologist at Roosevelt University in Chicago, Illinois. "It forces them to be more organized with their lives."[21]

Also, Carmichael's research reveals the cost of not engaging enough young people in sports and recreation:

- A study by the University of Toronto and York University looked at seven diseases and concluded that physical inactivity among Canadians amounted to $2.1 billion in health costs in 1999.
- More than half of the 5- to 17-year-olds in Canada are not physically active enough for optimal health and development
- Obesity among children ages 7 to 13 more than doubled in the period from 1981 to 1999.[22]

Dr. Bruce Svare, a professor of psychology at the University at Albany (SUNY) and director of the National Institute for Sports Reform, has similar statistics for children in the United States:

- Nearly half of American youths ages 12 to 21 years are not vigorously active on a regular basis.
- About 14 percent of young people report no recent physical activity.

- Participation in all types of physical activity dramatically declines as age or grade in school increases.
- Only 19 percent of all high school students are physically active for 20 minutes or more, five days a week, in physical education classes.
- Illinois is the only state that requires physical education and only 26 percent of the U.S. high schools offer daily physical education.
- Forty percent of high school students are never enrolled in a gym class. For high school seniors, the percentage is 75 percent.
- Over 60 million people are overweight, with childhood obesity becoming an epidemic.[23]

Dr. Svare compiled his research in an attempt to prove "the value of school-based sports as mainstream education is a myth; it grew from a tradition that is no longer relevant." Svare sees the lack of interest in high school sports as a reason to cut athletic programs instead of academic programs in schools that are struggling with their budgets. His point is certainly valid in many ways. Sports should not receive more priority than education. Two-time NFL Pro Bowl player with the Minnesota Vikings and two-time NCAA All-American at The Ohio State University, Robert Smith, would agree whole-heartedly. He backed up this thinking with more than words—sitting out his sophomore season at Ohio State to concentrate on academics *and* stepping away from a successful NFL career following a season in which he ran more than 1,500 yards. In his prime, Smith's primary focus was not athletics. However, taking away athletics completely would likely cause the numbers for inactivity and obesity to increase. Cutting sports is not a solution to curing its woes. Schools must maintain a proper perspective when allotting funds for academics and athletics, but when done correctly, the benefits of sports outweigh the costs. Svare's statistics prove that there is a need to keep children attracted to and involved in sports. Again, a nationwide alliance that can help as many communities as possible become involved in an accredited education program is a giant step toward meeting this goal.

All of the above should serve as proof that an effective education plan for administrators, coaches, and parents can help adults construct the best plans for running successful youth sports leagues. The only question remaining is how children will follow these plans. Scientific research offers evidence that kids will absolutely learn and imitate positive sportsmanship when they are taught properly.

Sidebar 16.3: Ethics of Competition Education Should Be Mandatory in All Schools

Junior high students often are required to take home economics classes that offer instruction on making wreaths, pillowcases, and cookies. There is nothing wrong with requiring a diverse education, and frequently these classes spark lifelong careers or hobbies. At the very least, moms get a return on their school supplies investment with a memorable gift or two. But in many other cases people never use the skills they have developed. Nonetheless, they are required classes.

Some schools ask students to take basic money management courses—how to write checks, count back change to a customer, and so on. This instruction is useful to most people. Others may never work at a department store or need to keep an inventory of the snack bar at Little League games, but you can only benefit from the experience. And, in many cases, it is required by the school.

Consider, therefore, how useful it would be to teach these same junior high students the ethics of competition—the importance of following rules: the correct methods of training or practicing, setting goals and using teamwork to achieve success, as well as how to deal with success so as to not become braggadocios or overconfident. Consider how beneficial it would be to learn about the myriad of real dangers involved with cheating, whether it is plagiarism in a debate competition or improper training and drug abuse in an athletic competition. It is obvious how much young athletes and nonathletes could gain from this information. Dancers, piano players, or student council members are no different than quarterbacks, shortstops, and point guards. The rules of competition and the tools of leadership apply to life as much as they do sports.

The concept of learning life lessons through sport may seem overused, but its ancient roots lend it true credibility. Victorians saw sports as an opportunity to educate society on the importance of the rule of law, building character through fair competition. In Rudyard Kipling's poem "If," he exhorts, "If you can meet with triumph and disaster / And treat those two imposters just the same / . . . you'll be a Man, my son!"[1]

There is a reason so many successful athletes claim that sports teaches skills needed to succeed in life. They experience it. And children should be required to experience it. Why? There are two equally important reasons. First, parents and other authority figures can give children the ability to attain many of the benefits mentioned above and many more, because so many young people today are never taught these skills—at home or in school. Secondly, there are problems growing in number and severity both directly and indirectly associated with athletes and athletics that society can help solve if it understands who the enemy is—cheating, drug abuse, winning at all cost, preferential treatment, placing more importance on athletics than on academics. Getting the basics at the beginning of our competitive lives is a way to wipe out some of these problems, or at least a way to give children the best chance to avoid these problems. Enforcing the rules still requires a hardworking and caring parent who understands and can teach that athletes are not entitled to more than nonathletes. Jocks are not entitled to use their stature to seek gratification by any number of means, including sexual assault.

We (the authors) have spent our entire lives competing and succeeding in sports. All-Star games and special treatment by family members were the norm for both of us. And we both continue to participate and enjoy competitions and sports in every way we can. But we also see the numerous problems in sports and recognize the need for dramatic change to ensure that young athletes are provided the right tools and teaching to succeed the right way. For parents who insist their star athlete needs to bend the rules in order to gain a deserved scholarship, this education probably won't be administered, supported, or reinforced in the home. But imagine how many parents would embrace this education, support their young citizen's appreciation for ethics, and positively reinforce this behavior in a loving way. Sewing a wreath and counting back change are skills we may never use again once class is dismissed, but we are no worse for the wear. Ethics in competition education can provide so many very applicable lessons for sons and daughters, moms and dads, and brothers and sisters. Good sportsmanship, mental toughness in overcoming adversity, and the ability to determine strengths and weaknesses are qualities all parents should want their child to possess.

Why not give everyone what they want and require that these skills be taught to junior high students?

In her article entitled "Emphasizing Sportsmanship in Youth Sports," Dr. Lori Gano-Overway concludes the following:

> Children learn moral behavior from engaging with others, watching the behaviors of others, and/or being taught ethical behavior. . . . Being involved in sport alone is not sufficient to ensure that participants will learn sportsmanlike attitudes and behaviors. Rather it is the "social interactions that are fostered by the sport experience" that will determine the benefit of sport to athletes.[24] [Achieving that benefit] requires that designated leaders

within the sport take action to teach ethical and moral behavior in sport. . . . For example, two moral intervention programs were introduced at a youth sport camp. The first (structural developmental) involved teaching one moral concept a week (e.g., fairness, sharing, aggression) over five weeks. The instructors also exposed moral issues as they arose in play and coached children to appropriate resolutions of the issues. Children (ages 5 to 7) in this intervention program understood the differences between right and wrong better than those who did not receive such training. The second intervention involved the instructor just demonstrating moral behavior when appropriate. This group also did better than a control group (who only participated in the sport program); however, this intervention was slightly less effective than the first intervention.[25] Children, thus, learn moral (sportsmanlike) behavior directly from instruction and indirectly by observing the responses of coaches and parents.[26]

There is likely a large segment of the population that believes it is more advanced in this crucial education process than the average parent is. Research shows that this is not the case. It is important that all parents know they may not be doing as good of a job as they think. Fred Engh, president and founder of the Florida-based National Alliance for Youth Sports (NAYS), says most of the nation's 2.5 million volunteer coaches and youth recreation administrators are well meaning but poorly trained. His organization has created a campaign to help them with positive coaching techniques. Such a campaign is similar to the "Pursue Victory With Honor" program discussed earlier. In about 600 communities, the NAYS requires parents to attend a class in sportsmanlike behavior and healthy competition. Engh says, "It's a hard sell because parents don't understand what the program is. They see it as a program telling them how to be a good parent. . . . We're going to compete all of our lives. Do we have to learn at age 9 that it's OK to cheat? To play when injured? To taunt the other team? Winning at all costs is probably the ugliest thing we can teach children, yet we have many, many people—parents and coaches—who do that today."[27] "The mission of the nonprofit, nonpartisan Joseph and Edna Josephson Institute of Ethics is to improve the ethical quality of society by changing personal and organizational decision making and behavior."[28]

Michael Josephson provides further evidence of the power of teaching when he explains that ethics are a fundamental element of succeeding in any aspect of life. He says teaching and modeling are crucial components of developing a high standard of ethics. "We use an acronym T.E.A.M—Teach, Enforce, Advocate, Model—and the notion is that all four of those things are critical. If you have three out of four, it does not work as well. But of all the four, modeling is the most absolutely essential. If you do the other three but you do not model—you teach, enforce and advocate but you don't represent them—the likelihood that it will be successful is very small."[29] Josephson's Web site—www.josephsoninstitute.org—can be a great starting point for anyone looking for a trusted authority on which to base any size sportsmanship program.

Though winning should never be the focal point of the teaching and modeling process, educating youngsters on *how* to win and how to *lose* is an underrated lesson. Losing, after all, can be a precursor to winning. As Walter Anderson writes in his book *The Confidence Course*, "True success is always the last of a string of failed attempts to get it right." Boston-based sports psychologist Harvey Dulberg, Ph.D., supports this notion by saying, "Let's face it, after a win, you're too impressed with yourself to hear anything. Guys who win all the time may not reach their potential if they never step out of their comfort zone and challenge themselves."[30]

SOLUTIONS IN COLLEGIATE SPORTS

One of the worst college sports recruiting scandals in our nation's history has produced one of the most effective actions toward reform in the history of the NCAA. Colorado's football program will never be the same, but neither will the programs and policies on hundreds of other campuses after the swift and strict measures adopted by the NCAA's Board of Directors in the summer of 2004. The use of sex and alcohol in trying to lure the country's top football prospects shook the foundation of a sport with a past filled with scandals. Whether these "extra benefits" violations were committed by upperclassmen throwing parties exclusively for these recruits, or if they were done in slightly less obvious but no less-structured fashion (nightclubbing with flirting females, introductions to promiscuous co-eds, or joining seniors in sauntering to strip clubs), the discovery at Colorado University was enough to move an organization criticized in the past for not moving fast or far enough. As discussed in chapter 14, even this action probably came too late considering the many examples of similar behavior occurring prior to 2004. From 2000–2003, Florida, Alabama, Oregon, Minnesota, and Alabama State all had recruits involved in publicized incidents that included the improper use of either alcohol or marijuana, as well as the use of sex or strippers, as an enticement to join the program. And no incident involved a recruit with as high a profile as Michigan and Mateen Cleaves in 1996. Still, the NCAA's 2004 actions—overdue or not—are real and were effective from their outset.

According to the NCAA, the following changes were approved in an emergency July 2004 vote and took effect immediately:

- Campuses must develop written policies that specifically prohibit inappropriate or illegal behavior in recruiting. Policies must be approved by campus presidents or chancellors by December 1st, and be on file with conference offices. The current policies of member institutions must be on file in their conference office (or the NCAA for independent institutions) prior to bringing any prospect to campus for an official visit in the 2004–2005 academic year.

The issues that must be addressed in the document include:

1. Specific, school-imposed penalties for violations. The NCAA also could sanction violators if infractions rise to a level that is "fundamentally contrary" to the school's stated policy.
2. A prohibition of underage drinking, sex, drug use, gambling or gaming activities, and the use of strippers during campus visits.
3. Statements about curfews, if any, and on- and off-campus entertainment.
4. An explanation of how head coaches will discuss the policy with prospects.

- Institutions cannot use private or chartered airplanes when transporting prospects; instead, they must use commercial air travel at coach-class fares.
- Campuses must use standard vehicles to transport prospective student-athletes and those accompanying them on official visits.
- Prospects and their parents or legal guardians must be housed in

standard lodging and offered standard meals similar to those offered on campus.

- Student hosts must be current student-athletes or students who conduct visits or tours as part of the admissions process. Gender-specific groups will be allowed if they are organized consistent with an institution's overall campus visit program.
- Institutions cannot use personalized recruiting aides (such as jerseys or scoreboard presentations) or game-day simulations during campus visits. Prospects can visit the locker room before or after a game or stand on the sidelines during pre-game activities under this measure.

"There are a couple of issues that must be addressed," NCAA president Myles Brand said after the drastic policy changes were approved. "First, there is a culture of entitlement, a sense that there are no holds barred and that anything goes. That has to change. The second is accountability. Who is accountable for assuring neither drugs, nor sex, nor alcohol will be a part of that process?"[31]

Another positive light shining amid the darkness behind the Boulder, Colorado, controversy is the effect it had on the nation's athletic directors and presidents, who were forced to look closely at their own situations. At Colorado, meanwhile, the school's Independent Investigative Commission, a panel appointed by the Colorado Board of Regents, found that school president Betsy Hoffman was responsible for a lack of control over her athletic department. The commission wrote: "As the university's chief administrator, Hoffman failed to exercise sufficient oversight until pressured by the governor and lawmakers. The university's leadership must be held accountable for systemic failings that jeopardized students' safety and allowed for ongoing misconduct in the football recruiting program."[32]

While this is an example of the NCAA's ability to do an effective job by addressing a serious problem, it highlights one of the organization's biggest weaknesses: a lack of significant punishment. By not imposing substantial mandatory penalties for violating the above policy, the NCAA is once again covering a blemish with a band-aid. There is no army of party police proficient enough to enforce these new guidelines. Instead, when ink on the honor policy is drying and the recruits are supposedly sleeping, the outcome of this emergency solution will once again be in the hands of hormone-driven young men, many of whom are either rebels, immature, or both. If an unethical system existed for decades under unwritten rules, what protection will a piece of paper offer unless it is held in place by a stone in which the consequences for breaking the rules are set?

The appearance of being soft amid an undeniable crisis is reason to doubt one's effectiveness. Considering the NCAA is often unable to prove many of the varying accusations brought against its member institutions, there is little reason to put faith in the patchwork covering the predicament of academic fraud or other utterly unacceptable cracks in the foundation of higher learning. Since they are understaffed and ultimately overwhelmed, there cannot be great expectations placed on those charged with monitoring the morality of well-established, well-protected powerhouse athletic programs. Again, the question of questionable punishment arises. If only a fraction of the crooked are caught, why not multiply the punishment severity to discourage cheating?

The NCAA has toughened its stance on academics recently under the direction of Myles Brand, the former president of the University of Indiana. As of the writing of this book, the NCAA was considering a solution for the academic failures of so many college athletic departments. The solution included giving schools credit for having players who are eligible and steadily work toward degrees, and punishing those schools that regularly do not graduate their players. Players who finish their senior year of eligibility will be required to have completed 80 percent of their requisite academic hours. Schools that fall below a certain percentage of available credits—80 to 85 percent among its athletes—will be given a public reprimand. If the trend continues, scholarships will be taken away, and ultimately a team might not be allowed to participate in postseason play.

Christine Plonsky, chairwoman of the NCAA's Management Council and women's athletic director at Texas, says schools will be required to furnish information for the NCAA's Committee on Academic Performance for the current year (2003–2004), but that the results will be used only to tell those programs not meeting the prescribed guidelines to get their houses in order.[33]

An even more important solution, however, would be to follow through on the first solution listed above. The Knight Commission on

Intercollegiate Athletics, a 14-member commission created in 1989 to recommend academic reform, once recommended that teams failing to graduate at least half of their athletes shouldn't be allowed to participate in the NCAA tournament. If those recommendations were followed, only 21 of the 65 basketball teams would have been eligible this season.[34] Challenging the sport to reach this goal, even if in five years most of the top 65 basketball teams are not playing in the tournament because the players are not meeting their graduation obligations, is another way to give this measure a sharp set of teeth. Raising academic standards and performances should be an unmatched priority. Only when we disregard excuses, follow through on penalties for those who fail to meet requirements, and reward those schools who compete *and* graduate their athletes will we show future generations that athletics do not take a higher precedence over academics.

Terry Holland cannot wait for that day, but he doubts it can happen under the current system. The former University of Virginia coaching great and ex-athletic director for the Cavaliers believes there are other problems in college sports that will actually cause more incidents of academic fraud by teams failing to reach the new education requirements. In his February 2003 presentation to the Knight Commission, Holland pleaded with college presidents to pursue two of his suggested proposals aggressively. Holland writes:

1. SAY WHAT YOU MEAN AND MEAN WHAT YOU SAY: If you [the presidents] believe that academics are our first priority, then simply demand that athletes attend every class as the minimal requirement to conduct an athletic program on the campus of every institution. I coached nationally competitive basketball teams in the ACC for 16 years and our players rarely missed a class for regular season games—we did, however, miss a huge amount of class for ACC and NCAA tournaments since we had no control over the scheduling of those events. Only men's basketball will have actual problems meeting such a mandate and, even in the short term, careful scheduling can eliminate 70 to 80 percent of the current missed classes in men's basketball without affecting the television contracts already in place. Our athletes can never believe that academics are important as long as athletic competitions are scheduled during their classes, their exams, and even during their graduation ceremonies.

2. PUT YOUR MONEY WHERE YOUR MOUTH IS: If you really want our institutions to recruit football and basketball players who can, and will, succeed academically, then provide financial and competitive rewards to those institutions who award scholarships to athletes with academic credentials similar to those of their classmates. This would at least allow institutions to choose between trying to succeed financially simply by doing whatever it takes to win or to succeed financially by recruiting athletes who fit the institution's academic profile. It is a simple fact of life that every institution cannot have a winning record in any given year but it is possible for every institution to recruit athletes who fit that institution's academic profile every single year—if we can eventually provide sufficient motivation for them to do so.

If the NCAA does not commit itself to reducing the number of classes players must miss because of their travel schedules, Holland says the corruption will continue. "Mainly," he says, "academic fraud in order [for players] to qualify and then to retain eligibility since athletes will continue to miss more and more class time in order to play 'national schedules' and to be on television. This will begin to occur in all sports, not just the so-called revenue sports" (see sidebar 16.4: "Q&A with Terry Holland").

Since problem solving is the root of the Knight Commission's existence, the NCAA should rely on it as a source of solutions. In 2001 the commission said that sports "threatens to overwhelm the university . . . the threat has grown rather than diminished." The commission suggested making efforts to minimize commercialization and bring coaches' salaries "into line with prevailing norms across the institution."[35] Coaches subsequently argued that salaries in other businesses are not limited in this way. However, collegiate sports should not be compared to other businesses. They may never again be viewed as simply an extracurricular activity for students. Capping salaries is one way for universities to reestablish that athletics are not more important than academics. Devoting so much money for coaches' salaries is no different from asking players to devote more time to travel than study—it creates the wrong perception. When coaches reach their salary ceiling, let them jump to the professional ranks if they are so motivated. Brand says, "Student-athletes are first. The NCAA has

Sidebar 16.4: Q&A with Terry Holland[1]

Question: Have we seen the worst yet?

Answer: Unless we act to help the 98 percent of athletes who want to do well in the classroom, we will see a continuing decline and increasing outrageous and irresponsible behaviors (of athletes, coaches, athletic administrators, governing board members, and college presidents, all of whom Holland implicated as a part of the problem when he spoke to the Knight Commission in February 2003).

Q: Are there some problems that will never go away (e.g., a coach/academic advisor/booster/tutor helping commit academic fraud)?

A: There will always be people who will cut corners to win but the measurement should be "is that percentage increasing or decreasing each year?" If we are "playing a losing game"—and there is every indication that athletics on any individual campus could go into "free fall" at any time, so we are definitely playing a losing game—it is imperative that the leadership of the NCAA and our presidents take action. They are unwilling to take any action that represents risk to them or their jobs, so we are stuck with a failing system.

Q: Are people behind the scenes working as hard as they need to be (e.g., the Knight Commission) to combat problems that appear to be even worse than most realize?

A: There are groups outside of the NCAA and the presidents who are calling for substantive reforms (such as the Knight Commission, the Drake Group, etc.) but the leadership has responded by tweaking a broken machine instead of providing leadership.

Q: Who is doing good things to solve these problems? And what are they doing?

A: Faculty groups (not the faculty athletic representatives as they are co-opted by the many perks they receive from their positions) are beginning to speak out, but there are several instances of whistle blowers losing their jobs as our current NCAA leadership does not even have the guts to protect those faculty members who report academic fraud.

Q: Who is doing nothing (or worse trying to cover things up)?

A: Most presidents and AD's are very good people who simply try to be optimistic by seeing the glass as half full rather than half empty, but if you cut to the chase, they are simply doing what they are being paid to do while rationalizing the irrational and defending the indefensible, in most cases.

Q: Who else needs to do more?

A: This can only be solved if the presidents are willing to stand up and do the right thing. Unfortunately, more and more presidents are directly interfering with admissions processes, hiring coaches with tainted records, etc., so they must act before the quicksand pulls them under.

Q: Are we failing to stop the bleeding with our band-aids?

A: The tweaking of a broken machine will guarantee that the bleeding will increase!

Q: In regard to the two ideas for reform you presented to the Knight Commission—say what you mean and put your money where your mouth is—are the recent reforms approved by the NCAA enough of a move (e.g., awarding scholarships for those who graduate their players)?

A: No. Emphasis on increasing graduation rates without addressing the fact that many of those not graduating are under-prepared and unmotivated guarantees increased academic fraud!

Q: You said: "careful scheduling can eliminate 70 to 80 percent of the current missed classes in men's basketball without affecting the television contracts already in place." Does this mean playing home games or nearby road games during the week and saving longer trips for weekends? What other scheduling considerations can help?

A: Yes. If ADs and coaches made class attendance a priority, they could easily schedule games during the week against teams that are located close by. I did it as a coach of a nationally ranked program in the ACC.

We could also play two games on a weekend (Saturday and Sunday). We often did this when I coached—sometimes playing a home game on Saturday (at Virginia) and flying to Ohio State or Missouri for a Sunday game. It can be done. It is just a matter of what your priorities are.

And teams that played back-to-back games won at least the same percentage of road games that teams today are winning (often traveling a day in advance of a game), so there is little or no effect on performance on the court. I remember one game when N.C. State ran into weather while traveling on game day. They finally got a private aircraft to carry the head coach and six players to nationally ranked Georgia Tech. The players walked onto the court with no warm-up and won the game! The remaining players and coaches arrived piecemeal during the game as aircraft became available, which had to be a huge distraction to the team members already playing. That is probably still the biggest win for N.C. State at Georgia Tech in the last 30 years.

Coaches and teams miss class to travel a day ahead simply to make their program look big time, and the players quickly buy into this seemingly "professional" attitude, but it has zero impact on winning and losing.

to be focused on student-athletes, focused on the conditions under which they play, but also on education."[36] It should not be impossible to recruit students who are also athletes. Brock Stratton, a former high school honor student who chose to play football at Texas Tech, says, "It can be tough at times, but as a student-athlete you have to remember what you are."[37]

SOLUTIONS TO THE WINNING-AT-ALL-COST MENTALITY

Svare, who in addition to being a professor and an expert on ethics in sport, is an avid sports fan. He wants to cut all athletic scholarships, hardly a realistic solution. But his aggressive, radical thinking is what is necessary to attack the issues affecting all levels of sport. Svare agrees with the need to gain help from the government to regain control of all levels of sports. Svare wants to create a federally funded national sports commission to "oversee the entire spectrum of sports from the promotion of health and fitness for all to the training of Olympic athletes." Its goals would include helping to elevate sports funding and "encourage the formation of a club system of athletics for the entire life span of our population."[38]

Svare's suggestion to remove the athlete entirely from the student-athlete equation is not limited to the collegiate level. Svare believes that high schools should cut sports programs when budget reductions threaten to weaken a school's educational mission. In his June 2004 article in the *(Albany) Times Union*, he argues, "The United States is the only country in the world that supports competitive sports through its educational system. The value of school-based sports as mainstream education is a myth; it grew from a tradition that is no longer relevant. . . . Shouldn't we think more seriously about placing competitive sports in the hands of outside clubs that have proliferated in our present sports culture and can serve the same needs without costing our public schools precious time and scarce resources?"[39]

Another proponent of government involvement is Dr. Frank Uryasz, president of the National Center for Drug Free Sport, and the NCAA's director of sports sciences. He says, "The U.S. Federal Government channels some funds through the U.S. Anti-Doping Agency, but otherwise there really aren't any significant sources of funding [for research]. Organizations like the IOC [need to invest more in testing]. Sure they spend a lot of money, but the Olympics still make a lot of money. There's no question they can put some resources behind research. . . . I think it's an appropriate role for the government to play. Research funding has a role to play. The professional leagues and certainly the IOC."[40]

Michael Josephson, founder and director of the Josephson Institute of Ethics, agrees that government can have a substantial and positive impact, but he believes this involvement should not be mandated.

> I think government should give permission to teach principles of morality, but not necessarily in the context of religion or a particularly narrow perspective. I don't think they should encourage any particular perspective on abortion or capital punishment or cloning, etc. I think they should encourage the teaching of, first of all, ethical reasoning, which includes the big controversial issues. And I think they should do everything possible to give permission or to encourage schools to teach character. We [the Institute] always benefit when it's mandated, because we're the largest character development organization in the country by a long way, and every time it's mandated we get more programs, but it also invites the shallowness of approach. You have to be careful that people aren't just waving a banner; they're just not accomplishing anything.
>
> We need proficiency in teaching character, just as we need proficiency in teaching literacy. Not everyone knows how to teach reading. I know how to read, but I don't know how to teach it. That's also true for character development. We need to denote this proficiency and create enough of a demand from the parents themselves who want it and the communities that want it—I think they do. Trying to mandate it turns into a legislative process that can be counterproductive.

Legislators may appear to be working toward solutions, but they often lack the proficiency Dr. Josephson speaks of as a primary ingredient to solving problems. Legislators, even if they remain in office for more than one or two terms, appear to be disconnected from the problems affecting sports. They lack critical information or ignore valuable opinions needed to make thorough decisions. If they do invest time in these issues—such as John McCain's senate hearings into the steroid issue in baseball—they are criticized by the public for delving into "light or soft" sports topics. *Aren't there bigger issues they should be dealing with?* Perhaps not, if you can draw the logical connection between professional baseball players who operate with no drug policy and influential teens who use drugs in an attempt to become their idols, that is, to become big, strong, successful pro ball players. There is no bigger problem than children who use illegal drugs. And by combating steroid use, the ATLAS program has shown (in chapter 7), you combat drug use as a whole, drinking and driving, and other issues related to the world's crumbling character.

But as is the case with any solution a politician seeks to implement, effective research and efficient action are needed. Steroids in sports is a perfect example of how some legislators who are hoping to take credit for acting on a hot topic (before another lawmaker beats them to it) will rush to draw up a bill that mandates steroid tests—tests that most research claims do not work and are therefore unworthy of the high cost. Testing will always be a deterrent, but no valuable research indicates it has any success in permanently changing a person's decision to abuse drugs. If it did, the percentage of users in professional sports would decrease, and athletes would not be searching for undetectable methods. Testing, like locking your back door, keeps honest people out of trouble. Cheaters will cheat until they're caught.

Are legislators limited in their resources or unwilling to listen? Dr. Lynn Goldberg, who created ATLAS, was asked for his opinion on the subject by Sen. Jackie Speier (D- California, San Mateo/San Francisco). Goldberg has proof that his peer-based education program works. Speier has decided not to invest taxpayer's money in a proven solution, but instead is seeking money for drug testing. Speier and other legislators whose efforts are well intended should be praised for actively being a very necessary part of the solution to problems in sports today. But there is much work to be done. Fortunately there is reason to believe that the positive hard work by many individuals and small groups across the country—many mentioned above and many more that are not—can begin to cause a serious shift in society's understanding of these problems. The key is to combine efforts as much as possible to help facilitate the transformation of society's willingness to solve these problems.

> "Never doubt that a small group of thoughtful, committed citizens can change the world. Indeed, it's the only thing that ever has."
>
> —Margaret Meade

17

More Solutions: Athletes Doing the Right Thing

Mike Hall could bench press 400 pounds when he was 16 years old. He lived his entire life as a giant, enduring ridicule as a kid, and overcoming much more than that as he grew into a 6-foot-2, 410-pound mountain of muscle. By the time he retired from the sport of powerlifting in 1991, he owned 10 national championships, five world titles, and two gold medals in the Pan-American Games—all of them earned drug free, an amazing feat considering he did so in a heavily drug-infested sport. There is no question that Hall is a special, gifted individual, perfectly suited for his chosen sport. His size may be his biggest visible advantage—his wrists were 10 inches in diameter and his ring finger as thick as a quarter—but his faith in God and his determination to succeed without steroids lifted him to heights his size and strength alone could not reach.

A number of factors make Hall's accomplishments impressive, including the pressure of using widely accepted and, at the time, legal performance-enhancing drugs. As the evidence chronicled in this book shows, young athletes are highly susceptible to these and other drugs. Steroids were prevalent when Hall was growing up in the small town of Dagsboro, Delaware. He was only 17 when he was first offered steroids in the U.S. Marine Corps, shortly after being asked to join the weightlifting team.

"Sir, no one told the private he had to do steroids to be a champion," Hall remembers telling the acting coach of the team—his superior officer.

"Then you'll never become a champion. You'll never become anyone. Get out of the gym."[1]

So Hall, in one of his lowest moments, walked away, not sure what to feel moments after one of his greatest joys was seemingly taken from him. But before he reached the door he stopped, did an about face, and said respectfully but confidently: "Sir, the private will be somebody one day." He did another about face, walked away from drugs and toward an unprecedented career. "I knew what I told that sergeant had to come from God. That was a big emotional cut in my heart. I know now the things God let me do. I had to have more than a desire to succeed. I had to have Him."

Hall eventually returned to the Marine Corps weightlifting team when the coach was reassigned overseas and replaced with a new one. And while he says the negative effects of his former coach's words remained with him, they also motivated him. "That hurt me. And every time I heard about someone who took steroids, I was possessed to show them I didn't need them." Hall won his first world championship in 1986, leading the U.S. team to a title in Amsterdam, Holland. A year later he earned the title of the world's strongest drug-free man when he benched, squatted, and deadlifted a combined 2,340 pounds—the highest drug-free total in history—at the world championships in Oslo, Norway. Hall won the 1988 international championships in Hawaii and won a third consecutive super-heavyweight world title in Australia. At one time, he held every lifting record for super heavyweights. And his 2,340-pound performance in 1987 remains unmatched.

Hall's success is remarkable considering that the sport's history is littered with performance-enhancing drug abusers. From the questions surrounding the 1952 Soviet Union weightlifting team to the 11 weightlifters testing positive or otherwise violating the antidoping policies during or before the 2004 Athens Summer Games, doping and weightlifting have been inseparable. (See chapter 4, "BALCO and Beyond," for more on the more than two dozen athletes sanctioned for using banned substances in Athens.)

That Hall was offered drugs by a branch of the U.S. armed services is not surprising. Organized doping in the 1970s was and would continue for decades to be a part of sports. The evidence of this (provided in chapter 2) is hefty: the Soviets (beginning in the 1950s); the East Germans (1960s and 1970s); the unofficial 68 percent of all athletes polled unscientifically prior to the 1972 games in Munich, Germany; the 20 medal winners in the 1984 Olympic Games in Los Angeles who were provided steroids by Dr. Robert Kerr; the University of South Carolina football team in the late 1980s; the six Chinese athletes who had drug-related suspensions at the world championships in Australia in 1998 (bringing the total of Chinese suspensions in the 1990s to 28); and the recent BALCO case in which it is alleged that numerous NFL football players and U.S. track-and-field athletes were provided the designer steroid THG by the Bay Area Laboratory Co-operative (see chapter 4 for more details). For Hall, the biggest challenge was overcoming an organized Marine Corps system that encouraged or required weightlifters to dope. And because the coach was a ranking officer, Hall did not want to disobey.

The fact that his professional competition was doping and getting away with it made the temptation even greater. In 2003 the U.S. Anti-Doping Agency conducted 6,890 drug tests. Only six (0.09 percent) were positive. Yet there was much evidence to show that far more athletes were doping (see evidence listed in chapter 1 and chapter 3). Hall, however, stood firm in his quest to remain clean. He maintained his resolve despite a backlash by his steroid-using world-class competitors. "You've offended them because they spend a lot of money on strength-inducing drugs and they're defeated by a drug-free guy. They didn't like that. I was such a threat to the weightlifting world. . . . I was making a lot of enemies. . . . If they thought they could have knocked me off, they would have done it. Eventually I started receiving threatening phone calls. The thing that drove me most was remembering what happened to me when I was 17 years old [in the Marine Corps]. And my motivation became the [next generation of weightlifters]."

Hall also said an external strength carried him through his most difficult moments. "I was an ugly child, I stuttered, was in special-ed classes, I was poor, the kids called me 'Baby Huey' [after the chubby cartoon character] when I was little. But it doesn't matter where you are in life, God has a plan for you."

Hall says he never had a human coach, but he remembers doing an interview before becoming a Christian and telling a reporter: "I want to thank my coach. His name is God. . . . Even though I said that, I didn't emphasize it. But when I became saved, I was desperate to mention Him."

An injury once presented the toughest mental challenge in Hall's career. Needing a quick recovery and to regain the strength he had lost while he was recuperating, "the evil thought was sitting on my shoulder—take steroids."

"Steroids were still legal at the time. I had made a choice—even when they were legal—to not use them. But when I was injured I thought, 'everyone else does, no one will care.' Two things scared me: No. 1 was the vow I made to God. . . . And No. 2 was the kids. I wore 'drug free' as a medal of honor. That was a great test for me. My weakness was that I didn't want to lose.

"When I decided I wasn't going to use steroids, I had to train like I never had before. I told myself that the greatest gift we have is who we are. Who made me? God. Why go to some thing that's temporary? Why take something out of a bottle when I can go to the one who made what's in that bottle?"

Today Hall wishes to carry that message beyond the state where he was born and still lives. "The message was not just meant for Delaware; it was meant for the whole world. Something out there wants me to do this. God wants me to do this. The word has to get out."

There are many more athletes who share Hall's desire to spread the word that competing drug free is not only the cool thing to do, it's the only thing to do if you wish to become a true champion. Below are the stories of some of these athletes—Olympians, role models, and true champions:

- John Godina, 1996 silver medalist in the shot put, 2000 bronze medalist in the shot put, and an Olympian in discus in 1996: "Track's different than a lot of sports; you can't hide behind teammates. . . . You know cut and dry how good you are. The biggest thing (to tell kids) is to go out and have fun, work hard and try your hardest. If someone is better than you, don't try to cheat. There's a good chance they are clean. . . .

  "Track reveals your shortcomings; no one wins all the time in track. People need to learn to accept that someone can be better than you. It makes you work hard to be your best and be satisfied with that. . . . In track there is often one winner and thousands of losers; it's one of the few sports where winning isn't everything. Improving yourself is what's important."[2]
- Tara Cunningham, 2000 gold medalist in weightlifting, 48 kg (106 lbs), and 2004 Olympian: "Our society is such that winning is ev-

erything. I think that is a big reason that kids turn to performance-enhancing drugs. Kids feel that if they win, no matter how they get there, they will be someone. Sports should be a place to build character, not destroy it.

"I am not sure kids should be encouraged to become Olympic champions, but instead should be encouraged to work to reach their highest potential. If their highest potential is last place at the Olympics then they should be able to stand proud knowing that they gave it their all."[3]

- Alison Dunlap, mountain bike world champion and two-time Olympian: "I know that ever since I was a little girl I wanted to be an Olympian. No one ever told me how to accomplish this goal. I never knew how I would do it, just that I would some day.

"I think you can tell kids that if they really want to be an Olympian more than anything, then they can achieve their goal with lots of hard work, dedication, a huge amount of passion, and a burning desire to be the best. This applies to any and all sports.

"Kids also need to know that the only way to become a true champion is to compete drug free. Athletes that cheat are never true champions. They will always carry a huge amount of guilt with them for the rest of their lives. Becoming an Olympian happens only through years and years of hard work. You have to be willing to sacrifice a lot of things. You have to be willing to handle setbacks, injuries, and defeats. An Olympian is someone who has overcome all the odds, all the people who said they couldn't do it, all the injuries and all the other competitors in their sport. Becoming an Olympian is the pinnacle of sport.

"To become an Olympian in cycling is no different from other sports. You need to train hard, work with a coach, eat right, and most of all have fun. Kids won't make it unless they enjoy what they are doing. Having fun in sports is the most important thing. Of course there is always a little bit of luck involved. But that's how life is."[4]

- Steve Holman, 1992 U.S. Olympian and two-time national champion in track and field (1,500 meters and indoor mile): "Physically, [aspiring track Olympians should not] do too much too soon. There are countless youth and high school superstars that never made it to the next level because of injuries, burnout, and excessive expectations. I don't think kids should really train that hard until their bodies can handle it—and that usually isn't until their late teens. I had great coaches in high school who taught me to love the sport, and they pushed me to work hard. I probably could have run much faster in high school, but I think my high school coaches held back not to sacrifice my long term potential. It was a very unselfish act, and I remain grateful.

"Mentally, to be successful, you have to enjoy—no, love—what you are doing. If you hate working out and races make you sick with anxiety, you might want to consider doing something else. Why pursue something that makes you miserable?

"Morally, I think the concept of being a sportsman/woman has been eclipsed by the need to win. Being a sportsman is to maintain your integrity in victory and defeat. Being a sportsman obviously means that you won't cheat to get ahead, but it also means dedication to your sport, respect for your opponents, modesty in victory, and grace in defeat. Sounds very naive and nineteenth centuryish, but I think if we did a better job of instilling those values from the beginning for what sports are really about, maybe things might be different."[5]

- Kenta Bell, 2004 U.S. Olympian, track-and-field triple jump: "The No. 1 approach athletes should have—in any sport—is to learn all fundamentals. Too many people try to skip steps. . . . Miles Davis, once he learned all fundamentals, only then did he popularize jazz music. You also have to be knowledgeable. Too many people depend upon coaches, and they might not necessarily have enough skills to coach. A lot of times [a coach] is doing it on the side. As an athlete don't be dependent on coaches to know everything. We need to educate ourselves and get a better understanding of the sport and the training philosophy of the sport, so when coaches teach a new theory, we can grasp it.

  "If I was talking to a kid, I would recommend to stay away from all the protein supplements, weight gainers, Andro, and so on. I'd recommend a healthy diet. You can eat most of these foods by eating the brightest colors—tomatoes, carrots, and so on. They flush the kidney and liver. They're loaded with antioxidants, B6 and B12, and vitamins C and E. They keep your immune system functioning at its peak. . . . One in five supplements test positive for something that's banned. Avoid that whole situation. Physically you'll feel better and mentally you'll definitely feel better about yourself when you know you did it the right way. What's done in dark comes to light."[6]

"Rowdy" Roddy Piper is not afraid to speak of the dark world he once lived in. For many years he was a professional wrestler America loved to hate. Years since his retirement, he is outspoken about the destruction steroids can cause—physiologically and emotionally:

> When I first started taking steroids, the government told us a blatant lie. It said steroids do nothing to enhance your performance. Now we know that steroids might not enhance talent, but they make your bench press go from 450 to 500, so it absolutely enhances your performance.
>
> The biggest and most dangerous impact steroids has on a person is that it increases your aggressiveness. I'd hit the turnbuckle with such force that I'd tear up my body. That's the biggest downfall of steroids, how hard it makes you go. The harder you go, the harder you work to better yourself, the more damage you can do. I was on top for 30 years. But I had my right hip replaced with titanium.[7]

Piper wants to believe the drug problems in elite sports can be turned around. His experiences, however, are an indication of how difficult that will be.

> There is a mind-set with the professional athlete that you have to do whatever it takes to stay on top. For me, once I got past 25 or 26, I became a lifer. At that point you don't allow anyone to get into your medicine cabinet, so to speak. A lot of people don't know what it's like to have to say, "I'm doing this for my family." I wouldn't be interested in anyone telling me to stop taking steroids.

This mind-set, Piper agrees, is why stopping steroid use as early as possible is crucial to gaining an edge on a growing problem. Piper offers a suggestion for a solution: Telling kids the facts, which include how successful you can be without steroids and how disabled you can become when your playing days are over if you abuse them.

> All the steroids in the world are not going to help you if you don't have the talent. You need talent, you need power, and you need hard work. I was probably the smallest of big-league wrestlers in stature, but I learned how to present myself large. If someone would have come up to me and con-

vinced me that it takes talent, not steroids, I would have been so much better off. There are some great examples of people who have passed on that took steroids that never became the main-eventers. And I rest my case on that.

These kids need to know that you might be able to run faster now, but in 10 years you're not going to be able to walk; you're going to have a titanium hip and things are going to look different when you can't run and your buddies are still running. They need to look at the long term.

As one of the kings of bad-guy wrestlers, Piper welcomed wrestling fans into *The Piper's Pit* every week. It was wrestling's daytime TV talk show. His guests were a mix of good and bad guys, but Piper's demeanor was consistently deranged. He helped publicize the professional wrestler's rage on camera. His personality was perfectly suited to explode into spitting and stuttering rants, madly hollering at his opponents, and often bringing the stage act to a violent conclusion right there on the set. This was the fake part of wrestling. His titanium hip is evidence of the sport's reality. His hissing and biting tongue are not quite as venomous these days, but his passion is evident and his frustration is real when he discusses steroids.

> I could tell my hip was deteriorating, and I was told the same thing by doctors maybe five years before the replacement. I actually . . . This is so stupid now. I. Please. I-I-This is not a. I . . . Stupid is the word.
>
> I actually said to myself, if it's going to cost me a hip to get my family where I need them to go, I was willing to do that. And sure enough it cost me a hip. That just shows you the ignorant mind-set I was in at the time.

This shows how addicting the success of professional sports can be. It is an addiction that threatens so many of our younger athletes who seek to accomplish what, for so many, is next to impossible. The never-before-seen financial rewards—or for aging veterans, the need to prolong a fading career—fuel this addiction. Money is the root of this evil.

> You were wrestling one night, and the next night you didn't have a job if you're not drawing crowds and money. There was no insurance, no health care. Most of the wrestlers in my day didn't know what you were getting paid until the promoter gave you your check. And if you didn't like it . . . tough. I had one promoter who would tell me, "There are six roads out of here. You can be on any one of them." There was a paranoia of keeping a

job. If you did start selling out arenas, the only way you could keep your value up was to keep selling out, because there was nowhere to go but downhill after that. That's a huge piece of pressure on you. Plus the guys in the opening matches (the undercard), who are getting paid by the count of the house, if you're not selling out, you're letting them down also. And then you're letting your family down. You're letting everybody down except yourself, and you put yourself in the category of "it doesn't matter, as long as they [are provided for]." And that's not good thinking.

I used my family as justification, but it still doesn't make it right. Possibly I could have gone out and became something else, but I couldn't see it back then. I was a wrestler, the way I was broken in—old school—they used to beat you up and try to make you leave they'd beat you up so bad. You get so course and so rough, going town to town, you get such a rough, hard, pirate mentality. I had such a reckless abandonment, that it was just about impossible to get through to me [to convince me to quit]. If I did think about getting out, somebody would say to me, "You know how many people are out there? Fourteen thousand. So what's your problem." The money was there so the conversation would come to an end.

So how can this problem be attacked in any sport where money is an incredibly powerful lure and the jagged consequences do not seem real enough to serve as a deterrent?

Get honest. People like myself, saying, "Do you want your hips gone? Do you want your joints gone? Do you want to die? Are you really willing to put death on the line night after night with not much light at the end of the tunnel?" For professional athletes today—and I'm not knocking anybody—but the amount of pressure from coaches and the public that is on these guys is just enormous. You're getting paid $15 million, you better score a touchdown. However, the guys who are doing the designer steroids now, they need to step forward, whether or not they're using them now. They can't be worried about that. They need to step forward and tell our young people the truth.

My kids look at what happened to me and they say, "I'm not touching that garbage." Because they see what happened to their dad. We need to—we being the body of athletes who have done steroids—we need to come out right now with the truth. And if we're in the NFL and we come out and say something, the NFL can't come down on them—and before you know it you're selling life insurance.

There are ways to do it, where we can tell these kids this is the way it is when you use steroids and this is the way it can be without them. I really believe I would have done just as well without steroids. Other than giving me a little more power, steroids gave me a little more water weight so I looked bigger. But I had the tenacity. I had the refuse-to-give-up attitude. In hindsight, I really believe nothing would have changed had I not taken the 'roids. And we need to tell these kids that.

Schools today have sex education, and it's co-ed. They'll show all the sexually-transmitted diseases that are out of control and it's important for kids to watch out for if you want to keep a life. It's the same thing with all the kids in sports. Most young kids are involved in some kind of sport. You must have some caring for people who look up to you when you're in the spotlight.

We have a responsibility to the youth who look up to us to show them what's right and wrong. So kids need to have this kind of education. Knowledge is power. The kids don't believe the people they're hearing it from. They need to hear it from the people who have been there. Kids are the same today as I was when I was a kid—young, dumb, and full of confidence. I wasn't afraid of nothing, until I found out how dumb I was. Now I'm afraid of everything—especially my wife. The youth mentality needs to be broken by someone like myself who will tell them, "Sit down and shut up. You don't know what you're talking about."

I would go to the school football team, the track team, find kids who weren't on steroids who are successful and prove to kids that steroids don't make the difference; talent does. I would tell them their bodies are not used to that much extra power. The damage you're doing to your body on the tackle, on the run, on the block, on the body slam, whatever it might be; the fact that it allows you to push your body so hard, your body does harm to itself. That's the worse part about steroids.

I could feel it every day—I had no cartilage the last two years (before hip-replacement surgery). I know without a doubt it was because of how hard I hit and how tenacious the steroids made me and that extra will not to give up. I'm one of those guys who believed in no retreat, no surrender. And that's a neat phrase, but there's another one—come back to fight another day. That's a neat phrase, too. It's OK to lose once in a while, especially if you're saving yourself.

Notes

CHAPTER 1   REALITY CHECK: KIDS ARE USING STEROIDS

1. Charles E. Yesalis, *The Steroids Game* (Champaign, IL: Human Kinetics Publishing, 1998).

2. Michael Bahrke and Charles E. Yesalis, *Performance Enhancing Substances in Sport and Exercise*, (Champaign, IL: Human Kinetics Publishing, 2002).

3. Dr. Charles Yesalis, telephone interview (December 6, 2004).

4. "For Athletes, Drug Test Is an Easy Opponent," *Los Angeles Times* (January 19, 1984), sec. 3. p. 14.

5. Dr. Kalinski first received the document detailing the Soviet Union's performance-enhancing drug program in 1979. He defected in 1990 and waited until 2003, when he became a U.S. citizen and had reestablished his academic career following the fall of communism, to reveal the documentation. See Janet Rae Brooks, "Former Sports Scientist Reveals Soviet Steroid Program for Athletes," *The Salt Lake Tribune* (August 31, 2003), 1C.

6. A San Francisco–area company known as BALCO (Bay Area Laboratory Co-Operative) is being investigated by the U.S. government on suspicion of steroid distribution. Barry Bonds' trainer, Greg Anderson, and BALCO owner, Victor Conte, whom Bonds calls his nutritionist, along with two other Bay-area men have been indicted on steroid conspiracy charges. They are suspected of distributing the anabolic steroid known as THG to an unknown number of elite athletes including Major League Baseball players Bonds, Jason Giambi, Gary Sheffield, Marvin Bernard, Benito Santiago, and Randy Velarde.

7. Steven Ungerleider, *Faust's Gold: Inside The East German Doping Machine* (New York: St. Martin's Press, 2001), 1.

8. Two East German doctors and four coaches were charged with causing bodily harm to 19 young swimmers by giving them anabolic steroids without informing them or their parents. The women suffered from such problems as unnatural body hair, excessive muscle growth, voice changes, or severe acne. The six men—former sports doctors Dieter Binus and Bernd Pansold, and former coaches Rolf Glaeser, Volker Frischke, Dieter Lindemann, and Dieter Krause—were each fined. Pansold was hit with the heaviest fine—$8,200 in American currency, while the other defendants received fines ranging from $1,750 to $5,300. See "Former East German sports doctor fined for giving steroids," *Associated Press* (December 7, 1998), BC cycle.

9. Brigitte Berendonk and Werner Franke, "Hormonal doping and andro-genization of athletes: A secret program of the German Democratic Republic government," *Clinical Chemistry* 43 (1997): 1262–79.

10. Before dying in 1984, Ziegler realized the harmful impact he had made on sports. "I wish to God I'd never done it," he said. "I'd like to go back and take that whole chapter out of my life." See M. A. Mehta, "Steroid Scandals Come to a Head After Long History," *Newark Star-Ledger* (March 17, 2004), Sports.

11. Charles Yesalis and Michael Bahrke, "Where There Is a Will to Gain an Edge, Athletes Find a Way," *New York Times News Service* (March 6, 2004), Sports section, p. 10.

12. James E. Wright, *Anabolic Steroids and Sport* (Natick, MA: Sports Science Consultants, 1982), 2:119.

13. Powerlifter Terry Todd reported in a 1983 *Sports Illustrated* article that Kerr had 10,000 steroids patients. See Terry Todd, "The Steroid Predicament," *Sports Illustrated* (August 1, 1983): 70–73.

14. Kerr, who died of a heart attack January 3, 2001, at age 65, steadfastly denied being an advocate of steroids, saying instead that if athletes were going to choose to take steroids, they should do so under the care of a physician. He discontinued his prescriptions to athletes when he said some were taking additional steroids obtained on the black market. When asked on CBS's *60 Minutes* about the ethics of helping athletes cheat, Kerr responded: "This is not cheating—not when everyone does it." Quoted here from Steve Woodward, "Reputation Led Athletes to 'Steroid Guru,'" *USA Today* (April 6, 1989), 10C.

15. "Names in the Game," *The Associated Press* (November 4, 2004), BC cycle.

16. Craig Lord, "China Drug Fears Increase," *The Times* (of London) (February 20, 1998), Sports section.

17. Tetrahydrogestrinone (THG) is an anabolic steroid that has been altered by chemists to avoid detection by normal doping tests. The world's sporting community and the general public learned of THG's existence only after an anonymous athletics coach contacted the U.S. Anti-Doping Agency (USADA) with claims that several top athletes were using it. The coach then provided a syringe containing THG, which was used by the USADA to develop a test that could detect the substance. See Pete Carey and Lisa Krieger, "Suspected Steroid Lies in Legal Limbo," *San Jose Mercury News* (October 22, 2003), 1C www.mercury news.com/mld/mercurynews/sports/7073588.htm?1c (accessed April 13, 2004).

18. The list of athletes to test positive for THG as of the writing of this book are: four Oakland Raiders—defensive tackle Dana Stubblefield, center Barret Robbins, linebacker Bill Romanowski, and defensive tackle Chris Cooper; and four U.S. track athletes who tested positive during the June 2003 U.S. national championships at Stanford University—Regina Jacobs, the 2003 U.S. 1,500 meters champ who forfeited her title shortly after accepting a four-year ban from USADA and has since retired from the sport; Kevin Toth, a shot-putter currently receiving a two-year ban from USADA, John McEwen, a hammer thrower serving a two-year ban from USADA; and Melissa Price, a hammer thrower also serving a two-year ban. See "Who's Who: A List of Those Implicated in the BALCO

Investigation by a federal grand jury in San Francisco," *Washington Post* (December 4, 2004), D11.

19. See www.ncaa.org/library/research/substance_use_habits/2001/substance _use_habits.pdf (accessed April 13, 2004).

20. Brian McCallum, "La. Teens No. 1 in Steroid Use," *Shreveport Times* (August 19, 2001), 1A.

21. Brian McCallum, "Survey: Local Kids Take Steroids," *Shreveport Times* (August 19, 2001), 1C. This survey was conducted and published as a part of the investigative series "Shortcut to Power," written by Brian McCallum, which won first place in the largest newspaper circulation category for sports enterprise in the 2002 Louisiana Sports Writers Association contest, the state's top sports writing prize. It was one of three consecutive projects edited and directed by John McCloskey to win state or national awards during his tenure as sports editor in Shreveport. The other two award-winning projects were titled "Caring for youth sports," written by Brian Vernellis in 2000, and "Winning at all costs," written primarily by McCallum in 2002.

22. Rob Gloster, "Half of Calif. prep boys know someone taking steroids, supplements," *Associated Press* (March 24, 2004), BC cycle.

23. Monitoring The Future is conducted at the Survey Research Center in the Institute for Social Research at the University of Michigan, www.monitoringthe future.org (accessed April 13, 2004).

24. See www.thesportjournal.org/2002Journal/Vol5-No3/anabolic-steroids .asp (accessed April 13, 2004).

25. Rob Gloster, "High schools struggling with rising steroid use," *Associated Press* (March 26, 2004), BC cycle.

26. CNN, "Teens and Steroids," August 9, 2001. www.ironmagazineforums .com/showthread.php?threadid=21830 (accessed April 21, 2004).

27. Dennis L. Breo, "Foul Play: Janus-Faced Sports Policy Makes Drug Testing an Idle Threat," *Physician's Weekly* 18, no. 4 (January 22, 2001).

28. Three were arrested, 12 others contributed. On a team of 54 students, 15 students represent 28 percent.

29. ESPN.com comprehensively detailed the ease with which steroids can be purchased. See Tom Farrey, "Yesterday's drug makes comeback," ESPN.com. espn.go.com/gen/s/2000/1207/929174.html (accessed December 20, 2000).

30. Monitoring The Future Survey at www.monitoringthefuture.org/data/ 03data/pr03t1.pdf (accessed May 2, 2004).

31. Brian McCallum, "La. teens No. 1 in steroid use," 1A.

32. Rick Cantu, "Schools Say Steroids Not a Problem in Texas," *Austin American-Statesman* (October 22, 2002), C1.

33. Rick Ryan, "Steroids not an issue for area athletes," *Charleston (W.Va.) Gazette* (July 19, 2002), 1B.

34. Anita Manning, "Kids and Steroids Don't Mix," *USA Today* (July 9, 2002), 14C.

35. Frank Uryasz, telephone interview, April 1, 2004.

36. Aynsley Smith quoted here from CNN, "Teens and Steroids."

37. Edward Morgan quoted here from Brian McCallum, "Parents Roles Vary On Tender Issues," *Shreveport Times* (August 21, 2001), 1C.

38. Nicholas DiNubile quoted here from Anita Manning, "Kids and Steroids Don't Mix," *USA Today* (July 9, 2002), 14C.

39. John McCloskey, "Fight against steroid use must be aggressive," *Shreveport Times* (August 23, 2001), 1C.

40. Rob Gloster, "Half of Calif prep boys know someone taking steroids, supplements," BC cycle.

41. Frank Uryasz quoted here from Jon L. Wertheim, Luis F. Llosa, and Lester Munson, "Jolt of Reality: Following the Lead of Elite Athletes, Teenagers are Increasingly Juicing Their Workouts With Pills and Powders—Sometimes with Tragic Results," *Sports Illustrated* (April 7, 2003), 68.

Sidebar 1.1   Survival of the Fittest?

1. Jim Loehr and Tony Schwartz, "The Making of a Corporate Athlete," *Harvard Business Review* (January 2001), 120.

2. Chris Redden quoted here from Brian McCallum, "Medical student insists steroids help quality of life," *Shreveport Times* (August 23, 2001), 1C.

3. Redden quoted here from McCallum, 1C.

4. Redden quoted here from McCallum, 1C.

CHAPTER 2   FOLLOW THE LEADER: KIDS NEED BETTOR MENTORS, HEROES

1. Charles Barkley, *I May Be Wrong But I Doubt It* (New York: Random House, 2002).

2. J. C. Watts, "Society Needs a Wakeup Call," *The Sporting News* 228, no. 11 (March 15, 2004): 8.

3. Bridget Maher, *The Family Portrait*, Family Research Council (2002), www.frc.org/get.cfm?i = BK04C01 (accessed December 20, 2004).

4. President's Council of Economic Advisors, "Families and the Labor Market, 1969–1999: Analyzing the 'Time Crunch.'" The report found that U.S. workers now spend more time on the job than workers in any other developed country. It also highlighted the finding that American parents have 22 fewer hours per week to spend at home compared with the average in 1969.

5. Michael Josephson, telephone interview, June 2, 2004.

6. John Leavens, telephone interview, May 5, 2004.

7. "Dad," Father's Day Sermon (June 15, 2002) from St. Paul's United Methodist Church, www.saintpauls-umc.com/sermons/2002/dad.htm (accessed June 13, 2004).

8. "Spirituality and Religion reduce risk of Substance Abuse," The National Center on Addiction and Substance Abuse at Columbia University, November 14, 2001, http://www.casacolumbia.org/absolutenm/templates/PressReleases.asp ?articleid = 115&zoneid = 48 (accessed June 9, 2004).

9. Michael Josephson, telephone interview, June 2, 2004.

10. Bridget Maher, *The Family Portrait*.

11. Maher, *The Family Portrait*.

12. Daniel Patrick Moynihan quoted here from Bridget Maher, *The Family Portrait*. "Despite the difficulty of proving causation in the social sciences, the

weight of evidence increasingly supports the conclusion that fatherlessness is a primary generator of violence among young men" (David Blankenhorn, *Fatherless America* [New York: Basic Books, 1995]).

13. William J. Bennett, John J. DiIulio Jr., and John P. Walters, quoted here from Maher, *The Family Portrait*.

14. Maher, *The Family Portrait*.

15. Charles Barkley, telephone interview (May 10, 2004).

16. Johnette McCrery, e-mail interview (May 31, 2004).

17. Michael Josephson, Biographical Information, http://www.character counts.org/mj-bio.htm (accessed May 7, 2004).

18. Michael Josephson, telephone interview (June 2, 2004).

19. Judith Rich Harris, *The Nurture Assumption: Why Children Turn Out the Way They Do* (New York: Free Press, 1998).

20. Close to 90 percent of kids 8 to 12 years old prefer to act in a group than on their own, and 90 percent of kids' brand decisions are heavily influenced by their peers, according to Martin Lidstrom and Patricia B. Seybold, *Brandchild* (London: Kogan Page Ltd., 2003), 320.

21. Kimberly Zola, et al., "Adolescence: Change and Continuity," Insidebard-.com (Bard University), inside.bard.edu/academic/specialproj/darling/adpeer3 .htm (accessed May 22, 2004). Zola writes: "There are problems affiliated with being involved in a peer group whether popular or rejected. These problems consist of youth unemployment, teenage suicide, juvenile crime, delinquency, drug and alcohol use and premarital pregnancy. These problems have increased dramatically since the 1940's, due to the rise and power of peer groups." (Dr. Laurence Steinberg, psychology professor at Temple University, wrote a book entitled *Beyond the Classroom: Why School Reform Has Failed and What Parents Need to Do* [New York Simon and Schuster, 1996], contending that parents have become "seriously disengaged" from their children's lives.) Some feel these problems have become more severe due to the isolation of adolescents from adults during this period.

22. Gordon Neufeld and Gabor Mate, *Hold on to Your Kids: Why Parents Matter* (Toronto: Knopf, 2004).

23. Brian Bethune, "Does Peer Group Trump Family?" *Maclean's* (March 1, 2004): 33.

24. Michael Josephson, telephone interview (June 2, 2004).

25. Eugen Tomiuc, "Doping—'Muscle Mania' Poses Risk of Steroids Abuse Among Youths," Radio Free Europe/Radio Liberty (March 26, 2004), www.rferl .org/featuresarticle/2004/03/cc344a87-3bbd-4c99-9522-b2b8b62687f7.html.

26. "Blue Cross and Blue Shield Association Survey Projects 1.1 Million Teens Have Used Potentially Dangerous Sports Supplements and Drugs," www .Healthycompetition.org (accessed May 20, 2004).

27. Charles Yesalis, "Cardiovascular Disease: Man Expects Years of Steroid Use to Kill Him," *Sex Weekly* (March 30, 1998): 4–5.

Sidebar 2.1   Q&A with Jack Nicklaus

1. Jack Nicklaus quoted here from an interview with Scott Tolley, Nicklaus' director of communications (August 29, 2004).

Sidebar 2.2   A Word to Parents

1. Arthur W. Pink quoted here from Grace Online Library, http://www
.graceonlinelibrary.org/full.asp?ID = 474 (accessed April 17, 2004).

CHAPTER 3   ATHLETES TO KIDS:
DO AS WE SAY, NOT AS WE DO

1. Charles Barkley, telephone interview (May 10, 2004).

2. Rich Wanninger, e-mail interview (October 1, 2004).

3. Michael Bahrke and Charles Yesalis, "Where There Is a Will to Gain an Edge, Athletes Find a Way," *New York Times* (March 6, 2004)), Sports section, p. 10.

4. An example of one athlete's doping supervised by three different doctors: "Canadian sprinter, Angela Issakenko, testified to the [Dubin] Commission that she obtained her first prescription for Dianabol in 1979 from Dr. Gunther Koch, a physician practicing in Toronto. In 1983 she went on a different drug program following a visit to Dr. Robert Kerr in San Gabriel, California, while from the autumn of 1983 until 1988, her drug program was supervised by Dr. Jamie Astaphan, who also supervised the drug use of Ben Johnson." See Ivan Waddington, "Doping in Sport: Some Issues for Medical Practitioners," www.play-the-game .org/nyart/artikel.php?i = 361 (accessed March 31, 2004).

5. Waddington, "Doping in Sport."

6. Carl Lewis quoted here from Amy Shipley, "With Drug Tests, Answers Are Few," *Washington Post* (September 22, 1999), D1.

7. Robert O. Voy quoted here from Dennis L. Breo, "Foul Play: Janus-Faced Sports Policy Makes Drug Testing an Idle Threat," *Physician's Weekly* 18, no. 4 (January 22, 2001).

8. Scott. M. Reid, "IOC Won't Punish USOC for Its Drug-Case Handling," *Orange County Register* (May 18, 2004), Sports.

9. Elliott Pellman quoted here from William Sherman, "Growing Nightmare of Steroid Abuse: Athletes' Cocktail Big in Nation's Gyms," *New York Daily News* (July 28, 2002), 4.

10. Charles Yesalis quoted here from Jeff Schultz, "New Doping Fight's Time Has Arrived . . . Too Late," *Atlanta Journal-Constitution* (May 19, 2004), 1C.

11. Gerhard Treutlein, "From word to action: The ambivalence of western anti-doping," www.play-the-game.org/nyart/artikel.php?i = 409 (accessed June 8, 2004).

12. Yesalis quoted here from Rob Gloster, "Experts Face Long Road in Fighting Drugs in Sports," *The Associated Press* (October 25, 2003), AM Cycles.

13. Charles Barkley, telephone interview (May 10, 2004).

14. Breo, "Foul Play."

15. Gene Upshaw quoted here from Charles Chandler, "Substance Abuse Policy Unchanged," *Charlotte Observer* (July 4, 2003), 6C.

16. Charles Chandler, "Substances Policy Unchanged: NFLPA Pushed to Get Four-Game Suspension for First Positive Test Reduced," *Charlotte Observer* (July 4, 2003), 6C.

17. Frank Orr, "Drug Testing Pro Sports' Hottest Issue," *Toronto Star* (November 8, 1986), D1.

18. Sandy Padwe, "Drugs in Sports; Symptoms of a Deeper Malaise," *The Nation* 243 (September 27, 1986): 276.

19. George Allen quoted here from Padwe, "Drugs in Sports."

20. George Allen, "Other Voices: Strength Isn't From a Bottle," *(Newport News) Daily Press* (April 23, 2004), A15.

21. Raffaele Guariniello quoted here from Eamonn O'Hara, "Italian Football Rocked by Nerve Disease Findings," *Irish News* (February 26, 2003), 28.

22. Eugen Tomiuc, "Doping: Performance-Enhancing Drugs a Threat to Health and Ethics," Radio Free Europe/Radio Liberty, www.rferl.org/features article/2004/03/0258fb1a-dded-4481-b329-12a0f6dd3fdf.html (accessed March 26, 2004).

23. Jon Swartz, "Behind Fun Facade, Professional Wrestling Sees 65 Deaths in 7 Years," *USA Today* (March 12, 2004), 1C.

24. Terry Todd, "Anabolic Steroids: The Gremlins of Sport," *Journal of Sport History* 14, no. 1 (Spring 1987). The following three items in this bulleted list were not among those in Terry Todd's 1987 work, but occurred late in 1986, perhaps after his research for this timely article was complete.

25. This list is a very condensed version of Maher's work, without the many events, rumors, details of investigations, etc.—the article is nearly four times as long in its entirety. See John Maher, "The Year on Drugs," *Austin American-Statesman* (December 29, 1998), C4.

26. See August 30, 2003, USADA press release, "U.S. Cyclist Receives Lifetime Ban from USADA for Positive Drug Test," www.usantidoping.org/files/active/resources/press_releases/PressRelease_8_30_2002_d.pdf (accessed October 1, 2004).

27. Korey Stringer died from heat stroke at age 27. The 335-pound lineman was practicing in temperatures above 90 degrees and a heat index even higher. He had been taking a supplement containing ephedra, though it was not known how much or when he last used the supplement.

28. Elliott Almond and Mark Emmons, "Pushing The Steroid Issue: Anti-Doping Movement Depends on Public Getting Aboard," *San Jose Mercury News* (December 2, 2003), A1.

29. Paul Kelso quoted here from Eugen Tomiuc, "Doping—'Muscle Mania' Poses Risk of Steroids Abuse Among Youth," Radio Free Europe/Radio Liberty, http://www.rferl.org/featuresarticle/2004/03/cc344a87-3bbd-4c99-9522-b2b8b62687f7.html (accessed March 26, 2004).

30. Nicholas DiNubile quoted here from Anita Manning, "Kids, Steroids Don't Mix," *USA Today* (July 9, 2002), 1C.

31. "Teen Athletes 'Juicing' Says High-school Student Survey." State of California Senate Majority Caucus, democrats.sen.ca.gov/servlet/gov.ca.senate .democrats.pub.press.View?ID = 2103 (accessed March 31, 2004).

32. Charles Yesalis quoted here from Gwen Knapp, "Dangers of Doping Trickle Down to Kids," *San Francisco Chronicle* (November 2, 2003), B2.

33. Ben Arnold quoted here from Carl Dubois, "Supplement gains skeptics: Creatine's popularity has doctors worried," *Shreveport Times* (July 12, 1998).

34. Gary Wadler quoted here from M. A. Mehta, "Steroid Scandals Come to a Head After Long History," *Newark Star-Ledger* (March 17, 2004), Sports.

35. "Teen Athletes 'Juicing.'"

36. Allan Korn quoted from "Androstenedione: Groups Ask Ball Players to Halt Use," *American Health Line* (March 27, 2004), Trends and Timelines section.

37. Bud Selig quoted from "Androstenedione."

38. Robert Kerr quoted here from Steve Woodward, "Reputation Led Athletes to 'Steroid Guru,'" *USA Today* (April 6, 1989), 10C.

39. Werner Reiterer, "A Star's Descent to Drugs," *The Age* (July 5, 2000), 4.

40. Gerhard Treutlein, Author's biography at www.play-the-game.org/nyart/artikel.php?i=409 (accessed June 8, 2004).

41. "Comments on the Report of the Dubin Inquiry," collection.nlc-bnc.ca/100/200/300/ccsa-cclat/comments_dubin_inquiry/dubin.htm (accessed June 20, 2004).

42. Sophie Goodchild, "Aids Fear as Clubbers Inject New Bodybuilding Drug," *The Independent (London)* (July 2, 2000), 10.

43. The study was conducted by Dr. Harrison G. Pope Jr. and his colleagues at Harvard Medical School in Boston. They reviewed histories of patients at a private drug-abuse treatment facility in New Jersey. Eighteen of the former steroid users said they had started using opioid drugs to counteract steroid-induced insomnia and irritability; 14 said they used opioids to counteract the depression that accompanied withdrawal from anabolic steroids. See "Steroid Abusers May Go on to Abuse Opioids, Too," *NIDA (National Institute on Drug Abuse) Notes* www.nida.nih.gov/NIDA_Notes/NNVol15N6/BBoard.html#Steroid (accessed June 16, 2004).

44. Allan Korn, "Blue Cross and Blue Shield Association Survey Projects 1.1 Million Teens Have Used Potentially Dangerous Sports Supplements and Drugs," www.Healthycompetition.org. (accessed July 7, 2004).

Sidebar 3.1 Truth and Lies behind the NFL's "Exemplary" Drug-Testing Plan

1. Richard W. Pound, *Inside the Olympics* (Montreal, Canada: Wiley, 2004), 65.

2. Pound, 59.

3. Steve Courson quoted here from his position paper, "Performance-Enhancing Drugs, Image vs. Reality," June 24, 2004.

4. Courson, "Performance-Enhancing Drugs."

CHAPTER 4 BALCO AND BEYOND: THE BIGGEST DOPING SCANDAL IN SPORTS HISTORY

1. Don Walker and Mark Maley, "Bonds' Brilliance Has Asterisk," *Milwaukee Journal Sentinel* (March 28, 2004), 1C.

2. Mark Fainaru-Wada and Lance Williams, "Bonds Got Steroids, Feds Were Told; Slugger's Trainer Said to Have Given Substances to Several Athletes," *San Francisco Chronicle* (March 2, 2004), A1.

3. Mark Fainaru-Wada and Lance Williams, "Giambi Admitted Taking Steroids," *San Francisco Chronicle* (December 2, 2004), 1A.

4. Mark Fainaru-Wada and Lance Williams, "What Bonds Told BALCO Grand Jury," *San Francisco Chronicle* (December 3, 2004), 1A.

5. Mark Fainaru-Wada and Lance Williams "Track star's testimony linked Bonds to steroid use," *San Francisco Chronicle* (June 24, 2004), A16.

6. The Court of Arbitration for Sport has said it will hear the case of American sprinter Tim Montgomery on June 6 in San Francisco and Chryste Gaines on July 10 in New York. Both are suspected of using THG. It is not known when or if the U.S. Government will bring criminal charges on athletes involved in the BALCO scandal.

7. See "BALCO Timeline," *San Jose Mercury News* www.mercurynews.com/mld/mercurynews/sports/9220625.htm?1c (accessed August 20, 2004, December 4, 2004).

8. President Bush quoted here from "George W. Bush Delivers the State of the Union Address," FDCH Political Transcripts (January 20, 2004).

9. Pete Carey, "Bodybuilder with BALCO Indicted in Steroids Case," *San Jose Mercury News* (November 22, 2004), wire service.

10. John Shea, "Union Backs Toughening Baseball's Drug Rules," *San Francisco Chronicle* (December 8, 2004), A1.

11. ESPNradio.com poll, www.espnradio.com (accessed September 16, 2004).

12. Carol Pogash, "Federal Investigators Seized Vials From Bonds' Trainer, Document Says," *New York Times News Service* (April 29, 2004), D3.

13. Mark Fainaru-Wada and Lance Williams, "Bonds Used Steroids in 2003, Trainer Says on Secret Recording," *San Francisco Chronicle* (October 16, 2004), A1.

14. Fainaru-Wada and Williams, "What Bonds Told BALCO," A1.

15. Charles Elmore, "Steroids: Muscle Means Power in Baseball," *Palm Beach Post* (March 6, 2004), 8B.

16. Jim Schmaltz, "The King of Swing: what fuels baseball superhitter Barry Bonds?" *Muscle & Fitness* (June 1, 2003): 170.

17. Fainaru-Wada and Williams, "What Bonds Told BALCO."

18. Schmaltz, "The King of Swing."

19. Reggie Jackson quoted here from Terrance Moore, "Can't Silence Mr. October About Steroids," *Atlanta Journal-Constitution* (March 11, 2004), 2E.

20. Hank Aaron quoted here from Bill Madden, "Aaron: I'm Sad For Baseball," *(New York) Daily News* (February 29, 2004), 62.

21. Andy Van Syke quoted here from *Sporting News Radio* cited by Mark Fainaru-Wada, "Steroid Issue Has Divided Baseball Like No Other," *San Francisco Chronicle* (March 28, 2004), C1.

22. John Holway quoted here from Mark Maley and Don Walker, "Bonds' Brilliance Has Asterisk; Game's Biggest Slugger at Center of Steroids Storm," *Milwaukee Journal-Sentinel* (March 28, 2004), 1C.

23. Mark Whicker, "Steroids Offer No Help in Hitting Baseball," *Orange County Register* (March 6, 2004).

24. Erin McClam, "Effects of drugs ruled cause of death for Caminiti," *Associated Press* (November 1, 2004), BC cycle.

25. Amy Shipley, "Baseball Players Say Steroid Use Is Heavy," *Washington Post* (May 29, 2002), D1.

26. Richard W. Pound, *Inside the Olympics* (Montreal, Canada: Wiley, 2004), 64.

27. Pound, 60–61.

28. Pound, 59.

29. Pound, 66.

30. U.S. Anti-Doping Agency spokesman Rich Wanninger, e-mail interview (October 1, 2004).

31. "World Anti-Doping Code: Summary of Provisions," Genomics Gateway, www.bradford.ac.uk/acad/sbtwc/gateway/DRUGS/doping_code.htm (accessed December 8, 2004).

32. Jeff Greenfield, "Can the Government Clean Up the Game?" *Sports Illustrated* (March 15, 2004): 44.

Sidebar 4.1   What Keeps Barry Swinging

1. Jim Schmaltz, "The King of Swing: what fuels baseball superhitter Barry Bonds?" *Muscle & Fitness* (June 1, 2003): 170.

Sidebar 4.2   Summary of Doping in Athens

1. "Fact Boxes on Athletes Charged with Doping in Athens," *Reuters* (August 28, 2004); and "Doping Cases at the Athens Games," *Associated Press* (August 28, 2004).

2. "Russian Olympic Committee Asks CAS to Strip Hamilton's Gold," *Associated Press* (October 20, 2004), BC cycle.

CHAPTER 5   STEROIDS AND DESIGNER DRUGS

1. A. A. Berthold, "Transplantation der Hoden," *Arch. Anat. Phys. wiss. Med.* 16:42. 1849.

2. M. S. Bahrke and C. E. Yesalis, eds., *Performance-Enhancing Substances in Sport and Exercise* (Champaign, IL: Human Kinetics 2002).

3. C. E. Yesalis, M. S. Bahrke, "History of doping in sport," in M. S. Bahrke and C. E. Yesalis, eds., *Performance-Enhancing Substances in Sport and Exercise* (Champaign, IL: Human Kinetics, 2002), 1–20.

4. C. Francis, *Speed Trap* (New York: St Martin's Press, 1990).

5. N. Wade, "Anabolic steroids: Doctors denounce them, but athletes aren't listening," *Science* 176 (1972): 1399–403.

6. C. E. Yesalis and M. S. Bahrke, "History of doping in sport," in M. S. Bahrke and C. E. Yesalis, eds., *Performance Enhancing Substances in Sport and Exercise* (Champaign, IL: Human Kinetics, 2002), 1–20.

7. L. Silvester, "Anabolic steroids at the 1972 Olympics," *Scholastic Coach* 43 (1973): 90–92.

8. C. E. Yesalis, S. P. Courson, and J. E. Wright, "History of anabolic steroid use in sport and exercise," in C. E. Yesalis, ed., *Anabolic Steroids in Sport and Exercise*, 2d ed. (Champaign, IL: Human Kinetics, 2000), 51–71.

9. C. E. Yesalis, C. K. Barsukiewicz, A. N. Kopstein, and M. S. Bahrke, "Trends in anabolic-androgenic steroid use among adolescents," *Archives of Pediatric and Adolescent Medicine* 151 (1997): 1197–206.

10. C. Yesalis, W. Buckley, W. Anderson, M. O. Wang, J. H. Norwig, G. Ott, J .C. Puffer, and R. H. Strauss, "Athletes' projections of anabolic steroid use," *Clinical Sports Medicine* 2 (1990): 155–111.

11. M. S. Bahrke and C. E. Yesalis, eds., "Anabolic-androgenic steroids," *Sports Medicine* 19, no. 5 (1995): 326–40; *Performance-Enhancing Substances in Sport and Exercise*, 326–40.

12. C. S. Ballantyne, S. M. Phillips, J. R. MacDonald, M. A. Tarnopolsky, and J. D. MacDougall, "The acute effects of androstenedione supplementation in healthy young males," *Can J Appl Physiol* 25, no. 1 (2000): 68–78.

13. M. Myhal and D. R. Lamb, "Hormones as performance enhancing drugs," in M. P. Warren and N. W. Constantini, eds., *Sports Endocrinology* (Totowa, NJ: Humana Press, 2000), 433–76.

14. K. E. Friedl, "Effect of anabolic steroid use on body composition and physical performance," in C. E. Yesalis, ed., *Anabolic Steroids in Sport and Exercise*, 2nd ed. (Champaign, IL: Human Kinetics, 2000), 139–74.

15. S. Ungerleider, *Faust's Gold* (New York: Thomas Dunne Books/St. Martin's Press, 2001).

16. Yesalis and Bahrke, "Anabolic-androgenic steroids," 326–40.

17. G. S. Lynch, D. G. Stephenson, and D. A. Williams, "Analysis of Ca2 + and Sr2 + activation characteristics in skinned muscle fibre preparations with different proportions of myofibrillar isoforms," *Journal of Muscle Research and Cell Motility* 16 (1995): 65–78.

18. Y. S. Kim and R. D. Sainz, "ß-adrenergic agonists and hypertrophy of skeletal muscles," *Life Sciences* 50 (1992): 397–407.

19. See P. Embleton and G. Thorne, "Anabolic primer," *Muscle Mag International* (1998); and I. D. Prather, D. E. Brown, P. North, and J. R. Wilson, "Clenbuterol: a substitute for anabolic steroids," *Medicine and Science in Sports and Exercise* 27 (1995), 1118–21.

20. G. S. Lynch, "Beta-2 Agonists," in M. S. Bahrke and C. E. Yesalis, eds., *Performance-Enhancing Substances in Sport and Exercise* (Champaign, IL: Human Kinetics, 2002), 47–64.

21. K. E. Yarasheski, J. J. Zachweija, J. A. Campbell, and D. M. Bier, "Effect of growth hormone on muscle growth and strength in older men," *American Journal of Physiology* 268 (1995): E268–76.

22. S. Brownlee, "Moms in the fast lane," *Sports Illustrated* (May 30, 1988), www.findarticles.com/p/articles/mi_hb292/is_198805/ai_n5539506 (accessed December 2004).

23. S. B. Karch, "Stimulants," in M. S. Bahrke and C. E. Yesalis, eds., *Performance-Enhancing Substances in Sport and Exercise* (Champaign, IL: Human Kinetics, 2002), 257–65.

24. R. Gloster, "USOC: Toth tested positive for THG, modafinil," SignOnSan Diego.com/pt/cpt (accessed February 16, 2004).

25. "Trainer says banned stimulant was used," *USA Today* (May 15, 2002); "Gwynn says 'Greenies' a problem in baseball," *USA Today* (April 23, 2003).

26. S. Wilson, "British sprinter tests positive for THG," *AP Online* (October 22, 2003).

27. S. K. Ritter, "Designer Steroid Rocks Sports World," *Science and Technology* 81 (2003): 66–69.

28. M. Bertrand, R. Masse, and R. Dugal, "GC-MS: approach for the detection and characterization of anabolic steroids and their metabolites in biological fluids at major international sporting events," *Farmaceutische Tijdschrift Voor Belgie.* 55, no. 3 (1978): 85–101.

29. R. de la Torre, J. Segura, A. Polettini, and M. Montagna, "Detection of testosterone esters in human plasma," *Journal of Mass Spectrometry* 30 (1995): 1393–404.

30. R. Masse, C. Lalibert, l. Tremblay, and R. Dugal, "Gas chromatographic/mass spectrometric analysis of 19-nortestosterone urinary metabolites in man," *Biomedical Mass Spectrometry,* 12, no. 3 (1985): 115.

31. L. Dehennin and A. M. Matsumoto, "Long-term administration of testosterone enanthate to normal men: alterations of the urinary profile of androgen metabolites potentially useful for detection of testosterone misuse in sports," *Journal of Steroid Biochemistry and Molecular Biology* 44 (1993): 179–89.

32. See H. Oftebro, "Evaluating an abnormal urinary steroid profile," *Lancet* 359 (1992): 941–42; and E. Raynaud, M. Audran, J. F. Brun, C. Fedou, J. L. Chanal, and A. Orsetti, "False-positive cases in detection of testosterone doping," *Lancet* 340, no. 8833 (December 12, 1992): 1468–69.

33. R. C. Kammerer, "Drug Testing in Sport and Exercise," in M. S. Bahrke and C. E. Yesalis, eds., *Performance-Enhancing Substances in Sport and Exercise* (Champaign, IL: Human Kinetics, 2002), 323–39.

34. R. Pound, *Inside the Olympics: A Behind-the-Scenes Look at the Politics, the Scandals, and the Glory of the Games* (Etobicoke, Ontario, Canada: John Wiley & Sons, 2004).

CHAPTER 6   SUPPLEMENT BOOM: BIG BUSINESS SPURS BIG TROUBLE

1. Scotty Romans quoted here from Kristen Go, "Larger Athletes a Growing Concern; Supplement Use Part of the Trend," *The Arizona Republic* (September 22, 2002), 1C.

2. Harlan Malamud quoted here from Jamie Malernee and Rhonda Miller, "Drug Use on the Rise for Physical Perfection," *(Fort Lauderdale, Fla.) Sun-Sentinel* (June 8, 2003), 1A.

3. L. B. Jeter quoted here from Carl Dubois, "Supplement Gains Skeptics: Creatine's popularity has doctors worried," *Shreveport Times* (July 12, 1998), 1C.

4. Dubois, "Supplement Gains Skeptics," 1C.

5. Ralph W. Hale, "Increased Penalties for Anabolic Steroid Offenses," *Federal Document Clearing House Congressional Testimony* (March 16, 2004).

6. Go, 1C.

7. Madelyn H. Fernstrom quoted here from Christopher Snowbeck, "Ban Signals Supplement Crackdown," *Pittsburgh Post-Gazette* (April 12, 2004), A1.

8. Joan Ryan, "It isn't a scandal in kid sports; Supplements help boost performance," *San Francisco Chronicle* (March 16, 2004), B1.

9. Brian McCallum, "Teens Powering the Supplement Industry Surge," *Shreveport Times* (Auguest 19, 2001), 1C.

10. Go, 1C.

11. Virginia Anderson, "Body builders?: Supplements are $16 Billion Industry, But Researchers Doubt Their Worth," *Atlanta Journal-Constitution* (February 24, 2004), 4E.

12. McCallum, 1C.

13. "Dangerous Supplements Still At Large," *Consumer Reports* 69, no. 5 (May 2002): 12.

14. "Drug Abuse: Survey Projects 1.1M Teens Have Used Sports Supplements, Drugs," *Health and Medicine Week* (November 23, 2003), 234.

15. "Drug Abuse," 234. Also see www.healthycompetition.org.

16. Jim Rueda, "To Gain an Edge, High School Athletes Turn to Protein Supplements," *Associated Press* (November 8, 2003), PM cycles.

17. Richard Kreider quoted here from Dubois, 1C.

18. Rick Collins quoted here from McCallum, 1C.

19. I (John McCloskey) began taking creatine regularly roughly one year after graduating from college in 1995. Within months, and after a consistent, strenuous, weight-training regimen, my bench press increased from the 185-pound level it had peaked at throughout my high school and college years to 255 pounds. I suffered the typical side effect of using creatine—regular cramping in my calves during pick-up basketball games as well as diarrhea, but the latter side effect occurred only when "loading," which involves taking much heavier amounts—up to three times the normal dose—of the supplement for the first week at the beginning of a six-week or longer "cycle." Nearly all makers of creatine initially recommended loading, but many experts now argue that it is unnecessary.

20. "Dangerous Supplements Still At Large," 12.

21. Mike Perko quoted here from Katy Hawes, "The Culture of Supplements: Pills, Powders and Potions Have Been Ingrained In Athletes' Way of Life," *The NCAA News* (June 3, 2003).

22. Etzel quoted here from Hawes, "The Culture of Supplements."

23. Etzel quoted here from Hawes, "The Culture of Supplements."

24. Stephen Barrett quoted here from Malernee and Miller, 1A.

25. "Quackery Targets Teens: Steroids and Growth Hormone," U.S. Food and Drug Administration, www.cfsan.fda.gov/~dms/wh-teen2.html (accessed May 15, 2004).

26. Troy Potter quoted here from Dubois, C1.

27. NFSHSA policy statement quoted here from Dubois, C1.

28. Glenn Cecchini quoted here from Brian McCallum, "Strength training helps programs stand out," *Shreveport Times* (August 20, 2001), 1C.

29. Ryan, B1.

Sidebar 6.1   Fearless Youth: Why They Use Supplements

1. Katy Hawes, "The Culture of Supplements: Pills, Powders and Potions Have Been Ingrained In Athletes' Way of Life," *The NCAA News* (June 3, 2003).

CHAPTER 7   SOLUTIONS TO THE OUT-OF-CONTROL DRUG PROBLEM IN SPORTS

1. Dr. Lynn Goldberg, telephone interview (April 23, 2004).

2. Goldberg, telephone interview.

3. Timothy Condin quoted here from "Salt Lake City Student-Athletes Turning Away From Drugs Thanks to New Prevention Program," Oregon Health and Science University, Salt Lake City School District, Salt Lake City Mayor's Office press release (March 5, 2002).

4. Goldberg, telephone interview.

5. Kevin Will quoted here from the Associated Press, "High Schools Struggling With Rising Steroid Use" (March 26, 2004).

6. Randall R. Wroble, Michael Gray, and Joseph A. Rodrigo, "Anabolic Steroids and Pre-Adolescent Athletes: Prevalence, Knowledge, and Attitudes," *The Sport Journal*, www.thesportjournal.org/2002Journal/Vol5-No3/anabolic-steroids.asp, (May 29, 2004).

7. Wroble, et al., "Anabolic Steroids and Pre-Adolescent Athletes."

8. See www.healthycompetition.org/hc/news/adult_survey_103103.html (accessed December 2004).

9. See www.healthycompetition.org/hc/news/supplement_survey.html. (accessed December 2004).

10. Brian McCallum, "Teens Powering the Supplement Industry Surge," *Shreveport Times* (August 19, 2001), 1C.

11. Goldberg, telephone interview.

12. Jeff Scudder quoted here from Jamie Malernee and Rhonda Miller, "Drug Use on the Rise for Physical Perfection," *(Fort Lauderdale, Fla.) Sun-Sentinel* (June 8, 2003), 1A.

13. See www.consumerreports.org (accessed May 21, 2004).

14. See www.casper207.com/files/HR3866.pdf (accessed July 7, 2004).

15. See www.casper207.com/files/S2195Biden.pdf (accessed July 7, 2004); the Anabolic Steroid Control Act of 2004 passed through the House of Representatives and the Senate and was signed into law by President Bush in October 2000.

16. U.S. Anti-Doping Agency spokesman Rich Wanninger, e-mail interview (October 1, 2004).

17. Terry Madden, e-mail interview (October 1, 2004).

18. Frank Uryasz, telephone interview, April 1, 2004.

19. Richard W. Pound, *Inside the Olympics* (Montreal, Canada: Wiley, 2004), 82.

20. William Llewellyn quoted here from Rob Gloster, "Easily Obtained Ste-

roids Focus of Debate on Drugs in Sports," *Associated Press* (November 29, 2003).

21. Neil Roth quoted here from William Sherman, "Growing Nightmare of Steroid Abuse: Athletes' Cocktail Big in Nation's Gyms," *New York Daily News* (July 28, 2002), 4.

22. Sherman, 4.

23. Stuart Stevens, "My Life As a Drug Cheat," *Telegraph Magazine* (December 14, 2003), 16.

24. John P. Lopez, "Steroid Problem at Your Fingertips," *Houston Chronicle* (March 18, 2004), 1C.

25. Terry Todd, "Anabolic Steroids: The Gremlins of Sport," *Journal of Sport History* 14, no. 1 (Spring 1987).

26. Dr. Frank Uryasz, telephone interview (April 1, 2004).

27. Pound, 64.

28. Pound, 65.

29. Elliott Almond, "New guidelines will target athletes' support staff, too," *San Jose Mercury News* (December 20, 2003), Sports section.

30. Ray Seals quoted here from Jeff Jenkins, "Getting noticed: Incoming juniors, seniors attend player program," *Houston Chronicle—This Week* (June 12, 2003), 13.

31. Paul Tagliabue quoted here from Nick Cafardo, "Patriots Notebook," *Boston Globe* (March 9, 2004).

32. Robert Voy quoted here from Dennis L. Breo, "Foul Play: Janus-Faced Sports Policy Makes Drug Testing an Idle Threat," *Physician's Weekly* 18, no. 4 (January 22, 2001).

33. Voy quoted here from Breo, "Foul Play."

34. Mark McGwire and Barry R. McCaffrey quoted here from Carl Dubois, "Popular Supplements May Harm Youngsters," *Shreveport Times* (August 29, 1999), C1.

Sidebar 7.2   Q&A with Dr. Frank Uryasz

1. Dr. Frank Uryasz, telephone interview (April 1, 2004). Dr. Uryasz is president of the National Center for Drug Free Sport, Inc., and the NCAA's director of sports sciences, which is responsible for the Association's sports medicine and education division.

Sidebar 7.3   Steroid and Supplement Legislation

1. See chapter 7, "Solutions to the Out-of-Control Drug Problem in Sports," for more information about the Anabolic Steroid Control Act of 2004, which President Bush signed into law in October 2004.

2. Actual summary of the bill: "This bill prohibits students from participation in high school sports unless they agree not to use performance-enhancing dietary supplements and steroids, and requires each school district to test for use of these supplements once the district has determined that there are funds to pay for the tests. This bill also requires each high school sports coach to complete and pay for a coaching education program on the use of such supplements."

See info.sen.ca.gov/pub/bill/sen/sb_1601-1650/sb_1630_cfa_20040426_160958 _sen_comm.html (accessed June 3, 2004).

3. Jim Sanders and Kevin Yamamura, "Energy Bill Makes Way to Governor," *Sacramento Bee* (August 28, 2004), A3.

4. A California Interscholastic Federation (CIF) bylaw recommends that schools have a policy regarding anabolic steroids and performance-enhancing drugs, and the California Education Code encourages schools to provide instruction in grades 7 through 12, but neither recommendation is mandatory.

5. From September 1998 to November 2001, the CIF sponsored training, which included drug education, of more than 10,000 coaches. But the program that was paid for by the state was then cut. Now school districts must pay for the program, and several, including San Juan Unified, have dropped it.

6. Actual summary of the bill: "This bill gives law enforcement the tools it needs to enforce a law banning the sale of dangerous pro-hormones to minors. Pro-hormones are one chemical step away from anabolic steroids, and may have some of the same harmful side-effects of their chemical cousins. A prior Speier bill (SB 1884) outlawed the sale of pro-hormones to minors, but because the term 'pro-hormone' was never defined, the state has been unable to enforce it so far. This bill would define the term, and specifically include androstenedione (andro) on the list of prohibited substances." See democrats.sen.ca.gov/servlet/gov.ca .senate.democrats.pub.members.memDisplaySpotlightFeature?district = sd08& ID = 2917 (accessed July 7, 2004).

7. Utah Sen. Orrin G. Hatch, who cowrote the Dietary Supplement Health and Education Act, has been the biggest financial beneficiary from supplement lobbyists. From 1994 to January 2002, the supplement industry contributed $143,950 to Hatch, $41,750 of it during his last re-election campaign. Hatch is now cosponsoring two bills that have the backing of the supplement industry. One would provide more funding to the FDA, and the other would declare supplements that contain steroid-like substances as controlled drugs.

8. It wasn't until 2002, when a Justice Department investigation forced Metabolife to turn over about 16,000 consumer complaints about its flagship ephedra product, that the extent of the problem became public. Then the death in 2003 of Baltimore Orioles pitcher Steve Bechler, whose heatstroke death was linked to the use of New Jersey–based Cytodyne Technologies' Xenadrine RFA-1 ephedra pill, increased the pressure on the FDA to take action. In December, after most of the major ephedra supplement companies had already pulled their ephedra products, the FDA announced it would ban them. See Penni Crabtree, "Critics want sharper teeth in rules on supplements," *Copley News Service* (April 13, 2004).

CHAPTER 8   DEAD SERIOUS: CATASTROPHIC AND FATAL INJURIES IN SPORTS

1. B. J. Maron, T. B. Gohrman, and D. Aeppli, "Prevalence of sudden cardiac death during competitive sports activities in Minnesota high school athletes," *Journal of the American College of Cardiology* 32 (1998): 1881–84.

2. A. P. Burke, A. Farb, R. Virmani, J. Goodin, and J. E. Smialek, "Sports-

related and non-sports-related sudden cardiac death in young adults," *American Heart Journal* 121 (1991): 568–75.

3. B. J. Maron, "Sudden death in young athletes," *New England Journal of Medicine* 349, no. 11 (2003): 1064–75.

4. See Burke et al., 568–75; Maron, 1064–75; and D. Corrado, G. Thiene, A. Nava, L. Rossi, and N. Pennelli, "Sudden death in young competitive athletes: clinicopathologic correlations in 22 cases," *American Journal of Medicine* 89 (1990): 588–96.

5. Maron, 1064–75; B. J. Maron, L. C. Poliac, J. A. Kaplan, and F. O. Mueller, "Blunt impact to the chest leading to sudden death from cardiac arrest during sports activities," *New England Journal of Medicine* 333 (1995): 337–43; and M. S. Link, P. J. Wang, N. G. Pandian, et al., "An experimental model of a sudden death due to low-energy chest-wall impact (commotio cordis)," *New England Journal of Medicine* 338 (1998): 1805–11.

6. Maron, 1064–75.

7. "Centers for Disease Control and Prevention: Sports-related recurrent brain injuries, United States," *Morbidity and Mortality Weekly Reports* 46 (1997): 224–27.

8. H. Ingemarson, S. Grevsten, and L. Thoren, "Lethal horse-riding injuries" *Journal of Trauma* 29 (1989): 25–30.

9. "Centers for Disease Control and Prevention: Alcohol use and horseback-riding-associated fatalities—North Carolina, 1979–1989," *Morbidity and Mortality Weekly Reports* 41, no. 19 (1992): 335.

10. J. Retsky, D. Jaffe, and K. Christoffel, "Skateboarding injuries in children: A second wave," *American Journal of Diseases of Children* 145 (1991): 188–93.

11. E. C. Powell and R. R. Tang, "In-line skate and roller skate injuries in childhood," *Pediatric Emergency Care* 12 (1996): 259–62.

12. B. D. Weiss, "Bicycle-related head injuries," *Clinics in Sports Medicine* 13, no. 99 (1994): 112; and J. E. Bailes and R. C. Cantu, "Head injury in athletes," *Neurosurgery* 48 (2001): 26–46.

13. T. G. Friermood, D. G. Messner, J. L. Brugman, and R. Brennan, "Save the trees: A comparative review of skier-tree collisions," *Journal of Orthopaedic Trauma* 8 (1994): 116–18; and J. B. Harris, "Neurological injuries in winter sports," *Physicians and Sports Medicine* 11 (1983): 110–22.

14. J. E. Bailes, J. M. Herman, M. R. Quigley, L. I. Cerullo, and P. R. Meyer Jr., "Diving injuries of the cervical spine," *Surgical Neurology* 34 (1990): 155–58.

15. A. M. Carr, J. E. Bailes, J. C. Helmkamp, C. L. Rosen, and V. J. Miele, "Neurological injury and death in all-terrain vehicle crashes in West Virginia: A 10-year retrospective review," *Neurosurgery* 54, no. 4 (2004): 861–86.

16. Bailes and Cantu, 26–46.

17. B. C. Barnes, L. Cooper, D. T. Kirkendall, T. P. McDermott, B. D. Jordan, and W. E. Garrett Jr., "Concussion history in elite male and female soccer players," *American Journal of Sports Medicine* 26 (1998): 433–38.

18. Bailes and Cantu, 26–46; and P. I. Bishop, R. W. Norman, M. Pierrynowski, and J. Kozey, "The ice hockey helmet: How effective is it?" *Physicians and Sports Medicine* 7 (1979): 97–106.

19. Bailes and Cantu, 26–46.

20. J. E. Bailes, M. N. Hadley, M. R. Quigley, V. K. Sonntag, and L. J. Cerullo, "Management of athletic injuries of the cervical spine and spinal cord," *Neurosurgery* 29, no. 4 (1991): 491–97.

21. Bailes et al., "Management of athletic injuries," 491–97.

22. Bailes et al., "Diving injuries of the cervical spine," 155–58.

CHAPTER 9   THE HEAT IS ON: HEAT STROKE CONTINUES TO KILL

1. J. P. Knochel, "Dog days and siriasis: How to kill a football player," *Journal of the American Medical Association* 233 (1975): 513–15; and M. Millard-Stafford, "Fluid replacement during exercise in the heat: Review and recommendations," *Sports Medicine* 13 (1992): 223–33.

2. J. E. Bailes, R. C. Cantu, and A. L. Day, "The neurosurgeon in sport: awareness of the risks of heatstroke and dietary supplements," *Neurosurgery* 51, no. 2 (2002): 283–86.

3. E. W. Schmidt and C. G. Nichols, "Heat and sun-related illnesses," in A. L. Harwood-Nuss, C. H. Linden, R. C. Luten, S. M. Shepherd, A. B. Wolfson, eds., *The Clinical Practice of Emergency Medicine*, 2nd ed. (Philadelphia: Lippincott-Raven, 1996), 1473–76.

4. O. Richards, R. Richards, P. I. Schofield, V. Ross, J. R. Sutton, "Management of heat exhaustion in Sydney's the Sun City-to-Surf run runners," *The Medical Journal of Australia* 2 (1979): 457–61; and L. E. Armstrong and C. M. Maresh, "The induction and decay of heat acclimatization in trained athletes," *Sports Medicine* 12 (1991): 302–12.

5. Millard-Stafford, 223–33; Richards et al., 457–61; and Schmidt and Nichols, 1473–76.

6. L. R. Bucci, "Selected herbals and human exercise performance," *American Journal of Clinical Nutrition*, 2nd supplement, 72 (2000): 624S–636S; and M. A. Pecci and J. A. Lombardo, "Performance-enhancing supplements," *Physical Medicine and Rehabilitation Clinics of North America* 11 (2000): 949–60.

7. Pecci and Lombardo, 949–60; B. I. Gurley, S. F. Gardner, and M. A. Hubbard, "Content versus label claims in ephedra-containing dietary supplements," *American Journal of Health-System Pharm* 57 (2000): 963–69.

8. E. A. Applegate and L. E. Grivetti: "Search for the competitive edge: A history of dietary fads and supplements," *Journal of Nutrition*, 5th supplement, 127 (1997): 869S–873S; and M. Bamberger, "The magic potion: Dietary supplement creatine," *Sports Illustrated* 87 (April 20, 1998): 58–61.

9. M. LaBotz and B. W. Smith, "Creatine supplement use in an NCAA Division I athletic program," *Clinical Journal of Sport Medicine: Official Journal of the Canadian Academy of Sport Medicine* 9 (1999): 167–69; and T. A. McGuine, J. C. Sullivan, and D. T. Bernhardt, "Creatine supplementation in high school football players," *Clinical Journal of Sport Medicine: Official Journal of the Canadian Academy of Sport Medicine* 11, no. 4 (2001): 247–53.

10. T. L. Jones, "Dangerously revved: Ephedrine misuse poses health hazards," *Texas Medicine* 92 (1996): 52–53.

11. A. Bruno, K. B. Nolte, and J. Chapin, "Stroke associated with ephedrine use," *Neurology* 43 (1993): 1313–16; and C. A. Haller and N. L. Benowitz, "Adverse cardiovascular and central nervous system events associated with dietary supplements containing ephedra alkaloids," *New England Journal of Medicine* 343 (2000): 1833–38.

12. Haller and Benowitz, 1833–38; and W. N. Kernan, C. M. Viscoli, L. M. Brass, J. P. Broderick, T. Brott, E. Feldmann, L. B. Morgenstern, J. L. Wilterdink, and R. I. Horwitz, "Phenylpropanolamine and the risk of hemorrhagic stroke," *New England Journal of Medicine* 343 (2000): 1826–32.

13. Haller and Benowitz, 1833–38; and E. Savdie, H. Prevedoros, A. Irish, C. Vickers, A. Concannon, P. Darveniza, and J. R. Sutton, "Heat stroke following Rugby League football," *The Medical Journal of Australia* 155 (1991): 636–39.

14. Savdie et al., 636–39; and N. D. Gill, A. Shield, A. J. Blazevich, S. Zhou, and R. P. Weatherby, "Muscular and cardiorespiratory effects of pseudoephedrine in human athletes," *British Journal of Clinical Pharmacology* 50, no. 3 (2000): 205–13.

15. Savdie et al., 636–39.

16. Knochel, 223–33; and Savdie et al., 636–39.

17. National Collegiate Athletic Association, "2000–2001 NCAA Sports Medicine Handbook: Guideline 2j-Nutritional ergogenic aids" (rev. July 2000), www.ncaa.org/library/sports_sciences/sports_med_handbook/2oo0-01/2j.pdf (accessed May 14, 2002).

18. C. P. Bolotte, "Creatine supplementation in athletes: Benefits and potential risks," *Journal of the Louisiana State Medical Society* 150 (1998): 325–27; A. S. Graham and R. C. Hatton, "Creatine: A review of efficacy and safety," *Journal of the American Pharmaceutical Association* 39 (1999): 803–10, quiz 875–77; W. I. Kraemer and J. S. Volek, "Creatine supplementation: Its role in human performance," *Clinical Journal of Sport Medicine: Official Journal of the Canadian Academy of Sport Medicine* 18 (1999): 651–66; and Pecci and Lombardo, 949–60.

19. T. W. Demant and E. C. Rhodes, "Effects of creatine supplementation on exercise performance," *Sports Medicine* 28 (1999): 49–60.

20. M. Greenwood, J. Farris, R. Kreider, L. Greenwood, and A. Byars, "Creatine supplementation patterns and perceived effects in select Division I collegiate athletes," *Clinical Journal of Sport Medicine: Official Journal of the Canadian Academy of Sport Medicine* 10 (2000): 191–94; Pecci and Lombardo, 949–60; Kraemer and Volek, 651–66; J. R. Poortmans and M. Francaux, "Adverse effects of creatine supplementation: Fact or fiction?" *Sports Medicine* 30 (2000): 155–70; and M. D. Silver, "Use of ergogenic aids by athletes," *Journal of the American Academy of Orthopedic Surgery* 9 (2001): 61–70.

21. Bolotte, 325–27; and Pecci and Lombardo, 949–60.

22. McGuine, Sullivan, and Bernhardt, 247–53.

23. Poortmans and Francaux, 155–70.

24. Haller and Benowitz, 1833–38; and Knochel, 513–15.

25. Bruno, Nolte, and Chapin, 1313–16.

26. Armstrong and Maresh, 302–12; Knochel, 513–15; Millard-Stafford, 223–33; and Savdie et al., 636–39.

27. Millard-Stafford, 223–33; and D. L. Costill, "Water and electrolyte requirements during exercise," *Clinical Journal of Sport Medicine: Official Journal of the Canadian Academy of Sport Medicine* 3 (1984): 639–48.

28. S. S. Jonnalagadda, C. A. Rosenbloom, and R. Skinner, "Dietary practices, attitudes, and physiological status of collegiate freshman football players." *Journal of Strength and Conditioning Research / National Strength & Conditioning Association* 15: 507–13.

29. Applegate and Grivetti, 869S–873S; Haller and Benowitz, 1833–38; and Bailes, Cantu, and Day, 283–86.

30. Bamberger, 58–61.

31. S. J. Massad, N. W. Shier, D. M. Koceja, and N. T. Ellis, "High school athletes and nutritional supplements: A study of knowledge and use," *International Journal of Sport Nutrition* 5 (1995): 232–45.

CHAPTER 10   BRAIN INJURY: SCIENCE WAGING WAR ON CONCUSSIONS

1. P. R. Yarnell and S. Lynch, "The 'ding': Amnestic states in football trauma," *Neurology* 23 (1973): 196–97.

2. J. T. Barth, S. N. Macciocchi, B. Giordani, R. Rimel, I. Jane, and T. Boll, "Neuropsychological sequelae of minor head injury," *Neurosurgery* 13 (1983): 529–33; D. Gronwall and P. Wrightson, "Time off work and symptoms after minor head injury," *Injury* 12 (1981): 445–54; and A. T. Tysvaer and E. A. Lochen, "Soccer injuries to the brain: A neuropsychological study of former soccer players," *American Journal of Sports Medicine* 19 (1991): 56–60.

3. Barth et al., 529–33.

4. Gronwall and Wrightson, 445–54; H. Hugenholtz, D. T. Stuss, L. L. Stethem, and M. T. Richard, "How long does it take to recover from a mild concussion?" *Neurosurgery* 22 (1988): 853–58; and H. Merskey and J. M. Woodforde, "Psychiatric sequelae of minor head injury," *Brain* 95 (1972): 521–28.

5. D. Gronwall and P. Wrightson, "Cumulative effects of concussion," *Lancet* 2 (1975): 995–97; M. W. Collins, S. H. Grindel, M. R. Lovell, D. E. Dede, D. J. Moser, B. R. Phalin, S. Nogle, M. Wasik, D. Cordry, M. K. Daugherty, S. F. Sears, G. Nicolette, P. Indelicato, and D. B. McKeag, "Relationship between concussion and neuropsychological performance in college football players," *Journal of the American Medical Association* 282 (1999): 964–70.

6. Gronwall and Wrightson, "Cumulative effects of concussion," 995–97; and K. M. Guskiewicz, M. McCrea, S. W. Marshall, et al., "Cumulative effects associated with recurrent concussion in collegiate football players: The NCAA Concussion Study," *Journal of the American Medical Association* 390, no. 19 (2003): 2549–555.

7. S. G. Gerberich, J. D. Priest, J. R. Boen, C. P. Straub, and R. E. Maxwell, "Concussion incidences and severity in secondary school varsity football players," *American Journal of Public Health* 73 (1983): 1370–75, 1983.

8. Collins et al., "Relationship between concussion and neuropsychological performance," 964–70.

9. Merril Hoge quoted here from J. Bailes, M. R. Lovell, and J. Maroon, eds.,

Sports-Related Concussion (St. Louis, MO: Quality Medical Publishers, 1999), 237.

10. Gerberich et al., "Concussion incidences," 1370–75.

11. Bailes, Lovell, and Maroon, eds., *Sports-Related Concussion*, 234.

12. I. Barth, W. Alves, T. Ryan, S. Macciocchi, R. Rimel, J. Jane, and W. Nelson, "Mild head injury in sports: Neuropsychological sequelae and recovery of function," in H. Levin, H. Eisenberg, and A. Benton, eds. *Mild Head Injury* (New York: Oxford Press, 1989), 257–75; and M. McCrea, J. P. Kelly, J. Kluge, B. Ackley, and C. Randolph, "Standardized assessment of concussion in football players," *Neurology* 48 (1997): 536–38.

13. J. W. Powell and K. D. Barber-Foss, "Traumatic brain injury in high school athletes," *JAMA* 282 (1999): 958–63.

14. Y. Tegner and R. Lorentzon, "Concussion among Swedish elite ice hockey players," *British Journal of Sports Medicine* 30 (1996): 251–55.

15. Tegner and Lorentzon, 251–55.

16. J. T. Matser, A. G. Kessels, M. D. Lezak, B. D. Jordan, J. Troost, "Neuropsychological impairment in amateur soccer players," *Journal of the American Medical Association* 282 (1999): 971–73.

17. B. C. Barnes, L. Cooper, D. T. Kirkendall, T. P. McDermott, B. D. Jordan, W. E. Garrett Jr., "Concussion history in elite male and female soccer players," *American Journal of Sports Medicine* 26 (1998): 433–38.

18. Mark Kelso quoted here from Bailes, Lovell, and Maroon, eds., *Sports-Related Concussion*, 234.

19. J. S. Delaney, V. J. Lacroix, S. Leclerc, and K. M. Johnston, "Concussions during the 1997 Canadian Football League season," *Clinical Journal of Sport Medicine: Official Journal of the Canadian Academy of Sport Medicine* 10 (2000): 9–14.

20. W. Langburt, B. Cohen, N. Akhthar, K. O'Neill, and J. Lee, "Incidence of concussion in high school football players of Ohio and Pennsylvania," *Journal of Child Neurology* 16, no. 2 (February 2001): 83–85; and J. S. Delaney, V. J. Lacroix, S. Leclerc, K. M. Johnston, "Concussion among university football players and soccer players," *Clinical Journal of Sport Medicine: Official Journal of the Canadian Academy of Sport Medicine* 12, no. 6 (November 2002): 331–38.

21. Centers for Disease Control and Prevention, "Injuries associated with soccer goalposts, United States, 1979–1993," *JAMA* 271 (1994): 1233–34.

22. Guskiewicz, McCrea, Marshall, et al., "Cumulative effects associated with recurrent concussion," 2549–55; and S. N. Macciocchi, J. T. Barth, W. Alves, R. W. Rimel, and J. A. Jane, "Neuropsychological functioning and recovery after mild head injury in college athletes," *Neurosurgery* 39 (1996): 510–14.

23. Barth, et al., "Neuropsychological sequelae," 529–33; L. M. Binder, "Persisting symptoms after mild head injury: A review of the post-concussive syndrome," *Journal of Clinical and Experimental Neuropsychology: Official Journal of the International Neuropsychological Society* 8 (1986): 323–46; and R. W. Rimel, M. A. Giordani, J. T. Barth, T. J. Boll, and J. A. Jane, "Disability caused by minor head injury," *Neurosurgery* 9 (1981): 221–28.

24. Bailes, Lovell, and Maroon, eds., *Sports-Related Concussion*.

25. Harry Carson quoted here from Bailes, Lovell, and Maroon, eds., *Sports-Related Concussion*, 244.

26. B. D. Jordan and J. E. Bailes, "Concussion history and current neurological symptoms among retired professional football players," presented at the 52nd Annual Meeting of the American Academy of Neurology, San Diego, California (May 6, 2000); and J. E. Bailes, *Neurology Reviews* 27 (June 2003).

27. Gronwall and Wrightson, "Cumulative effects of concussion," 995–97.

28. G. W. Roberts, D. Allsop, and C. Bruton, "The occult aftermath of boxing," *Journal of Neurology Neurosurgery and Psychiatry* 53 (1990): 373–78.

29. M. F. Mendez, "The neuropsychiatric aspects of boxing," *International Journal of Psychiatry* 25 (1995): 249–62.

30. A. H. Roberts, *Brain Damage in Boxers* (London: Pittman, 1969).

31. Y. Haglund and E. Eriksson, "Does amateur boxing lead to chronic brain damage? A review of some recent investigations," *American Journal of Sports Medicine* 21 (1993): 97–109; and M. Critchley, "Medical aspects of boxing, particularly from a neurological standpoint," *British Journal of Medicine* 1 (1957): 357–62.

32. B. D. Jordan, N. R. Relkin, L. D. Ravdin, A. R. Jacobs, A. Bennett, and S. Gandy, "Apolipoprotein E E4 associated with chronic traumatic brain injury in boxing," *JAMA* 278 (1997): 136–40.

33. Centers for Disease Control and Prevention, "Injuries associated with soccer goalposts," 1233–34.

34. G. M. Teasdale, J. A. R. Nicoll, G. Murray, and M. Fiddes, "Association of apolipoprotein E polymorphism with outcome after head injury," *Lancet* 350 (1997): 1069–71.

35. K. C. Kutner, D. M. Erlander, J. Tsai, B. Jordan, and N. R. Relkin, "Lower cognitive performance of older football players possessing Apolipoprotein E e4," *Neurosurgery* 47 (2000): 651–58.

36. J. T. Matser, A. G. Kessels, B. D. Jordan, M. D. Lezak, and J. Troost, "Chronic traumatic brain injury in professional soccer players," *Neurology* 51 (1998): 791–96.

37. O. Sortland and A. T. Tysvaer, "Brain damage in former association soccer players: An evaluation by cerebral computed tomography," *Neuroradiology* 31 (1989): 44–48.

38. R. C. Cantu, "Guidelines for return to contact sports after a cerebral concussion," *The Physician and Sportsmedicine* 14 (1986): 75–83; J. P. Kelly and J. H. Rosenberg, "Diagnosis and management of concussion in sports," *Neurology* 48 (1997): 575–80; and Report of the Sports Medicine Committee, *Guidelines for the Management of Concussion in Sports* (Denver, CO: Medical Society, 1991).

39. R. W. Rimel, M. A. Giordani, J. T. Barth, T. J. Boll, and J. A. Jane, "Disability caused by minor head injury," *Neurosurgery* 9 (1981): 221–28.

40. Kelly and Rosenberg, "Diagnosis and management," 575–80.

41. Rimel et al., "Disability caused by minor head injury," 221–28; and Kelly and Rosenberg, "Diagnosis and management," 575–80.

42. R. C. Cantu, "Second impact syndrome: A risk in any contact sport," *The Physician and Sportsmedicine* 23 (1995): 27–31.

43. J. T. Barth, R. Diamond, and A. Errico, "Mild head injury and post concussion syndrome: does anyone really suffer?" *Clinical EEG (electroencephalography)* 27 (1996): 183–86.

44. K. M. Guskiewicz, B. L. Riemann, D. H. Perrin, and L. M. Nashner, "Alternative approaches to the assessment of mild head injury in athletes," *Medicine and Science in Sports and Exercise* 29 (1997): 5213–21.

45. E. J. Pellman, J. W. Powell, D. C. Viano, I. R. Casson, A. M. Tucker, H. Feuer, M. Lovell, J. F. Waeckerle, and D. W. Robertson, "Concussion in professional football: epidemiological features of game injuries and review of the literature—part 3," *Neurosurgery* 54, no. 1 (January 2004): 81–94.

CHAPTER 11 CARING FOR YOUTH SPORTS: ARE WE OR NOT?

1. Dennis M. Docheff and James H. Conn, "It's no longer a spectator sport: Eight ways to get involved and help fight parental violence in youth sports," *Parks & Recreation* (March 1, 2004): 62.

2. Rick Wolff quoted here from Vicky Smith, "To Score or Not to Score: Toning Down Youth Sports," *Associated Press* (March 24, 2003).

3. Peter Cary, Randy Dotinga, and Avery Comarow, "Fixing Kids' Sports," *U.S. News & and World Report* (June 7, 2004): 44.

4. "Parents Want Programs to Focus Less on Winning," *Charlotte Observer* (August 24, 2003), 2A.

5. Barri Bronston, "Who'll Coach the Parents," *Times-Picayune (New Orleans, LA)* (November 4, 2002), Living section, page 1.

6. Scott Lancaster quoted here from Bronston, 1.

7. National Association of Sports Officials, www.naso.org/sportsmanship/badsports.html. (May 10, 2004).

8. Smith, "To Score or Not to Score."

9. Eleanor Sobel quoted here from Nick Sortal, "Bill Aims to Protect Sports Officials: Penalties for Assault Would Increase," *Sun-Sentinel (Fort Lauderdale, FL)* (February 14, 2004), 1B.

10. Carl Dubois, "When Do Parents Go Too Far," *Shreveport Times* (August 29, 1999), C1. Dubois' special report, "Building the Perfect Athlete," won the Louisiana Sports Writer's Association honor for best enterprise/investigative series in the state's highest newspaper classification. It was the first of four consecutive award-winning series during John McCloskey's tenure at the *Shreveport Times*, as assistant sports editor (1999) and sports editor (2000–2002).

11. Brian McCallum, "Parents Roles Vary on Tender Issues: Some Involved, Others Ignorant with Weight Training, Supplements," *Shreveport Times* (August 21, 2001), 1C.

12. Fred Engh quoted here from "Sports Overload? The Amount of Time and Money Families Spend on Sports is Soaring," *Time For Kids* (November 5, 1999), 4.

13. Mike Legarza quoted here from Bronston, 1.

14. Alan Tays, "Youth Leagues Losing Touch: The Decline of Sportsmanship," *Palm Beach Post* (December 24, 2002): 1C.

15. Cary et al., 44.

16. Greg Bach, "Youth Organizers Call Timeout!" *ASAP (National Recreation and Park Association)* (June 1, 2002), 60.

17. Cary et al., 44.

18. Barry Mano, telephone interview (May 7, 2004).

19. Cary et al., 44.

20. Martin Miller, "Painful sports lessons: Off the Field Pressures to Play Hard and to Win at all Costs Are Contributing to Young Athletes' Injuries," *Los Angeles Times* (May, 24, 2004), F7.

21. Len Remia quoted here from Nick Sortal, "A Call to Arms: Youth Sports Injuries Are on the Rise," *Sun-Sentinel (Fort Lauderdale, FL)* (February 8, 2004), 1D.

22. Sortal, 1D.

23. Sortal, 1D.

24. Elizabeth Simpson, "Young Athletes Face Rising Risk of Injury," *The Virginian-Pilot* (November 29, 2002), B1.

25. Miller, F7.

26. Carl Dubois, "Have Right Motivation for Sports," *Shreveport Times* (August 29, 1999), C1.

27. Jim Brown quoted here from Dubois, "Have Right Motivation," C1.

28. Mike McBath, telephone interview (May 28, 2004).

29. Miller, F7.

Sidebar 11.1   Top 10 Things Parents Don't Get About Kids and Sports

1. "Top 10 Things Parents Don't Get About Kids and Sports," *Sports Illustrated For Kids* (September 1996), 9.

Sidebar 11.2   Commentary: It's Inexcusable When a Youth Coach Breaks Rules, Our Trust

1. John McCloskey, "It's Inexcusable When a Youth Coach Breaks Rules, Our Trust," *Shreveport Times* (August 28, 2002), 1C.

CHAPTER 12   WINNING AT ALL COSTS: WHAT WE'RE DRIVEN TO DO AND WHY

1. Michael Josephson, telephone interview (June 2, 2004).

2. D. Stanley Eitzen, "Ethical Dilemmas in American Sports," Angelo State University 1995 Symposium on American Values, www.angelo.edu/events/university_symposium/1995/eitzen.htm (May 8, 2004).

3. Eitzen, "Ethical Dilemmas."

4. Eitzen, "Ethical Dilemmas."

5. Barry Mano, telephone interview (May 7, 2004).

6. Harry Edwards quoted here from Mark Emmons, "In Debate on Cheating, Even Sports Is Fair Game," *(San Jose) Mercury News,* www.mercurynews.com (June 27, 2004).

7. Jack Marshall quoted here from Emmons, "In Debate on Cheating."

8. Brenda Light Bredemeier quoted here from Robert Lipsyte, "Cheating Wends Way From Youth Sports to Business," *USA Today* (December 10, 2003), 23A.

9. Dr. Charles Yesalis, telephone interview (April 14, 2004).

10. Michael Josephson, telephone interview (June 2, 2004).

11. Becky Bartindale and Maya Suryaraman, "School Takes Action, but Pressure to Excel Remains," *(San Jose) Mercury News* (May 30, 2004), A1.

12. Hal Vogel quoted here from Kathleen Anderson, "Stewart Vow: I'll Be Back," *The Hollywood Reporter* (July 19, 2004).

13. Bartindale and Suryaraman, "School Takes Action," A1.

14. Brian McCallum, "Success Knows No Off-Season: Athletes Utilize Summer, Supplements to Build Strength and the Perfect Body," *Shreveport Times* (August 20, 2001), 1C.

15. McCallum, 1C.

16. McCallum, 1C.

17. Edd Wilbanks quoted here from Carl Dubois, "Have Right Motivation for Sports," *Shreveport Times* (August 29, 1999), 6C.

18. Dan Sileo quoted here from Michelle Kaufman, "Sports and the Fairer Sex," *Calgary Herald* (April 4, 2004), B4.

19. Jim Fitzpatrick quoted here from Kaufman, B4.

20. Tony Dorsett quoted here from "Glory Days: T.D. Always Had Fun in Big D," *Sporting News* (April 5, 2004), 8.

21. Rick Reilly, "Another Victim at Colorado," *Sports Illustrated* (February 23, 2004), 80.

22. "Timeline of events surrounding CU recruiting scandal," *Associated Press* (February 19, 2004), BC cycle.

23. Lynell Hamilton quoted here from "A National Issue: Colorado isn't the only school at which sex and recruiting have been linked in recent years," *Sports Illustrated* (February 23, 2004).

24. Malcolm Gillis quoted here from "A National Issue," *Sports Illustrated* (February 23, 2004), 67.

25. Chase McBride quoted here from Mike McGrane, "Santa Fe Christian soaring with section's elite," *San Diego Union-Tribune* (October 30, 2001), D1.

26. Martin Hickman quoted here from "Winning at All Costs in All 50 States," *Shreveport Times* (August 25, 2002), 6C.

27. "Winning at All Costs In All 50 States," 6C.

28. An investigation by the *Shreveport Times* revealed that five of the 35 players who played on Southwood's six state championship teams attended the school despite living in another district using the minority-to-majority transfer rule allowed by the Caddo school system. All five players were black, three of whom were members of the *Times'* All-City Basketball teams, including 1998 player of the year Krystal Jackson. The rule was implemented in 1981 following the consent decree, a court-ordered desegregation of schools. See Brian McCallum, "What Lies Beneath the Modern Dynasty: One Local School Fights Against Illegal Transfers," *Shreveport Times* (August 26, 2002), 1C.

29. Joey Hester, a parent of a football player at Evangel Christian Academy, a power at the state's largest classification despite an enrollment that matches that of one of the smallest classifications, said he tried to convince the son of the Caddo Parish Athletic Director to choose Evangel over Booker T. Washington, a predominantly black school. Hester admits he mentioned it to the player "every day. . . . I figured that was his best chance to play football in the future," Hester said. "I think there are schools that have athletes that are as good or better [than Evangel's] but they aren't getting the coaching. . . . When they say 'recruiting,' I've never seen [Evangel] coaches do it. Now dads, moms—yeah, they say to go to Evangel." The LHSAA prohibits the recruiting of high school athletes by coaches, other school employees, or active boosters. Most local coaches believe recruiting does go on in the area, whether by coaches or others working behind the scenes. Joey Hester quoted here from Brian McCallum, "Caddo Athletic Director: My Son Was Recruited," *Shreveport Times* (August 26, 2002), 1C.

30. Tommy Henry quoted here from McCallum, 1C.

31. Jim Page quoted here from Jason Pugh, "Winning At All Costs Has International Reach," *Shreveport Times* (August 27, 2002), 1C.

32. Mike Green quoted here from Brian McCallum, "Are Salary Bonuses an Incentive to Cheat? Caddo Will Reward Coaches for Winning," *Shreveport Times* (August 26, 2002), 6C.

33. Val McGyvers quoted here from McCallum, "Are Salary Bonuses an Incentive," 6C.

34. Leon Barmore quoted here from Jimmy Watson, "NCAA Concerned With Travel Issues," *Shreveport Times* (August 27, 2002), 5C.

35. Marco Cole quoted here from Jimmy Watson, "NCAA Concerned With Travel Issues," *Shreveport Times* (August 28, 2002), 5C.

36. Jane Jankowski quoted here from Watson, 5C.

Sidebar 12.1 Commentary: Winning At All Costs Is a Big Loss in Game of Life

1. James D. Nickel lives in Shreveport. This editorial originally ran in the *Shreveport Times* on September 1, 2002, the Sunday after the *Times*' "Winning at all Costs" series began.

Sidebar 12.2 A Senior Season Lost at a Burger King

1. Brian McCallum, "Ruling Costs Harris His Senior Season," *Shreveport Times* (August 25, 2002), 1A.

CHAPTER 13 RECURRENT UNEXPLAINED DEATHS IN SPORTS

1. G. I. Wadler and B. Hainline, *Drugs and the Athlete* (Philadelphia, PA: F. A. Davis Co., 1989).

2. J. Hoberman, *Mortal Engines* (New York, NY: Free Press, 1992).

3. Hoberman, *Mortal Engines*.

4. A. Sands and E. Poole, "Wrestling champ British Bulldog dies," *Ottawa*

Citizen (May 20, 2002); J. E. Bailes, R. C. Cantu, and A. L. Day, "The neurosurgeon in sport: awareness of the risks of heatstroke and dietary supplements," *Neurosurgery* 51, no. 2 (2002): 283–86; "Ephedra use under fire," *Physician and Sportsmedicine* 31 (2003): 13–15; and "Soccer Italy deaths," *Time* (May 5, 2003).

5. B. Goldman, *Death in the Locker Room: Steroids, Cocaine and Sports* (Berkley, CA, and Tucson, AZ: The Body Press, 1987).

6. L. Pugmire, "Ultimate takedown: For some wrestlers, the pressure to perform exacts a toll," *Los Angeles Times* (March 29, 2003); and "Roids wrestling deaths," *Los Angeles Times* (March 29, 2003).

7. J. Swartz, "High death rate lingers behind fun facade of pro wrestling," *USA Today* (March 12, 2004). http://www.usatoday.com/sports/2004-03-12-pro-wrestling_x.htm (accessed December 7, 2004).

8. Pugmire, "Ultimate takedown."

9. M. Fish, "Florence Griffith Joyner dies," *Atlanta Journal and Constitution* (September 22, 1998).

10. E. Tomiuc, "World: Doping-performance-enhancing drugs a threat to health and ethics," Radio Free Europe/Radio Liberty (March 26, 2004).

11. "Cyclist admits drug use," *Agence France Presse* (April 6, 2004).

12. Bailes, Cantu, and Day, 283–86.

13. "Ephedra use under fire," 13–15.

14. Hoberman, *Mortal Engines*.

CHAPTER 14   WHO'S IN CHARGE? ADMINISTRATION IS PART OF THE PROBLEM

1. John Calvin quoted here from "The Fifth Commandment," Providence Baptist Ministries www.pbministries.org/books/pink/Commandments/command _05.htm (accessed July 17, 2004).

2. L. Jon. Wertheim, "Good Job. You're Fired: Even Highly Successful Coaches Have Learned That Winning Doesn't Guarantee Security," *Sports Illustrated* (May 3, 2004), 54.

3. George Karl quoted here from Wertheim, 54.

4. Ron Wilson quoted here from Wertheim, 54.

5. Dave Odom quoted here from Wertheim, 54.

6. Rick Wolff, *Coaching Kids for Dummies* (Foster City, CA: IDG, 2000); *Good Sports: A Concerned Parent's Guide to Little League and Other Competitive Youth Sports* (New York: Dell, 1993); and "Parents' Guide To Youth Sports," *Sports Illustrated* (2004), bimonthly.

7. Rick Wolff's "Parents' Guide To Youth Sports," sponsored by Chrysler Plymouth, was "one of the most successful advertorial campaigns *Sports Illustrated* has ever run," according to www.sportsparenting.com, (accessed June 1, 2004).

8. Mike Finger, "Hardly Class Acts: Academic Fraud Runs Rampant at Major Universities," *San Antonio Express-News* (September 21, 2003), 1C.

9. Welch Suggs, "NCAA Chief Picks His Battles," *Chronicle of Higher Education* (January 16, 2004), 37.

10. Finger, 1C.

11. Leonard Hamilton quoted here from Michelle Kaufman, "Who's in Charge Here?" *Miami Herald* (October 19, 2003), D1.

12. Mike Krzyzewski quoted here from Kaufman, D1.

13. Tom Izzo quoted here from Drew Sharp, "Basketball Coaches Summit a Farce," *Detroit Free Press* (October 16, 2003), Sports.

14. Tony Barnhart, "Harrick Probe: Cheating Coaches Put Fate in Hands of Kids," *Atlanta Journal-Constitution* (March 1, 2003), 1F.

15. Linda Bensel-Meyers quoted here from Finger, 1C.

16. Terry Holland, e-mail interview (August 8, 2004).

17. Holland interview (August 8, 2004).

18. James Duderstadt quoted here from Michelle Kaufman, "Sports and the Fairer Sex," *Calgary Herald* (April 4, 2004), B4.

19. John DiBiaggio quoted here from Jim Hughes and Chuck Plunkett, "Colo. Athletics Dept. Recruiting Scandal Has Already Resulted in Changes," *Denver Post* (May 7, 2004).

20. Terry Holland quoted here from David Teel, "Terry The Crusader; Holland Says College Athletics Need Major Reforms," *(Newport News, Va.) Daily Press* (February 8, 2004), C1.

21. William C. Friday quoted here from Welch Suggs, "When the President Is Part of the Problem," *Chronicle of Higher Education* (March 28, 2003), 34.

22. Michael F. Adams quoted here from Suggs, "When the President Is Part of the Problem," 34.

23. Suggs, "When the President Is Part of the Problem," 34.

24. Robert J. Wickenheiser quoted here from Suggs, "When the President Is Part of the Problem," 34.

25. Christopher White quoted here from Welch Suggs, "Gardner-Webb President, Enmeshed in Sports Scandal, Resigns," *Chronicle of Higher Education* (October 25, 2002), 41.

26. Terry Holland quoted here from David Teel, "Terry The Crusader; Holland Says College Athletics Need Major Reforms," *(Newport News, Va.) Daily Press* (February 8, 2004), C1.

27. Johnny Bench quoted here from Barry Lorge, "The Pressure Is on to 'Pop'; To Some the Ideal Is 'Higher, Higher,'" *Washington Post* (May 28, 1979), D1.

CHAPTER 15   STRUGGLE FOR SPORTSMANSHIP: THROUGH A REF'S EAGLE EYES: Q&A WITH BARRY MANO

1. Barry Mano, telephone interview (May 7, 2004).

CHAPTER 16   SOLUTIONS: WINNING WITHOUT LOSING PERSPECTIVE

1. J. E. Bailes, R. C. Cantu, and A. L. Day, "The Neurosurgeon in Sport: Awareness of the Risks of Heatstroke and Dietary Supplements," *Neurosurgery* 51, no. 2 (2002): 283–86.

2. "Heat Illness Prevention Goes High Tech," *Physician Sports Medicine* 31 (2003): 2–7.

3. Leslie Bonci quoted here from Carl Dubois, "Area Teenagers Use Creatine to Gain Edge in Competition," *Shreveport Times* (August 29, 1999), 3C.

4. Julie Hartley quoted here from Carl Dubois, "Popular supplements may harm youngsters," *Shreveport Times* (August 29, 1999), C1.

5. John Leavens, telephone interview (May 5, 2004).

6. Michael Josephson, telephone interview (June 2, 2004). A complete list of Character Counts delegates can be found at charactercounts.org. The 16-page "Gold Medal Standards" can be found at www.charactercounts.org/pdf/Gold MedalStandards-YouthSports-050202.pdf.

7. Elizabeth Simpson, "Young Athletes Face Rising Risk of Injury," *The Virginian-Pilot* (November 29, 2002), B1.

8. Simpson, B1.

9. Nick Sortal, "A Call to Arms: Youth Sports Injuries Are on the Rise," *Sun-Sentinel (Fort Lauderdale, FL)* (February 8, 2004), 1D.

10. Barri Bronston, "Who'll Coach the Parents," *Times-Picayune (New Orleans, LA)* (November 4, 2002), Living section, p. 1.

11. Bronston, 1.

12. Bronston, 1.

13. Amy Dickinson, "It's Only a Game!: How can parents encourage a kid to love sports and be a good sport too? Step 1: stop yelling," *Time* (May 24, 1999), 96.

14. Robert Reynolds and Bob Carter quoted here from Brian Vernellis, "Anger Diminishes in Youth Sports," *Shreveport Times* (August 28, 2002), 5C.

15. Don Fradley quoted here from Vernellis, 5C.

16. John Kernaghan, "Sports Offer Many Pluses; Good Coaches and Parents Can Have Positive Influences on Kids' Sports," *Hamilton Spectator* (August 23, 2001), CK6.

17. Chris Hirsch quoted here from Brian Vernellis, "Matching Kids, Sports Crucial: Parents Should Do Research Before Signing Up Children," *Shreveport Times* (July 14, 2002), 1C.

18. Vernellis, "Matching Kids, Sports Crucial," 1C.

19. Bill Cushing quoted here from Robert Lipsyte, "Cheating Wends Way From Youth Sports to Business," *USA Today* (December 10, 2003), 23A.

20. Kernaghan, CK6.

21. "Sports Overload? The Amount of Time and Money Families Spend on Sports is Soaring," *Time For Kids* (November 5, 1999), 4.

22. Kernaghan, CK6.

23. Bruce B. Svare, "Bad Sports: Public School Athletics Programs Serve the Few at the Expense of the Many," *The Times Union (Albany, NY)* (June 6, 2004), B1.

24. D. L. Shields and B. J. Bredemeier, *Character Development and Physical Activity* (Champaign, IL: Human Kinetics, 1995).

25. B. J. Bredemeier, M. R. Weiss, D. L. Shields, and R. M. Shewchuck, "Promoting Moral Growth in a Summer Sport Camp: The Implementation of Theoretically Grounded Instructional Strategies," *Journal of Moral Education* (1986): 212–20.

26. Lori Gano-Overway, "Emphasizing Sportsmanship in Youth Sports," *Education World*, www.education-world.com/a_curr/curr137.shtml (accessed May 7, 2004).

27. Fred Engh quoted here from Vicki Smith, "To Score or Not to Score? Toning Down Youth Sports," *Associated Press* (March 30, 2003), BC cycle.

28. See Josephson Institute of Ethics mission statement at www.character counts.org/pdf/about/FactSheet-JI-0903.pdf.

29. Josephson interview (June 2, 2004).

30. Harvey Dulberg quoted here from Sam Dunn, "Winning by losing," *Men's Fitness* (August 1998).

31. Myles Brand quoted here from Michael Marot, "NCAA approves tighter recruiting rules," *Associated Press* (August 5, 2004), BC cycle.

32. Independent Investigative Commission, "Report: UC Officials Failed to Oversee Athletics," *Associated Press* (May 18, 2004), BC cycle.

33. Don Markus, "NCAA Board Likely to Approve Package of Academic Reforms," *Baltimore Sun* (April 29, 2004), 2E.

34. Markus, 2E.

35. Pete DiPrimio, "Coaches Shrug Off the Salaries, Signage," *Fort Wayne News Sentinel* (July 22, 2004).

36. Myles Brand quoted here from Welch Suggs, "NCAA Chief Picks His Battles," *Chronicle of Higher Education* (January 16, 2004), 37.

37. Brock Stratton quoted here from Mike Finger, "Hardly Class Acts: Academic Fraud Runs Rampant at Major Universities," *San Antonio Express-News* (September 21, 2003), 1C.

38. Bruce Svare quoted here from Steve Wilstein, "Fixes On Way, More Needed After Latest College Scandals," *The Associated Press* (May 9, 2004), BC cycle.

39. Svare, B1.

40. Frank Uryasz, telephone interview (April 1, 2004).

Sidebar 16.1   Tips for Coaches, Parents, and Players

1. Scott Lancaster, "The 7 Guiding Principles of NFL Youth Programs," www.nflyouthfootball.com/exec/NFLYP/7principles.cfm?publicationID = 219 (accessed April 29, 2004).

2. Dr. Darrell J. Barnett, "Sideline Suggestions: 10 Things Kids Say They Don't Want Their Parents To Do." Provided via e-mail by Dr. Barnett (December 9, 2004). Dr. Burnett is a clinical psychologist and a certified sports psychologist specializing in youth sports. He has been in private practice for 20-plus years in Laguna Niguel, California. His book, *It's Just a Game! Youth, Sports, & Self Esteem: A Guide for Parents*, is described on his Web site, www.djburnett.com, along with his other books, booklets, and audio cassettes on youth sports and family life.

3. Carl Dubois, "When Do Parents Go Too Far," *Shreveport Times* (August 29, 1999), C1.

4. Dr. Darrell J. Barnett, "Being a Good Sport," Soccerclinics.com, www.soccerclinics.com/IPAGameDay.htm (accessed December 9, 2004).

Sidebar 16.2   Teaching Sportsmanship Tips

1. Brooke de Lench and Shane Murphy, "Five Ways For Sport Parents To Set A Good Example," MomsTeam.com, www.momsteam.com/alpha/features/cheersandtears/five-ways.shtml (accessed December 9, 2004).

Sidebar 16.3   Ethics of Competitive Education Should Be Mandatory in All Schools

1. Rudyard Kipling, "If," www.swarthmore.edu/~apreset1/docs/if.html (accessed December 9, 2004).

Sidebar 16.4   Q&A with Terry Holland

1. Terry Holland is former University of Virginia basketball coach and athletic director. This text is quoted here from an e-mail interview (August 4, 2004).

CHAPTER 17   MORE SOLUTIONS: ATHLETES DOING THE RIGHT THING

1. Mike Hall, telephone interview (May 15, 2004).
2. John Godina, telephone interview (July 24, 2004).
3. Tara Cunningham, e-mail interview (July 27, 2004).
4. Alison Dunlap, e-mail interview (July 27, 2004).
5. Steve Holman, e-mail interview (August 2, 2004).
6. Kenta Bell, telephone interview (July 23, 2004).
7. Roddy Piper, telephone interview (July 12, 2004).

Index

Aaron, Hank, 60, 70
abortion, teens and, 28
Abrams, Doug, 181
abstinence, 30
academic fraud, 3, 201–6, 236–37, 241; coaches and, 230–31
academic requirements, 279
acceleration-deceleration injury, 143
acromegaly, 90
active fluid replacement, 149
Adams, Michael F., 239
administration, 227–41
adults, recommendations for, 265–66
age, versus preparedness for competition, 194
Ah You, C. J., 210
Aikman, Troy, 164
alcohol use, 16
Aldactone, 66
Allen, George, 42, 46
Allen, James, 210
all-terrain vehicles: and injuries, 141; preventive measures for, 255
ALS (amyotrophic lateral sclerosis), 46
Alzheimer's disease, cumulative injury and, 166
amantadine, 94
amateur athletic federations, drug policies of, 75
American Academy of Neurology, 168
Amies-Winter, Joanne, 57
Ammouri, Wafa, 77
amphetamines, 82; characteristics of, 93–94; with ephedrine, 152

amyotrophic lateral sclerosis (ALS), 46
Anabolic Steroid Control Act, 88, 104, 124, 128
anabolic steroids: mechanism of action of, 85–86; medical indications for, 84; side effects of, 86; testing for, 99–100. See also steroids
anabolism, 84
Anadrol. See oxymetholone
Anderson, Brady, 73
Anderson, Greg, 60–62, 66–68, 297n6
Anderson, Walter, 276
Andro. See androstenedione
androgens, 83–84
androstene. See androstenedione
androstenedione, 14–15, 49, 104–6; ban on, 2, 55–56, 122–23; Mc-Gwire and, 50
androsterone, 83–84
Annus, Adrian, 77
anterior cruciate ligament tears, 191–92, 265
Anti-Drug Abuse Act, 88
arginine, 71
aristolochic acid, 123
Armstrong, Gary, 48
Arnold, Ben, 55
Asarum canadense, 123
Asian Games, 51
ass ear, 123
Astaphan, Jamie, 302n4
asthma weed, 123
ATHENA program. See Athletes Targeting Healthy Exercise and Nutrition Alternatives program

Athlete Ambassador program, 129
athletes: Mano on, 249–50; and prob-
    lems in sports, 37–57; recommen-
    dations for, 261–62; as role models,
    31–33, 53–56, 287–93; and solu-
    tions for sports, 287–96; and ste-
    roid use, 37–38
Athletes Targeting Healthy Exercise
    and Nutrition Alternatives
    (ATHENA) program, 20, 112, 114
Athletes Training and Learning to
    Avoid Steroids (ATLAS) program,
    20, 33, 111–15; curriculum con-
    tent, 113
authority figures: abuses by, 3; chal-
    lenges to, 227–28; recommenda-
    tions for, 133–36. See also coaches;
    parents
Autin, Eraste, 74, 107
Auverbuch, Gloria, 262
ava/awa. See kava

Bailes, Julian, 74
Baker, Dusty, 228
BALCO. See Bay Area Laboratory Co-
    Operative scandal
Banham, Charles, 199
banned substances: lists of, 122–24;
    Merode on, 50; Samaranch on, 49,
    79
Barkley, Charles, 21, 30–31, 37
Barmore, Leon, 220
Barnes, Randy, 49
Barnett, Gary, 208–9, 239
Barrett, Stephen, 108
Bay Area Laboratory Co-Operative
    (BALCO) scandal, 1, 13, 59–79,
    95, 297n6; and decline in achieve-
    ments, 65–68; timeline of, 60–66
Bechler, Steve, 74, 107, 225, 312n8
Bell, Kenta, 258, 292–93
Belle, Albert, 55
Beller, Jennifer, 199

Benard, Marvin, 60
Bench, Johnny, 241
Bennett, William J., 29
Bensel-Mayers, Linda, 236–37
Benton, Shannon, 210
Benzoylecgonine, 49
Berendonk, Brigitte, 10–11
Berman, Howard, 124
Bernard, Marvin, 297n6
Berthold, A. A., 83
beta-2 agonists, 88–89, 97
Biden, Joseph R., 124, 128
Binus, Dieter, 297n8
birthwort, 123
bishop's tea. See ephedrine
bitter orange, 123
black root/wort, 123
bladderpod, 123
Bliss, Dave, 230
blood doping, 91–92
blood tests, 98
blue pimpernel, 124
boldenone undecylenate, 87
Bonci, Leslie, 258
Bonds, Barry, 59–60, 62, 65, 297n6;
    case against, 66–70; nutrition regi-
    men of, 71–72
books, on youth sports and sports-
    manship, 262
Boozer, Carl, Sr., 231
Bosworth, Brian, 47–48
Bowers, Randy, 183–84
boxing: brain injuries in, 143, 166; in-
    juries in, 142; preventive measures
    for, 256
brain injury, 142–43, 157–75; bio-
    mechanics of, 143–45; cumulative,
    164–67; diffuse, 169
Brand, Myles, 278–79, 281–82
Brathwaite, Reynaldo, 210
Bredemeier, Brenda Light, 200
Breithaupt, Charles, 17
Brennan, Christine, 181

Bromantan, 94
Brown, Dale, 236
Brown, Eric, 2
Brown, Jim, 193
bruisewort, 123
Buchanan, Ray, 52
Buncker, L. K., 262
Bundrick, William S., 193
Burman, George, 42–43
Burnett, Darrell J., 260–62, 326n2
Bush, George W., 62, 75, 78, 124
Bush, Lew, 52

caffeine, 81, 94–95, 153
Callahan, David, 199–200
Caminiti, Ken, 72–73
Cantu classification, 168
Capel, John, 78
cardiopulmonary resuscitation (CPR):
    and spinal injury, 146; and sudden
    death, 138
caring, 32
Carlisle, Rick, 228
Carmichael, David, 271
Carson, Harry, 161, 165
Carter, Bob, 267–68
CASPER. *See* Coalition for Anabolic
    Steroid Precursor and Ephedra Reg-
    ulation
Catlin, Don, 61
cavum septum pellucidum, 166
Cecchini, Glenn, 109–10
Center for Sports Parenting, 229
Center for Study of Retired Athletes,
    165
Center for Substance Abuse Preven-
    tion, 114
Cesbron. *See* clenbuterol
Chaikin, Thomas, 12
Chambers, Dwain, 12, 61
Champion Nutrition, 105
Chan, K. M., 262
Chanu, Sanamacha, 76

chaparral, 123
character: ATLAS program and, 115;
    Josephson on, 25, 32, 268
Chauvin, Mac, 213, 216
cheating: coaches and, 187–88; versus
    strategy, 198. *See also* academic
    fraud
Chemox, 152
children. *See* youth
China, 12, 48–49
chi powder. *See* ephedrine
Chislean, Victor, 77
chondroitin sulfate, 72
Christian schools, 3, 25, 210–11
chromium, 71
Ciba Pharmaceuticals, 11, 84
citizenship, 32
Citizenship Through Sports Alliance
    (CTSA), 24, 259
Citrus aurantium, 123
Clarett, Maurice, 232
Cleaves, Mateen, 209, 238
clenbuterol, 76, 89, 99
clomiphene, 87
coaches: abuses by, 3; bonuses for,
    219–20; and cheating, 187–88; and
    denial of problem, 17–18, 42,
    234–35; lack of respect for,
    228–29; Mano on, 249; Nicklaus
    on, 23–24; and problems in sports,
    182–96, 229–30; recommendations
    for, 133–36, 260; salaries for, 229,
    281; and solutions in sports,
    115–17; and steroid use, 18–20;
    and supplement use, 109–10; and
    violence, 179
Coalition for Anabolic Steroid Precur-
    sor and Ephedra Regulation (CAS-
    PER), 125, 129
cocaine, 16, 57, 82
Cole, L. C., 209
Cole, Marco, 220
Cole, Tony, 235

collaboration, for solutions, 259, 264

collegiate sports, solutions in, 276–84

Collins, Michelle, 63–65

Collins, Rick, 106

collision sports, definition of, 158

Colorado guidelines, 168

Colorado scale, 168

colostrum, 71–72

comfrey, 123

commotio cordis, 139

competition: versus cheating, 204; and doping, 82; ethics of, education on, 273–74

concussion, 2, 157–75; classification of, 167–69; evolution of knowledge about, 158–63; ignoring, 190–91; incidence of, 161–63; management of, 173; signs and symptoms of, 169; tests for, 171–74. See also mild traumatic brain injury

Condin, Timothy, 115

conditioning, 257–58

Conseco, Jose, 73

Consolidae radix, 123

consound, 123

contact sports, definition of, 158

Conte, Victor, 61, 63–64, 68, 71, 297n6

control: of emotion, losing, 188–90; lack of, 237–38

Controlled Substances Act, 15, 88

Conyers, John, 124, 127–28

Cook, D., 262

Cooper, Chris, 298n18

Copenhagen Declaration on Anti-Doping in Sport, 78

copper, 71

Courson, Steve, 44–45, 134

CPR. See cardiopulmonary resuscitation

Crable, Bob, 212

Crawford, Darren, 48

creatine, 71, 103, 153–55, 258; personal accounts of, 309n19

creosote bush, 123

CTSA. See Citizenship Through Sports Alliance

Cunningham, Tara, 290–91

Cushing, Bill, 270

cutting phase, 87

cycles, 86–87

cycling, 11–12, 49–50; deaths in, 223–24; injuries in, 140

Daniels, Ann Michelle, 268

Davis, Susan, 127

DEA. See Drug Enforcement Administration

Dean, Bud, 217–18

deaths of athletes, 1–2, 11, 221–26; from heatstroke, 151–56; mysterious, 46; prevention of, 254–55; sudden, 138–39

Deca-durabolin. See nandrolone

dehydration, 149; and death, 224; mechanisms of, 155

de la Hoya, Oscar, 52

de Lench, Brooke, 269

dementia pugilistica, 166

denial of drug problems, 17–18; Allen and, 42; coaches and, 234–35

Dennehy, Patrick, 230

Department of Education, Safe and Drug Free Schools Program, 114

Depo-testosterone, 66

depression: in children, 28; concussions and, 2; steroid use and, 88, 304n43

designer drugs, 81–101; future, 96

deterrence, Uryasz on, 119

dextrose, 71

d-glucosamine sulfate, 72

DHT (dihydrotestosterone), 100

Dianabol. See methandrostenolone

DiBiaggio, John, 239

Dietary Supplements Health and Education Act, 151–52, 312n7

diffuse brain injury, 169
dihydrotestosterone (DHT), 100
DiIulio, John J., Jr., 29
dinged state, 157–58
dinitrophenol, 152
DiNubile, Nicholas, 19, 54–55
diuretics, 92–93. *See also* masking
   agents
diving: preventive measures for,
   255–56; spinal injury in, 146–47
Dokovic, Dejan, 211
dop, 81
doping: prevention of, 121–22; term,
   81–82
Dorgan, Byron, 127
Dorsett, Tony, 208
downhill skiing, injuries in, 140
Dressel, Birgit, 222
Drug Enforcement Administration
   (DEA), 88
drug policies: MLB, 70–72; recommendations for, 133
drug testing, 37–38, 96–101; criticism
   of, 39; effects of, 112; history of,
   85; issues in, 100–101; MLB and,
   44; NFL and, 41–45, 48, 85; rec-
   ommendations for, 135; Uryasz on,
   118
Dubois, Carl, 192–93
Duderstadt, James, 210, 238
Duhon, Chris, 231
Dulberg, Harvey, 276
Dungy, Tony, 228
Dunlap, Alison, 291
Durbin, Dick, 127–28
Dyazide, 66
Dye, Pat, 236
Dykes, Hart Lee, 236

Earl, Lester, 236
East Germany, 10–11, 86, 297n8
education: on cheating, 206; deficien-
   cies in, 7–8; effectiveness of, 73; on

ethics, 273–74; Piper on, 296; recommendations for, 116, 265–66;
   on sportsmanship, 269; Uryasz on,
   118–19; USADA and, 125; on winning, 276
Edwards, Harry, 200
Edwards, Torri, 77
Eitzen, D. Stanley, 198–99
EKG. *See* electrocardiogram
Ekimov, Vyacheslav, 78
electrocardiogram (EKG), 139, 166
Elliott, Diane, 111
emetic herb, 123
emotion, losing control of, 188–90
Engh, Fred, 186, 275
ephedra (*Ephedra equisetina*), 52, 74,
   94, 107; and heatstroke, 152–53
ephedra products, 312n8
ephedrine, 52, 54, 94; ban on, 2, 122;
   and death, 225; and heatstroke,
   152–53
EPO. *See* erythropoietin
equestrian sports: concussion in, 162;
   injuries in, 139–40
Equipoise, 87
erythropoietin (EPO), 12, 49, 91, 97;
   and death, 224
Escande, Jean Paul, 223–24
estrogen, 83
ethics, education on, 273–74
ethics in sports, 5, 25, 197–201; social
   value of, 66
Etzel, Ed, 108
Eustachy, Larry, 230
Eveland, Roland, 17
Evens, Jessie, 231
Exum, Wade, 39, 135

faculty groups, Holland on, 282
fairness, 32
Fazekas, Robert, 76
FDA. *See* Food and Drug Administration

Federal Food, Drug, and Cosmetic Act (FFDCA), 88
Federal International Football Association, 162
La Fédération Internationale de Natation (FINA), 12, 49
Feher, Miklos, 224
Fehr, Donald, 65
female athletes: anabolic steroids and, 86; ATHENA program for, 20, 112, 114; benefits for, 271; and pregnancy doping, 92
Fernstrom, Madelyn H., 105
FFDCA. See Federal Food, Drug, and Cosmetic Act
FINA. See Fédération Internationale de Natation, La
financial motives: and academic fraud, 236–38; and steroid use, 55, 294–95; and supplement use, 103–10
Fitzpatrick, Jim, 208
Fleck, S. J., 262
Flowers, Lee, 52
Foe, Marc-Vivien, 224
folic acid, 72
Fonseca, Mabel, 76
Food and Drug Administration (FDA), 61, 107
football: brain injuries in, 143; concussion in, 159, 161; heatstroke in, 149; injuries in, 141–42; spinal injury in, 146; steroid use in, 14, 84–85
Forman, Peter, 128
Foster, Todd, 215
Fradley, Don, 268
Francis, Charlie, 63
Franke, Werner, 10–11
Friday, William C., 239
Frischke, Volker, 297n8
fun, youth and, 186, 190, 261
furosemide, 76

gagroot, 123
Gaines, Chryste, 13, 63, 65, 305n6
Galkin, Anton, 76
Gano-Overway, Lori, 274–75
gea/gi. See kava
gene doping, 37, 96
Gent, Pete, 43
German Democratic Republic, 10–11, 86, 297n8
germander, 123
gestrinone, 12, 95
GHRH. See growth hormone-releasing hormone
Giambi, Jason, 59–60, 62, 65, 297n6
Gierke, Bill, 211
Gillis, Malcolm, 210
Gilman, Benjamin J., 128
Glaeser, Rolf, 297n8
Glover, Sandra, 13
glucocorticoids, 85
glutamine peptides, 71–72
glycogen, 87
Gobel, Bob, 17
Godina, John, 206, 290
Goldberg, Linn, 32–33, 111–12, 115, 122, 286
Goldstein, Mark, 271
Gould, D., 262
government: Josephson on, 285; Mano on, 351
Graham, DeMingo, 52
Graham, Trevor, 61, 63–64
greasewood, 123
Green, Mike, 219–20
Greenies, 94
green orange, 123
Grout, Jack, 23
growth hormone-releasing hormone (GHRH), 90
Guariniello, Raffaele, 46
gum plant, 123
Gyurkovics, Ferenc, 76

Haborak, Milan, 77
Hahn, Billy, 232
Hainline, B., 221
Hall, Mike, 287–90
Hamilton, Leonard, 234
Hamilton, Lynell, 209
Hamilton, Tyler, 78
Hammond, Michael, 262
Hanlon, T., 262
Harrick, Jim, 230, 239–40
Harrick, Jim, Jr., 230, 235
Harris, Carl, 215–19
Harris, Carlos, 215–19
Harris, Gloria, 217–18
Harris, Judith Rich, 33
Harrison, Alvin, 13, 63, 65–66
Harrison, Calvin, 13, 64–66
Hartley, Julie, 258
Haskins, Clem, 230
Hatch, Orrin, 124, 128, 312n7
heading, 143
head injury. See brain injury
healing herb, 123
health, of youth, recommendations for, 264–65
heat cramps, 150
heat exhaustion, 150–51
heatstroke, 74, 149–56; and death, 224; deaths from, causes of, 151–56; definition of, 151; mechanism of, 150–51; prevention of, 254–55; signs of, 155; trends in, 149–50
Hedeoma pulegioides, 123
hedionilla, 123
helmet flower, 124
helmet standards, 161, 257
hemoglobin, 91
Henry, Tommy, 213, 216–17
heroin, 57
Hester, Joey, 322n29
HGC. See human chorionic gonadotropin

HGH. See human growth hormone
Hickman, Martin, 211
high school sports: drug use in, 14; recruiting in, 210–13; Uryasz on, 119–20
Hirsch, Chris, 270
Hnida, Katie, 208
Hoberman, John, 47, 225
Hoffman, Betsy, 278
Hoffman, Bob, 8
Hoge, Merril, 160–61, 164
Holland, Terry, 237–39, 241, 280–83
Holloway, Seth, 207
Holman, Steve, 291–92
Holway, John, 70
hoodwort, 124
Höppner, Manfred, 11
hormones, tests for, 99
Horn, Joe, 247
Howell, Ronnie, 217–18
Hsieh, Shanje, 205
5-HTP, 72
Huffman, Joe, 218
Hughes, Bill, 128
human chorionic gonadotropin (HCG), 87
human growth hormone (HGH), 12, 37, 48, 89–91
Humphries, Stan, 165
Hunter, C. J., 63–64
Hunter, Javin, 52
hydration, 149
hypertrophic cardiomyopathy, 138

ice hockey: brain injuries in, 143; concussion in, 162; injuries in, 142
indian tobacco, 123
individualism, and problems in sports, 53
injuries in sports, 137–48; ignoring, 190–93; mechanisms and incidence of, 139–42; mind-set on, 162–63;

prevention of, 157–75; stigma of, 161
in-line skating, injuries in, 140
insulin, 86–87
Internal Revenue Service, 61
International Association of Athletics Federations, 13
International Olympic Committee (IOC), 124; and drug testing, 85, 97–98
intoxicating pepper. *See* kava
iron, 71
Issakenko, Angela, 302n4
Izzo, Tom, 234–35

Jackson, Krystal, 321n28
Jackson, Reggie, 70
Jacobs, Regina, 65, 298n18
Jadwin, Tom, 48
Jankowski, Jane, 220
jarilla, 123
Jekot, Walter, 47
Jelks, Gene, 235–36
Jensen, Knut, 94
Jeter, L. B., 103
johimbi. *See* yohimbe
Johnson, Ben, 11–12, 49–50, 97, 302n4
Johnson, Michael, 13
Jones, Marion, 63–65
Jordan, John, 212–13
Josephson, Michael: on athletes, 32; on collaboration, 264; on education, 275–76; on ethics, 197–98, 201; on government, 285; on parental influence, 22; on solutions, 34
Josephson Institute for Ethics, 197, 264, 268–69, 275
Joyner, Florence Griffith, 223
judges, abuses by, 3
juicing, term, 86

Kalinski, Michael, 8
kao. *See* kava
Karl, George, 228–29
kava, 106, 123
kavain. *See* kava
kawa-pfeffer. *See* kava
Kecskes, Zoltan, 77
Kelso, Mark, 162–63
Kelso, Paul, 34, 54
Kennard, Donald Ray, 128
Kenteris, Costas, 77
Kerr, Robert, 11, 38, 56, 287, 298n14, 302n4
kew. *See* kava
Khomich, Albina, 76
kijitsu, 123
Kipling, Rudyard, 273
Klein, Eugene, 43
Knight Commission on Intercollegiate Athletics, 237, 279–83
Knine, Nan Aye, 77
knitback/bone, 123
Koch, Gunther, 302n4
Korchemny, Remi, 13, 62
Korn, Allan, 56–57
Korzhanenko, Irina, 76
Kovacs, Zoltan, 77
Kraemer, W. J., 262
Krause, Kieter, 297n8
Krauss, Sara, 2
Kreider, Richard, 106
Krzyzewski, Mike, 231, 234
Kumari, Pratima, 77
Kurlovich, Alexander, 47

LaFontaine, Pat, 165
Lancaster, Scott, 178, 260, 267
Langham, Antonio, 235
Larrea divaricata, 123
larreastat, 123
leadership, recommendations for, 133–36

learning disabilities, and diagnosis of
    MTBI, 160
Leavens, John, 24, 29, 259
Legarza, Mike, 186, 267
Lesnichiy, Aleksey, 76
Levine, Mel, 128
Lewis, Carl, 11–12, 38
Liddell, Eric, 202–3
Lindemann, Dieter, 297n8
Little, Grady, 228
Little League elbow, 265
Little League Parent Syndrome, 177
Llewellyn, William, 130
Llorente, Marcelo, 126
Lobelia inflata, 123
LOC. *See* loss of consciousness
Lombardi, Vince, 53, 195
long pepper. *See* kava
Lopez, John P., 131
loss of consciousness (LOC), 144;
    briefest, 169
Lou Gehrig's disease, 46
Louisiana High School Sports Athletic
    Association, 213–14
Lower, Steve, 210
L-theonine, 72
lucid interval, 144–45
Lue, Daniel, 9–10
lurk-in-the-ditch, 123

Madden, Terry, 61, 129
mad-dog herb/weed, 124
Madsen, Steen, 51
mad weed, 124
magnesium, 72
magnesium creatine, 71
Maher, Bridget, 22, 25–29
Maher, John, 48
Ma Huang. *See* ephedra
Major League Baseball (MLB):
    BALCO scandal and, 59–79; and
    coaches, 228; drug policy, 70–72,
74; drug-testing policy, 41, 44, 85;
    recommendations for, 133
Makke, Kristjan, 211
Malamud, Harlan, 103
Maley, Mark, 59
malohu. *See* kava
maluk. *See* kava
Mandell, Arnold, 43
Mano, Barry, 189, 199, 243–51
marijuana, 16, 78
Marinovich, Todd, 183
Mariucci, Steve, 228
Marshall, Jack, 200
Martin, Jacques, 228
masking agents, 39, 48, 51, 66, 93;
    and testing, 97
mass-cutting phase, 87
Massie, Giddeon, 206
mass phase, 87
Mate, Gabor, 33
Maye, Jereme, 213
Maynor, Glenn, 207
Mays, Willie, 66
McBath, Mike, 194
McBride, Chase, 210
McCaffrey, Barry R., 135
McCain, John, 62–63, 127
McCallum, Brian, 184, 215–19,
    299n21
McCarthy, John, 267
McCloskey, John, 187–88, 309n19
McCollum, Bill, 128
McCrery, Johnette, 31–32
McEwen, John, 13, 62, 298n18
McGuire, R., 262
McGwire, Mark, 2, 50, 55, 105
McGyvers, Val, 220
McInally, P., 262
McSeveney, Greg, 48
Mead, Margaret, 286
media, 4; and cheating scandals,
    205–6; Mano on, 250–51; and
    PEDs, 40; and role models, 31–32

Megyesy, Dave, 43
men, as role models, 27–28
Merode, Alexandre de, 50
meruk. *See* kava
Metabolife. *See* ephedra
metandienone, 49
methamphetamine, 11, 16
methandrostenolone, 11, 84, 132, 302n4
methyltestosterone, 51
Meyer, Rick, 48
middle schools, steroid use in, 49
mild traumatic brain injury (MTBI), 139, 157; classification of, 167–69; evolution of knowledge about, 158–63; personal accounts of, 160–61. *See also* concussion
milik. *See* kava
Miller, John, 232
Mitchell, Dennis, 49
MLB. *See* Major League Baseball
modafinil, 13, 94
Mohnike, Kerry, 205
Monitoring the Future survey, 14–16, 299n21
Montgomery, Tim, 60, 63, 65, 206, 305n6
moral development, sports and, 199
Morgan, Edward, 19
mosquito plant, 123
Moynihan, Daniel Patrick, 29, 200
MTBI. *See* mild traumatic brain injury
Munyasia, David, 77
Murphy, Shane, 262, 269
Murtha, Lydon, 210
Muscle Milk. *See* ephedrine
muscle protein synthesis, growth hormone and, 90
mushrooms, 81

n-acetyl d-glucosamine, 72
nandrolone, 49, 51, 87, 99

National Alliance for Youth Sports (NAYS), 178, 275
National Basketball Association, 228
National Center for Drug Free Sport, 129
National Collegiate Athletic Association (NCAA), 85; and academic requirements, 279; and travel requirements, 220
National Federation of State High School Associations, 109
National Football League (NFL): and coaches, 228; drug-testing policy, 41–45, 48, 85; drug violations in, 53–54; High School Player Development Program camp, 134–35
National Hockey League (NHL), 48, 228
National Institute on Drug Abuse, 8, 114
National Safe Children Campaign, 191
NAYS. *See* National Alliance for Youth Sports
neroli oil, 123
Neufeld, Gordon, 33
Neuheisel, Rick, 230
NFL. *See* National Football League
NHL. *See* National Hockey League
Nickel, James D., 202–3
Nicklaus, Jack, 23–24
nitroglycerine, 82
Nitrophen, 152
norbolethone, 52
Novartis, 11, 84
Nowinski, Chris, 162
Nubain, 57
nutrition, 258, 292–93

Oakland Raiders, 95, 298n18
O'Bee, Kirk, 52
O'Brien, Jim, 232
Odom, Dave, 229
Okafor, Ivan, 2

Olander, Rachel, 104
Olefirenko, Olena, 76
Olympic Games: 1936, 84; 1960, 11; 1968, 94; 1972, 11; 1976, 11; 1984, 11, 38; 1988, 11–12; 1996, 94; 2000, 63; 2002, 214, 219; 2004, 64, 74–79
omega-3 fatty acids, 72
omega-6 fatty acids, 72
opioid drugs, 57, 304n43
Oral-Turinabol, 11
Osborne, Tom, 124, 127–28
Osgood-Schlatter's disease, 265
O'Toole, Tim, 233
overuse, 191–92
Owens, Terell, 247
oxanfrolone, 76
oxymetholone, 87

Page, Jim, 214, 219
Pan American Games, 11
Pansold, Bernd, 297n8
Pantani, Marco, 224
Parcells, Bill, 190
parents: abuses by, 3; influence of, 29–30, 33; Josephson on, 25; Mano on, 248–49; Pink on, 26; and problems in youth sports, 182–96; recommendations for, 133–36, 260–61; shortcomings of, 21–22; and solutions in sports, 121–22; and steroid use, 18–19; Uryasz on, 120; and violence, 177–80; Walsh on, 55; youth and, 184–86
Pausinystalia yohimbe. See yohimbe
PEDs. See performance-enhancing drugs
peers: and education, 33, 115, 286; and steroid use, 18
Pellman, Elliott, 38
penalties for drug use: criticism of, 53; policies on, 277; recommendations for, 133

pennyroyal oil, 123
people skills, Mano on, 246
Peppers, Julius, 52
Perata, Don, 126
Pereira, Mike, 250
performance-enhancing drugs (PEDs): control efforts, 124–30, 311n2, 312n6; cover-up on, 40; deaths from, 221–26; history of, 81–88; myths regarding, 45; Pound on, 5; and recreational drug use, 56–57; signs of use, 117–21. See also steroids
Perkins, Danny, 268
Perko, Mike, 107
phentermine, 52
phenylalanine, 71
phenylpropanolomine, 94
Phillips, Chris, 13
physical appearance: anabolic steroids and, 86; and steroid use, 34–35
physicians: and parents, 19; and steroid use, 11, 38
Pierce, Kyle, 192–93
Pierson, Carl, 216–17
Pink, Arthur W., 26
Piper, Roddy, 293–96
Piper methysticum. See kava
Pisarenko, Anatoly, 47
plateauing, term, 86
pliolerial, 123
Plonsky, Christine, 279
Plunknett, Ben, 97
pole vaulting: injuries in, 142; preventive measures for, 257
Pope, Harrison G., Jr., 304n43
Positive Coaching Alliance, 186
postconcussion syndrome, 163–64
Potteiger, Jeffrey A., 67
Potter, Troy, 104, 109
Pound, Richard, 5; on drug policies, 75; on drug testing, 100; on MLB, 74, 133; on NFL, 43; on penalties, 53; on supplements, 130

pregnancy, teen, 28
pregnancy doping, 92
presidents of academic institutions: Holland on, 280, 282–83; and problems in sports, 231, 239–40, 278
President's Council of Economic Advisors, 22
pressure: and academic fraud, 203; and steroid use, 15; and youth, 186
prevention, 157–75
Price, Melissa, 62, 298n18
Price, Mike, 229
Primabolin, 132
principals, recommendations for, 133–36
probenecid, 97
problems in sports, 1–2; administration and, 227–41; athletes and, 37–57; Holland on, 282; youth and, 1–2, 177–96
Project World Record, 63
protein, 103
Protovent. See clenbuterol
pseudoephedrine, 48, 94
pudding grass, 123
pukeweed, 123
pulegium, 123
Pursuing Victory with Honor program, 268–69
pushing youth: too early, 193; too hard, 183–84
Putting Youth Back Into Sports program, 268
pyramid, term, 86

Quackwatch, 108
quaker bonnet, 124
Quenneville, Joel, 228

Ramsey, Eric, 236
rape, 2, 208–9, 232
rauschpfeffer. See kava

recreational drug use, PEDs and, 56–57
recruiting methods, 3, 208–13, 322n29
red blood cells, 92
Redden, Chris, 9–10
referees. See sports officials
Reilly, Rick, 208
Reiterer, Werner, 56
religious beliefs: and drug use, 24–25; Hall on, 287–90
Remia, Len, 191
research: Uryasz on, 118; USADA and, 125
Resource Exchange Center, 129
respect, 32; lack of, 227–29
Respert, Jason, 209
responsibility, 32; Uryasz on, 120
return to play: with concussion, 171–74; with MTBI, 159–60; premature, 192; and second impact syndrome, 170
Reynolds, Robert, 267
Rieser, Otto, 84
Ripped Fuel. See ephedrine
Robbins, Barret, 298n18
Rogol, Alan, 67
role models: athletes as, 53–56, 287–93; importance of, 3, 27; male, 27–28; monitoring, 34; need for, 21–35; Nicklaus on, 23–24; recommendations for, 133–36
roller skating, injuries in, 140
Romanowski, Bill, 62, 298n18
Romans, Scotty, 103
Rotella, R. J., 262
Roth, Neil, 131
Rozelle, Pete, 42–43
rugby, 49–51
rules, Mano on, 246–47, 249–50
run-by-the-ground, 123
Rusley, Bobby Joe, 215, 217
Ruth, Babe, 60

sakau. *See* kava
Salanson, Fabrice, 224
Salisbury State (MD) University, 48
salsify, 123
Samaranch, Juan Antonio, 49, 79
Sampanis, Leonidas, 76
sangree root/sangrel, 123
Santiago, Benito, 60, 297n6
Saratoga High School (CA), 203–6
Sarcev, Milos, 63–64
Sbeih, Adham, 12
Schilling, Curt, 73
Schwarzenegger, Arnold, 126
science: on concussion, 157–75; and
    solutions in sports, 253–58
Scott, Byron, 228
Scudder, Jeff, 122
scullcap, 124
Scutellaria lateriflora, 124
Seals, Ray, 134–35
second impact syndrome (SIS), 170–71
selenium, 71
Selig, Bud, 56, 62
Sensenbrenner, F. James, Jr., 124, 127
Serostim, 66
serpentary/serpentaria, 123
Seville orange, 123
sexual assault, 210. *See also* rape
shangzhou zhiqiao, 123
Shchukina, Olga, 76
Sheffer, John B., III, 126
Sheffield, Gary, 59, 297n6
Sherman, William, 131
Sileo, Dan, 208
Simpson, Alan, 128
Simpson, Tom, 11, 94
Sipe, Brian, 211
SIS. *See* second impact syndrome
skateboarding, injuries in, 140
Skelos, Dean, 126
Slaughter, T. J., 52
slin, term, 86–87
slippery root, 123

Small, Eric, 262
Smith, Aynsley, 19
Smith, Gary, 207
Smith, Josh, 192
Smith, R. E., 262
Smith, Robert, 272
Smoll, F. L., 262
snakeroot/weed, 123
snowboarding, injuries in, 140
snowmobiling, injuries in, 140
Sobel, Eleanor, 181
soccer: brain injuries in, 143, 167; con-
    cussion in, 162; deaths in, 224;
    drug use in, 50; injuries in, 142
social problems, 21–22, 24–29; ethics
    and, 200; Mano on, 243–45
Solfo black, 152
solutions for sports, 1, 27, 111–36,
    253–86; athletes and, 287–96;
    Mano on, 246–47; time with youth
    and, 34
somatostatin, 90
somatotropin/Somatropin. *See* human
    growth hormone
sour orange, 123
Soviet Union, 8
spearing, 258
Speier, Jackie, 55, 126–27, 286
spinal injury, 145–47; types of, 147
Spiropent. *See* clenbuterol
sport rage, 177
sports concussion. *See* mild traumatic
    brain injury
sportsmanship: books on, 262; and
    coaches, 229; education on, 269;
    Nicklaus on, 24; official on,
    243–51; web sites on, 262–63
sports officials, 227–28; assaults on,
    177, 179–80, 188–90; personal ac-
    counts of, 243–51; protection for,
    181, 244–46; recommendations
    for, 264
squaw balm/mint, 123

stacking, term, 86
stanozolol, 50–51, 76, 87, 97
Stark, Pete, 128
Steinbrenner, George, 214
steroid precursors, side effects of, 105
steroids, 81–101; history of, 83–88; limiting ease of access to, 130–32; testing for, 97; trafficking in, 132. *See also* performance-enhancing drugs
steroid use: appearance and, 34–35; effects of, 67; Hall on, 287–90; in high school, 14–15; history of, 8–11; influence of, 54; magnitude of, 7–8, 15–16, 37–38, 72–73; in middle schools, 49; motives for, 53; personal accounts of, 9–10, 87–88, 293–96; youth and, 7–20
Stevens, Stuart, 131
Stewart, Martha, 204–5
stimulants: characteristics of, 93–95; testing for, 97
stinking balm, 123
Stoll, Sharon, 199
Stowers, Travis, 107
strategy, versus cheating, 198
Stratton, Brock, 284
stress, and diagnosis of MTBI, 160
Stringer, Korey, 54, 74, 107, 225, 303n27
strychnine, 81
Stubblefield, Dana, 298n18
substantia nigra, 166
Sudafed. *See* pseudoephedrine
sudden death, 138–39; prevention of, 254–55
suicide, teen, 28
Sule, Shabaz, 77
Sun, Lauren, 205
supplements, 103–10; Bell on, 292–93; Bonds and, 69; and heatstroke, 151–52; motivations for use of, 104; prevalence of use of, 104–5;

recommendations for, 258; regulation of, 107–8; Uryasz on, 129–30; web sites on, 263
Svare, Bruce, 271–72, 284
Svare, Harland, 43
Swarts, Art, 48
Swartz, Jon, 223
Sweeney, John, 124, 128
swimming, 12, 48, 50
Sydnocarb, 94
Sylvester, Jay, 11
Symphytum officinale, 123
Symphytum radix, 123

Tagliabue, Paul, 135
Tanoos, Dan, 211
Tarkanian, Jerry, 230, 240
Terrell, Jamil, 231
testosterone, 84; discovery of, 83; testing for, 11, 44, 49, 82, 97, 99–100
testosterone enanthate, 87
tetrahydrogestrinone (THG), 12–13, 37, 298nn17–18; BALCO scandal and, 59–79; ban on, and decline in achievements, 65–68; characteristics of, 95–96
Teucrium chamaedrys, 123
Thanou, Katerina, 77
THG. *See* tetrahydrogestrinone
Thomas, Eric, 13
Thomas, Tammy, 52
Thompson, J. M., 262
Thurmond, Strom, 128
tickweed, 123
Tien Chi. *See* ephedrine
Todd, Terry, 47
Tofler, Ian, 261
tonga. *See* kava
Toomay, Pat, 42
Toon, Al, 164–65
Toth, Kevin, 298n18
Tour de France, 11–12, 46, 50, 91
track and field, 49, 290–93

traumatic injury, 137
travel requirements, 220, 281, 283
trenbolone, 95, 99
Treutlein, Gerhard, 39
Triamterene, 12, 48–49
trustworthiness, 32
tyrosine, 71
Tzekos, Christos, 77

UCLA Olympic Analytical Laboratory, 61
UK Athletics, 12–13
Umeh, McCollins, 2
umpires. *See* sports officials
Ungerleider, Steven, 10, 86
United States Anti-Doping Agency (USADA), 13, 61, 125, 129
United States Department of Health and Human Services, and ATLAS program, 20, 33, 114–15
United States Marine Corps, 287–88
United States Olympic Committee (USOC), 3, 214; and doping, 38–39
University of Colorado, 208–9, 238–39, 277–78
University of Michigan: Institute for Social Research, 15; Monitoring the Future survey, 14–16, 299n21
Upshaw, Gene, 41
urine tests, 98
Uryasz, Frank, 118–20, 311n1; on coaches, 20; on education, 73, 117–19; and National Center for Drug Free Sport, 129; on NFL, 42–43; on parents, 19; on regulation, 132; on supplements, 129–30; on winning mentality, 284–85
USADA. *See* United States Anti-Doping Agency
USOC. *See* United States Olympic Committee

Vainio, Martti, 12
Valente, James J., 62

Vanderbilt University, 47
Van Slyke, Andy, 70
Vargas, Fernando, 52
Velarde, Randy, 60, 297n6
Vernacchia, R., 262
violence, 3, 188–90; incidents of, 178–80; parents and, 177–78; penalties for, 266; youth and, 28, 181–82
vitamins: A, 71; B_1, 71; B_2, 71; B_6, 71–72; B_{12}, 71; C, 71; D, 71; E, 71
Vogel, Hal, 205
vomit wort, 123
Voy, Robert O., 15, 38, 135

WADA. *See* World Anti-Doping Agency
Wadler, G. I., 221
Wadler, Gary, 55
Walker, Don, 59
wall germander, 123
wallwort, 123
Walsh, Bill, 55
Walters, John P., 29
Watts, J. C., 22
web sites: Josephson Institute, 276; on sportsmanship, 262–63; on supplements, 263
weightlifting, 11, 34, 50, 77, 84–85; Hall and, 287–90
weight training: popularity of, 207; for youth, 192–93
Weiss, M. R., 262
Welty, John D., 240
Wheeler, Rashidi, 74, 107, 225
whey protein, 71–72
Whicker, Mark, 70
White, Christopher, 233, 240
White, Kelli, 13, 63
Whitlock, Janine, 52
Wickenheiser, Robert J., 231, 240
Wiggins, Paul, 50

Wilbanks, Edd, 207
wild germander, 123
wild ginger, 123
wild tobacco, 123
Wilkins, Perriss, 52
Will, Kevin, 115–16
Williams, Michael David, 47
Williams, Willie, 209
Wilson, Ron, 229
winning: costs of, 197–220; Cunningham on, 290–91; education on, 276; Lombardi on, 195; Nickel on, 202–3; overemphasis on, 184–88
winning-at-all-cost mentality, solutions for, 284–86
Winstrol. *See* stanozolol
Wolff, Rick, 178, 229, 262
World Anti-Doping Agency (WADA), 12, 97, 124; and drug testing, 39; Uryasz on, 118
World Anti-Doping Code, 78
World Conference on Doping in Sport, 124
wrestling: brain injuries in, 143; deaths in, 46, 223; Piper on, 293–96
Wroble, Randall R., 15
wurzelstock. *See* kava

yagona/yangona. *See* kava
year-round participation, 191–92
Yesalis, Charles: on appearance, 35; on drug testing, 37–39; on ethics, 200–201; on fans, 40; on media, 4; on parental encouragement of steroid use, 18–19; on steroid use, 7–8; on youth, 55
yohimbe, 106, 124
Young, Jerome, 13, 65
youth: and parents, 184–86; problems of, 28–29; and role models, 31; and violence, 28, 181–82
youth sports: benefits of, 271; books on, 262; core values of, 182; problems in, 1–2, 177–96; solutions for, 253–86

Zelezniak, Joe, 48
Zeranol, 99
zhi oiao/xhi, 123
Ziegler, John, 11, 298n10
zinc, 72
ZMA, 72
Zola, Kimberly, 301n22